CAPD – A Decade of Experience

Contributions to Nephrology

Vol. 89

KARGER

Basel · München · Paris · London · New York · New Delhi · Bangkok · Singapore · Tokyo · Sydney

2nd European Symposium on Peritoneal Dialysis, Alicante, May 25–27, 1989

CAPD –
A Decade of Experience

Volume Editors

G. La Greca, Vicenza; *J. Olivares,* Alicante;
M. Feriani, Vicenza; *J. Passlick-Deetjen*, Oberursel/Taunus

63 figures and 90 tables, 1991

KARGER

Basel · München · Paris · London · New York · New Delhi · Bangkok · Singapore · Tokyo · Sydney

This publication was made possible by an educational grant from Fresenius AG.

Library of Congress Cataloging-in-Publication Data
European Symposium on Peritoneal Dialysis (2nd: 1989: Alicante, Spain)
CAPD – A decade of experience / 2nd European Symposium on Peritoneal Dialysis, Alicante,
May 25–27, 1989; volume editors, G. La Greca ... [et al.].
(Contributions to nephrology; vol. 89)
Includes bibliographical references and index.
1. Continuous ambulatory peritoneal dialysis – Congresses.   I. La Greca, G.   II. Title.
III. Series.   IV. Series: Contributions to nephrology; v. 89.
[DNLM: 1. Peritoneal Dialysis, Continuous Ambulatory – congresses.   2. Peritoneal Dialysis,
Continuous Ambulatory – methods – congresses.   3. Peritonitis – congresses.
W1 CO778UN v. 89 / WJ 378 E89c 1989]
RC901.7.P48E9   1989
617.4'61059 – dc20
ISBN 3–8055–5307–2

Bibliographic Indices
This publication is listed in bibliographic services, including Current Contents® and Index
Medicus.

Drug Dosage
The authors and the publisher have exerted every effort to ensure that drug selection and dosage
set forth in this text are in accord with current recommendations and practice at the time of
publication. However, in view of ongoing research, changes in government regulations, and the
constant flow of information relating to drug therapy and drug reactions, the reader is urged to
check the package insert for each drug for any change in indications and dosage and for added
warnings and precautions. This is particularly important when the recommended agent is a new
and/or infrequently employed drug.

Contents

Contents

Therapy of Peritonitis

Osmotic Agents

Transport Kinetics in Peritoneal Dialysis

Contents

Clinical Experiences in Peritoneal Dialysis

Differential Indications for Peritoneal Dialysis

Psychological, Social and Economic Aspects of Peritoneal Dialysis

Preface

This volume of *Contributions to Nephrology* reports on the 2nd European Symposium on Peritoneal Dialysis held in Alicante in May 1989.

Despite a dramatic increase of CAPD in the last 10 years there is still considerable debate going on about whether CAPD is a real long-term alternative to hemodialysis, particularly in terms of patient and technique survival.

The first part of the book devoted to the status of peritoneal dialysis deals with these problems in selected countries and selected patient groups, the results being presented by groups deeply involved and experienced in CAPD. The section confirms the recent view that CAPD and hemodialysis provide similar patient survival rates, while technique survival is still different.

Main factors affecting technique survival are presented in the following three chapters, dealing with different approaches to peritoneal access, prevention of peritonitis and therapy of peritonitis, since these problems still represent the most frequent causes of technical drop out. Comparisons of different strategies and suggestions to overcome these problems are reported in three separate sections by experts in the field.

Ultrafiltration loss and metabolic problems both linked to the use of glucose as the osmotic agent are other emerging causes of technical drop out. A special section deals with this topic presenting alternative osmotic agent studies and proposing new suitable substances.

New aspects of peritoneal transport kinetics, clinical experiences in the use of erythropoietin, first results of the use of vitamin D and a low calcium solution in CAPD patients, other facets of hyperparathyroidism, and experiences on the treatment of loss of ultrafiltration are reported in two other sections of this book.

Since the most important issue for the success of peritoneal dialysis is the adequate selection of patients, one special part is devoted to that problem.

Another very important topic, the psychological, social and economic aspect of CAPD, is developed in the last chapter.

This meeting of experts involved in the field of peritoneal dialysis research and clinical application would not have been possible without the generous support of Fresenius AG. We would also like to thank the staff of S. Karger AG for their efforts and advice in publishing these proceedings.

This book illustrates the significant contribution provided by CAPD, together with hemodialysis and transplantation, to the treatment of ESRD patients.

The Editors

Status of Peritoneal Dialysis

La Greca G, Olivares J, Feriani M, Passlick-Deetjen J (eds): CAPD – A Decade of Experience. Contrib Nephrol. Basel, Karger, 1991, vol 89, pp 1–5

CAPD in Europe

J. Olivares, J.M. Gas, M.C. Prados, F. Rivera, C. de Santiago,
L. Jiménez, A. Franco, F. Picazo, J. Perez-Contreras

Hospital Alicante Insalud, Department of Nephrology, Alicante, Spain

At present, CAPD is considered to be an effective method, together with transplantation and hemodialysis (HD), in the therapy of end-stage renal diseases (ESRD).

During the last 10 years there has been a significant worldwide spread of this technique so that, according to the available data, at the end of 1986 there were about 330,000 patients on renal replacement therapy: 70% on HD, 9% on peritoneal dialysis (PD; over 98% on CAPD) and the remaining 21% had functional kidney transplants. Thirty percent of these patients were treated in Europe, whereby the percentage of CAPD patients was comparable to that of the rest of the world [1]. Table 1 depicts the steady increase of PD patients in Europe [2–4] during the last decade.

The total number of PD patients increased proportionally to the total number of patients on regular dialysis treatment (RDT); thus the percentage of PD patients has reached a stable level of about 10% of the global RDT (table 2) [3].

The percentages of the different ESRD treatment modalities from 1976 to 1986 are shown in table 3 [5]. It can be noted that, while hospital HD has fallen slightly and home HD has dropped markedly, CAPD and transplantation have increased from 0 to 7% and from 18 to 27%, respectively.

These data are even more striking in ESRD patients with diabetic nephropathy. This is a clear consequence of the changes that have occurred in medical attitude towards this group of patients and which have led to a dramatic increase in renal replacement therapy in these patients. In fact, in 1976 only 3% of the new patients treated for ESRD were diabetics, while in 1985 this group accounted for 10.7% of the new patients accepted for RDT [6].

Table 1. PD patients in Europe: total number of patients on IPD and CAPD at the end of the year [2–4]

	1979	1983	1986	1988
UK	132	1,565	2,800	3,613
Italy	77	1,120	1,400	1,901
France	296	820	1,026	1,067
Spain	24	650	798	763
Germany	38	385	562	800
The Netherlands	5	290	484	663
Sweden	30	150	196	288
Switzerland	40	130	273	293
Denmark	36	60	234	211
Finland	11	150	203	206
Greece	0	110	174	274
Belgium	45	90	177	155
Ireland	0	20	64	90
Portugal	0	10	37	40
Norway	6	20	36	22
Austria	3	10	43	82
Total Europe	779	5,480	8,507	10,468

As can be seen in table 4, PD as the first method of treatment was chosen in a greater proportion of patients with diabetic nephropathy than in patients with other reasons for ESRD (table 3). A similar observation was made for patients alive on renal replacement therapy in 1985 (table 5). At this time the percentage for hospital HD was similar, while it was higher for home HD and transplantation [6].

The rate of peritonitis, the major complication of CAPD treatment, decreased significantly from 1.5 episodes per patient-year in 1979, 1.3 in 1983, and 1.0 in 1986 to 0.6 episodes per patient-year in 1988, mainly due to the improved CAPD systems and the broader experience in their use.

Despite the dramatic increase of CAPD, there is still a considerable debate about whether CAPD is a valid long-term alternative to HD, particularly in terms of patient and technique survival.

As far as patient survival is concerned, in 1988 Maiorca et al. [7] published a 5-year comparison of patients on CAPD and HD. Cox's proportional hazard regression model showed no difference in survival rate between the two groups when the pretreatment risk factors were taken into account.

Table 2. Dialysis in Europe 1988: total number of patients on different forms of renal replacement therapy at the end of 1988 [3]

	Total dialysis patients	HD patients[1]	PD patients[2]	% PD patients of total
UK	7,751	4,138	3,613	46.6
Sweden	1,399	1,111	288	20.6
Denmark	813	602	211	25.9
Norway	204	182	22	10.8
Finland	516	310	206	39.9
The Netherlands	2,953	2,290	663	22.5
Belgium	2,849	2,694	155	5.4
France	15,401	14,334	1,067	6.9
Germany	20,937	20,137	800	3.8
Switzerland	1,578	1,281	297	18.8
Spain	9,395	8,632	763	8.1
Italy	15,435	13,834	1,601	10.4
Portugal	2,663	2,623	40	1.5
Greece	1,835	1,561	274	14.9
Austria	1,901	1,819	82	4.3
Ireland	315	225	90	28.6
Total	85,945	75,773	10,172	11.8

[1] Hospital and home HD.
[2] IPD and CAPD.

Table 3. Growth of various treatment modalities in percent in Europe from 1976 to 1986 [5]

	1976	1981	1986
Hospital HD	65	63	61
Home HD	15	11	5
Transplantation	18	20	27
CAPD	0	4	7
IPD	1	1	1

However, a significantly better technique survival for HD patients was observed both in the above-mentioned study and in the United Kingdom Registry [8].

Table 4. First choice of treatment in patients with end-stage renal failure secondary to diabetes mellitus type I and II, who started renal replacement therapy in 1983–1985 [6]

	Diabetes type I	Diabetes type II
Total	4,568	1,622
HD, %	63	72
IPD, %	10	12
CAPD, %	25	16
Transplantation, %	2	<1

Table 5. Proportional distribution (%) of patients with diabetic nephropathy undergoing renal replacement therapy at the end of 1985, by treatment method [6]

Hospital HD	59
Home HD	1
IPD	2
CAPD	19
Transplantation	18

In summary, during the last 10 years the proportion of patients treated with home HD has notably decreased while an increase in CAPD and transplantation has been observed. There are clear geographical differences in the implementation of CAPD, perhaps due more to socioeconomic factors than to medical reasons.

Diabetic nephropathy has become one of the major causes of ESRD. PD is more often chosen in diabetic patients compared to patients with other causes of ESRD, and once again geographical differences are observed [6].

The patient survivals of CAPD and HD are statistically equivalent. However, the technique survival is currently better in HD [7, 8]. Obviously, a technical improvement of CAPD systems and solutions and a reduction of complications could lead to an improvement of the technique survival in CAPD as well, especially since improved CAPD systems and a broader experience in their use have considerably reduced the peritonitis rate.

Finally, we believe that both HD and CAPD should be complementary techniques, and should be offered impartially to all patients with ESRD.

References

1 Wing AJ, Broyer M, Brunner FP, et al: Registry report. Demography of dialysis and transplantation in Europe, in 1985 and 1986: Trends over the previous decade. Nephrol Dial Transplant 1986;3:714–727.
2 European Dialysis and Transplantation Association (EDTA): Combined Report on Regular Dialysis and Transplantation in Europe, XVIII, 1986.
3 European Dialysis and Transplantation Association Combined Report on Regular Dialysis and Transplantation in Europe, XIX, 1988. Nephrol Dial Transplant, 1989; 4(suppl 4):7.
4 Data for 1979 and 1983 were kindly made available by Nephro Control, Barcelona.
5 European and Dialysis Transplantation Association: Combined Report on Regular Dialysis and Transplantation in Europe, VIII, 1987.
6 Brunner FP, Brynger M, Challah S, et al: Registry Report. Renal replacement therapy in patients with diabetic nephropathy, 1980–1985. Report from the European Dialysis and Transplant Association Registry. Nephrol Dial Transplant 1988;3: 585–595.
7 Maiorca R, Vonesh E, Cancarini GC, et al: A six-year comparison of patients and technique survival in CAPD. Kidney Int 1988;34:518–524.
8 Gokal R, Jakubowski C, King J, et al: Outcome in patients on CAPD and haemodialysis: 4-year analysis of a prospective multicenter study. Lancet 1987;ii:1105–1109.

Dr. J. Olivares, Hospital Alicante Insalud, Nefrologia,
C/Maestro Alonso 109, E–03012 Alicante (Spain)

La Greca G, Olivares J, Feriani M, Passlick-Deetjen J (eds): CAPD – A Decade of Experience. Contrib Nephrol. Basel, Karger, 1991, vol 89, pp 6–10

CAPD in North America

Jose A. Diaz-Buxo

Metrolina Kidney Center, Charlotte, N.C., USA

The introduction of CAPD in 1976 and continuous cyclic peritoneal dialysis (CCPD) in 1981 renewed the interest in peritoneal dialysis as chronic renal substitution therapy worldwide and created a new medical industry [1, 2]. The simplicity and availability of CAPD has had variable impact in different countries. Where medical resources are limited the percentage of the end-stage renal disease (ESRD) population treated with CAPD often exceeds 50% (Mexico 74%), while in many industrialized countries the proportion remains less than 5% (Japan, FRG). In the USA and Canada the impact of CAPD has been intermediate. Approximately 16% of all ESRD patients receive CAPD/CCPD in the USA and 36% in Canada.

The data available on CAPD/CCPD in the USA are mostly provided by the National CAPD Registry of the National Institutes of Health. The Registry began operations in January of 1981 and closed in July of 1988. It was responsible for developing information regarding the number of patients receiving CAPD/CCPD, their demographic characteristics, the incidence of complications and the survival of patients. It also evaluated specific problems in samples of the CAPD population. The submission of data to the Registry was on a voluntary basis, with an approximate population coverage of 50%. Additional sources of information include the annual Health Care Financing Administration (HCFA) report and estimates from the dialysis industry. The primary source of information in Canada is the Canadian Renal Failure Register. The information contained herewith represents approximations based on these sources with the latest reports including the patient census as follows: National CAPD Registry – 1987, HCFA – 1986, Baxter Laboratories – 1987, and Canadian Register – 1986.

Approximately 15,000 patients undergo treatment with CAPD/CCPD in the USA, accounting for 15% of the total ESRD population (table 1). This number has more than tripled since 1981, but the total population of patients

Table 1. Dialysis in the USA[1] and Canada[2]

	USA		Canada	
	n	%	n	%
Hemodialysis				
Center	79,508	81	2,242	50
Home	3,580	4	682	15
IPD				
Center	441	–	200	5
Home	168	–	19	–
CAPD	12,995	13	1,264	28
CCPD	1,728	2	48	1
Total	98,420		4,462	

[1] Data from Health Care Financing Administration, 1987.
[2] Data from Canadian Renal Failure Register, 1985.

Table 2. Distribution of CAPD patients by etiology of renal disease according to year (percent of patients): modified from the USA CAPD Registry Report, 1988

Etiology	1981–1983	1984	1985	1986	1987
Diabetic glomerulosclerosis	21.4	25.6	28.0	29.7	31.5
Chronic glomerulonephritis	21.3	17.0	14.4	14.3	12.8
Arterial hypertension	16.0	14.2	14.5	15.7	15.7
Interstitial disease	6.6	8.7	8.7	8.3	7.7
Polycystic kidneys	7.5	6.3	5.6	5.5	5.4

at home has not changed accordingly due to the simultaneous reduction in home hemodialysis. In Canada, however, 29% of all ESRD patients undergo CAPD/CCPD while an additional 5% undergo other modalities of peritoneal dialysis.

The median age for CAPD/CCPD patients in the USA is 53 years with 33% of the patients above age 59 years. Fifty-five percent of the patients are male, 75% white and 19% black [3].

The proportion of diabetics among CAPD/CCPD patients has consistently increased in both countries accounting for 32% of all CAPD patients

Table 3. Complication rates for CAPD patients by year of registration (episodes per patient year): modified from the USA CAPD Registry, 1988

Complication	1981	1982	1983	1984	1985	1986	1987
Peritonitis	1.3	1.4	1.3	1.3	1.3	1.3	1.3
Exit site/tunnel infection	0.6	0.7	0.5	0.5	0.6	0.6	0.8
Catheter replacement	0.2	0.3	0.3	0.3	0.2	0.2	0.3

Table 4. Reasons for transfer from CAPD to hemodialysis: modified from the USA CAPD Registry, 1988

Reason for transfer	Percent	
Peritonitis	27	36
Exit site/tunnel infection	9	
Inadequate ultrafiltration	4	8
Inadequate solute removal	4	
Cather leaks/malfunctions	7	
Hernia	2	
Frequent hospitalizations	3	
Other medical complications	16	
Patient/family choice	17	
Visual/manual impairment	1	
Others	10	

in the USA and 24% in Canada. Diabetes is the leading growing cause of ESRD and is responsible for 32% of all ESRD cases in the USA in 1987 (table 2).

The complication rates for peritonitis, exit site/tunnel infection and catheter replacement by year of registration in the USA CAPD Registry are summarized in table 3. Despite the proliferation of connectology devices and techniques and catheter designs since 1981, no significant differences in the rate of occurrence of these complications are apparent.

Termination of CAPD/CCPD due to transfer to an alternate dialytic therapy remains relatively high. The cumulative probability of transfer from CAPD to hemodialysis, IPD, or off-dialysis, without return of renal function in the USA is 20, 34, 44 and 52% at 1, 2, 3 and 4 years, respectively [3]. Similar figures are reported for CCPD. The principal reasons for transfer to hemodialysis are summarized in table 4. Peritonitis and exit site/tunnel infections

Table 5. Technique survival by type of dialysis and age (excluding diabetics) in Canada

Age, years	Technique survival, %							
	CAPD				hemodialysis			
	1 year	2 years	3 years	4 years	1 year	2 years	3 years	4 years
15–44	79	58	41	36	88	86	84	84
45–64	78	65	54	44	78	76	70	68
≥ 65	83	72	61	55	74	72	66	65

Approximation based on Canadian Renal Failure Report, 1981–1985 [4].

Table 6. Cumulative probabilities of survival for CAPD/CCPD patients in the USA and Canada

	Patient survival, %			
	1 year	2 years	3 years	4 years
CAPD – USA[1]	83	69	58	49
CCPD – USA[1]	78	63	50	–
CAPD – Canada[2]				
All patients	82	70	62	56
Nondiabetic	83	72	66	60
Diabetic	74	58	45	39

[1] USA National CAPD Registry, 1988 [3].
[2] Canadian Renal Failure Register, 1985 [4].

remain the major cause of abandonment of therapy. The cumulative probability of discontinuing CAPD for any reason, including transplantation and death, is 41% after 1 year, 64% at 2 years and 84% at 4 years. The technique survival for CAPD appears to be lower than that of hemodialysis [4]. Table 5 provides the technique survival for CAPD and hemodialysis according to age groups based on the Canadian Register data. Although the technique survival is superior among hemodialysis patients for all age groups, the difference is largest among the younger patients.

Patient survival, however, has proven similar to that observed with hemodialysis [4]. Table 6 summarizes the cumulative patient survival for CAPD/CCPD patients in the USA and Canada. Although no significant differences were observed between the survival rates for CAPD and CCPD or between patients in the two countries, marked differences were noted between diabetic and nondiabetic patients. The lower survival among diabetics increases as a function of time on dialysis.

Significant progress has been made in the field of peritoneal dialysis. At present, the survival rates of patients treated with CAPD/CCPD are similar to those obtained with hemodialysis. Nonetheless, the high rate of dropout from peritoneal dialysis and the persistence of infectious complications deserve our interest.

References

1   Popovich RP, Moncrief JW, Decherd JF, et al: The definition of a novel portable/ wearable equilibrium peritoneal dialysis technique (abstract). Am Soc Artif Intern Organs 1976;5:64.
2   Diaz-Buxo JA, Farmer CD, Walker PJ, et al: Continuous cyclic peritoneal dialysis. A preliminary report. Artif Organs 1981;5:157–161.
3   Lindblad A, Novak JW, Nolph KD (eds): Continuous ambulatory peritoneal dialysis in the USA – Final Report of the National CAPD Registry 1981–1988. Dordrecht, Kluwer, 1989.
4   Posen GA, Arbus GS, Hutchinson T, et al: Dialysis in Canada; in LaGreca G, Chiaramonte S, Fabris A, Feriani M, Ronco C (eds): Peritoneal Dialysis. Milano, Wichtig Editore, 1988, pp 207–212.

Jose A. Diaz-Buxo, MD, FACP, Metrolina Kidney Center,
928 Baxter Street, Charlotte, NC 28204 (USA)

La Greca G, Olivares J, Feriani M, Passlick-Deetjen J (eds): CAPD – A Decade of Experience. Contrib Nephrol. Basel, Karger, 1991, vol 89, pp 11–15

Status of Peritoneal Dialysis in Latin America

J.C. Divino Filho

Nephrology Section, Hospital São Severino, Sorocaba, Brazil

One of the goals of the Latin American Society of Peritoneal Dialysis is the organization of a peritoneal dialysis (PD) registry.

In fact, up to now, the 'Best Demonstrated Practices', edited by Baxter-Brazil is the only available epidemiological source for PD in Latin America [1]. These data concern 20 CAPD units from different regions of Brazil.

Different health policies and dialysis realities affect PD programs in different countries in Latin America.

This report is based on the information of some leading nephrologists in the field of PD in Latin America and the data of Baxter International.

Aspects of Peritoneal Dialysis in Different Latin American Countries

In Latin America, intermittent peritoneal dialysis (IPD) was the only alternative to hemodialysis (HD) and in some countries the main modality of treatment from 1967 to 1980. The high costs of HD were the main reason for this choice.

However, the use of Deane prothesis and plastic bottles containing dialysis fluid led to a constant high peritonitis and drop-out rate. The use of the Tenckhoff catheter and the introduction of a new closed IPD system [2] into clinical practice greatly decreased the infections and drop-out.

Table 1 depicts the distribution of dialysis in Latin America in April 1989.

In Brazil a marked development of the PD program has taken place during the last 10 years. In 1984, less than 200 patients were on CAPD, while in 1989 this number has increased to 1,480. In addition, 794 patients were on

Table 1. Distribution of dialysis in Latin America in April 1989

Country	Total dialysis patients	HD patients	PD patients	% PD of total
Brazil	12,724	10,450	2,274	21
Argentina	4,000	3,920	80	2
Venezuela	1,100	500	600	55
Mexico	3,000	700	2,300	77
Colombia	1,000	750	250	25
Cuba	1,000	500	500	50
	22,824	16,820	6,204	

IPD at this time. This steady increase is probably due to economic reasons. Despite the fact that HD is still the most profitable dialysis modality for the majority of dialysis units, the high import taxes charged on HD equipment do not allow to meet the increasing demand by new patients. Though, in 1986 more than 1.6% of the Brazilian Health Care budget was assigned to the dialysis patients who represented only 0.008% of the population [3].

The analysis of dialysis costs per year of survival showed that CAPD is less expensive than HD and both are less expensive than transplantation [4].

In Mexico, one of the consequences of the recent earthquake was the destruction of the majority of the HD installations. This led to an increase of CAPD and IPD patients, so that 77% of the overall dialysis population is now treated by these modalities.

In Venezuela PD accounts for 55% of the overall dialysis population. The majority of PD patients are treated with CAPD (590 patients), while less than 1% (10 patients) are on IPD. The government reimburses the same amount for either HD or CAPD.

Although Argentina has been one of the first countries to introduce PD in Latin America, only 2% of the dialysis population are now treated with this modality. The most probable reason is that the government does not reimburse CAPD costs.

Colombia has a very effective program of CAPD which comprises 25% of the whole group of uremic dialyzed patients.

Only a few patients, mainly children, are on CAPD in Uruguay, while in Cuba 50% of dialyzed patients are on PD and all of them on IPD.

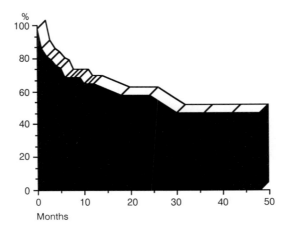

Fig. 1. Technique survival after 4 years of treatment.

Status of Peritoneal Dialysis in a Brazilian Hospital

The São Severino hospital is located in Sorocaba (400,000 inhabitants), 80 km away from São Paulo.

Ninety-three patients have been treated with CAPD since 1984, while IPD has mostly been used as a waiting treatment for CAPD.

Thus, 66% of the dialysis population are now on CAPD and 4% in IPD. The main reason for this proportion is likely due to the choice of the patients who had previously been on HD in other units and who live far away from the dialysis center.

The double-cuff Tenckhoff catheter is almost always implanted by the same surgeon and the break-in period is accomplished with IPD. The average training period is 2 weeks and the same nurse has been responsible for it since 1984.

Peritonitis is the most frequent complication with an incidence of 1.4 episodes/patient/year. The most frequent germ isolated is *Staphylococus aureus*, but 19% of the cultures are negative. Gentamycin is still the first choice antibiotic in peritonitis with a success rate of 69% and of 83% when a cephalosporin is added.

After 4 years of treatment, the technique survival amounted to 46.9% (fig. 1) while patient survival was 71.4% (fig. 2).

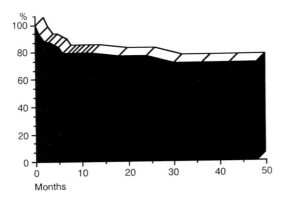

Fig. 2. Patient survival after 4 years of treatment.

In summary, PD has had a marked development in Latin America during the last 10 years, basically because of the introduction of CAPD.

A great part of the dialysis population in Brazil, Mexico, Venezuela and Colombia is already being treated with CAPD while Argentina and other countries are still waiting for a decision concerning the reimbursement from their governments to extend the CAPD program.

Many reports from different centers in Latin America present as good results by now as those from North America, Europe and Australia.

The main goal of the Latin American Society of Peritoneal Dialysis is to organize a registry for a more accurate evaluation of the CAPD status in this continent. On the other hand, IPD will continue to play its role as a simple and less expensive treatment for chronic renal failure.

The economic aspects of the dialysis therapy still play an important role in the choice of the available dialysis modalities in Latin America.

References

1   Best Demonstrated Practices (BPD): São Paulo, Baxter Labs, 1989.
2   Leitao Castro AC, Nascimento S, Huehara M, Vieira CC, de Gouveia MI, de Andrade AM, da Silva JA, Divino JC, Coelho MAC: Uma nova alternativa para tratamento da Insuficiencia Renal: A DPCI com cateter de permanencia e sistema fechado. J Bras Nefro 1985;7:33–38.

3   Dados do Instituto Nacional de Assistencia Medica da Previdencia Social n 9: Rio de Janeiro, INAMPS-Secretaria do Planejamento, 1986, pp 2–20.
4   Sesso R, Eisenberg JM, Stabile C, Draibe S, Ajzen H, Ramos O: Cost-effectiveness analysis of the treatment of end-stage renal disease in Brazil. Int J Technol Assess Health Care. In press.

Dr. J.C. Divino Filho, Hospital São Severino, Av. Roberto Simonsen, 987, 18090 Sorocaba-São Paulo (Brazil)

La Greca G, Olivares J, Feriani M, Passlick-Deetjen J (eds): CAPD – A Decade
of Experience. Contrib Nephrol. Basel, Karger, 1991, vol 89, pp 16–27

Outcome and Follow-Up on CAPD

J. Rottembourg, M. Allouache, B. Issad, R. Diab, A. Baumelou, C. Jacobs

Department of Nephrology, Hôpital de la Pitié, Paris, France

Continuous ambulatory peritoneal dialysis (CAPD) has emerged as one
of the most significant developments in the treatment of end-stage renal
disease (ESRD) in the past decade.

The number of ESRD patients treated by CAPD has increased exponentially during this first decade: as of December 1988 more than 35,000
patients were on CAPD around the world. 10,000 of them in Europe [1] and
1,500 in France [2]. The patients on CAPD comprise from 4 to 50% of the
population maintained on dialysis in various countries: 42% in the United
Kingdom, 33% in Denmark, 20% in Switzerland, 8% in France, 4% in
Germany.

The main advantages of CAPD are simplicity, promotion of home
dialysis, short training period and feasibility of long distance travel due to
freedom from dependency on machines. Despite its many advantages the
failure rate has remained high, probably because of inexperience with the
technical aspect of the procedure and inappropriate selection of patients for
this treatment [3]. Two different attitudes have emerged: as in the United
Kingdom, CAPD is preferred to hemodialysis as a temporary therapy prior
to a planned or early transplantation [4] or as CAPD is a new technique, it
should be given only to high-risk patients with poor survival on hemodialysis
[2]. This second attitude was predominantly selected in the Hôpital de la
Pitié during this first decade. This report describes the outcome and follow-
up of 305 patients and examines the risk factors that might contribute to
CAPD failure.

Table 1. Underlying renal diseases in 305 CAPD patients

	Number	Percentage
Glomerulonephritis	106	34
Diabetic nephropathy	86	28
Pyelonephritis	45	15
Nephroangiosclerosis	15	5
Polycystic kidney	10	3
Various or unknown nephropathies	46	15
Total	305	100

Patients and Methods

Patients

Between August 1978 and December 1988, 305 ESRD patients (185 males, 120 females) were trained for CAPD-CCPD in a special unit devoted to this task. Twenty-eight other patients did not succeed in the training and were transferred before completion to other modalities of dialysis and were not included in this report. Age of these CAPD-CCPD patients ranged from 18 to 89 years with an average of 58.2 ± 16.2 years. One hundred and three patients were aged more than 70 years at the start of CAPD. Two hundred and eighty patients were trained for CAPD and since 1981, twenty-five for continuous cyclic peritoneal dialysis (CCPD) [5]. The duration of CAPD-CCPD ranged from 1 to 116 months with an average of 24 ± 20 months per patient and a cumulative experience of 7,320 months (610 patient-years).

The underlying renal diseases are listed in table 1. Two hundred and thirty-six patients constituted a high-risk group because of diabetes, age, cardiovascular status or other severe associated diseases. Hypertension was present in 256 patients (85%). Cardiomegaly defined as a cardiothoracic ratio of more than 50% on the chest radiography was observed in 210 patients (69%). The major cardiovascular complicating factors present at start of CAPD were heart failure in 15% of the patients, angina in 25%, cardiac infarction in 13%, pulmonary edema in 13%, and cerebrovascular accident in 7%.

Training and Dialysis Techniques

As originally described all patients on CAPD-CCPD were dialyzed through an indwelling Tenckhoff catheter with the preferential use of the curled type [6]. Our training technique has been described in an earlier publication [7]. Most patients were dialyzed with four 2-liter exchanges per day; if on this regimen serum creatinine remained over 1,500 μmol/l, patients were advised to use five exchanges per day; on the other hand, when serum creatinine was less than 600 μmol/l, especially in patients with a substantial residual renal function, they were allowed to dialyze with three exchanges per day. Over the decade four different batches of commercially available bags were used with two different buffer solutions: acetate was abandoned in 1983 after the treatment of more than 120 patients and lactate solutions, introduced in 1981, were used for all patients thereafter [8]. Over time, eight different types of connections were used in order to

Table 2. Outcome of 305 CAPD patients

	Number	Percentage
Still on CAPD	45	15
Kidney transplantation	32	11
Recovery of renal function	11	4
Withdrawal of CAPD–CCPD	109	35
Death	108	35

prevent the occurrence of peritonitis. Chemical disinfection around the bag-spike of the luer lock connection was used during half of the entire observation time in 30% of the patients. Most of the diabetic patients were taught to use three to four times per day intraperitoneal injections of regular insulin to control their blood glucose levels [9]. Reasons and protocol for insulin administration were widely described [10]. For CCPD an automatic peritoneal cycler was required; commercial dialysates with different glucose concentrations were used [5]. Selection of dialysate was made by the patients according to their need for ultrafiltration: four to five short nocturnal cycles were completed during the daytime with one hypertonic exchange drained before the first nocturnal cycle.

Survival and Drop-Outs

In the present study, the terms 'discontinuation' and 'drop-out' were used synonymously and referred to cessation of CAPD for any reason. The term failure included death and withdrawal. The latter term was equivalent to all transfers to other dialysis modalities. Mortality on CAPD was defined as death occurring during CAPD treatment or death within 2 weeks after discontinuation of CAPD if the cause of death could be directly related to a complication of CAPD. In the determination of actuarial technique success rate, transplantation and recovery of renal function were considered as lost to follow-up whereas withdrawal and death were regarded as failure. These definitions of technique and patient survivals were in accordance with definitions used by others [11].

Results

Survival and Outcome

At the time of writing among the 305 patients (table 2) CAPD-CCPD was discontinued in 109, 32 received a kidney transplant, 11 recovered a kidney function allowing the discontinuation of the procedure, 108 patients died, while 45 continue on CAPD-CCPD. Figure 1 shows the cumulative actuarial patient survival and technique success rate for all 305 patients over a 5-year period. At 3 years cumulative patient survival was 74% and the percentage of those remaining on CAPD was 25%. During this entire follow-

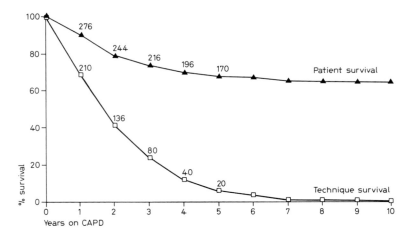

Fig. 1. Cumulative patient and technique survival in 305 CAPD–CCPD patients at the Hôpital de la Pitié.

up period 18 patients returned to their native countries including the West Indies, Algeria, Tunisia, Madagascar, Djibouti, and other African countries. The longest time on CAPD-CCPD is today 120 months (36 months on CAPD, 84 months on CCPD).

CAPD and Renal Transplantation

Thirty-two patients exclusively treated by CAPD received a kidney transplant while they were still on the technique. These patients (21 males, 11 females) mean age at start of CAPD 40.2 ± 9.5 years (range 21–52) received a cadaveric kidney in all cases except one. Eight of them were insulin-dependent diabetics, 3 were dialyzed in jail, 8 were Africans, 6 Asiatics. Mean time on CAPD was 22.1 ± 14 months (range 4–52 months). Kidney transplantation was performed during the first year of CAPD in 11 patients, during the second year in 12 patients and later in 9 patients. Mean peritonitis rate was low in this group: one episode every 24 months of treatment. Delay between end of peritonitis treatment and transplantation was requested to be over 4 weeks. The outcome after transplantation was as follows: 25 patients were living with their transplant from 3 months to 8 years; last mean creatinine level was 127 μmol/1. Three patients died on transplantation: 2 diabetics of cardiovascular complications and 1 patient of aplastic anemia. Four patients returned to dialysis: 3 to CAPD and 1 to hemodialysis.

Table 3. Reasons for drop-out in 109 CAPD patients

Abdominal complications	76
Peritonitis	39
Sclerosing peritonitis	11
Ultrafiltration failure	12
Intestinal perforation	8
Hernias	3
Tunnel infection	1
Abdominal and back pain	2
Patient's preference	22
Cachexia and malnutrition	8
Cardiovascular complication	2
Malignancy	1

CAPD and Recovery of Renal Function

Eleven patients (10 males, 1 female) mean age 65.8 ± 11.8 years (range 52–82) whose primary renal diseases were nephroangiosclerosis in 4 cases, interstitial nephropathies in 4, diabetic nephropathies in 2, and unknown nephropathy in 1, started CAPD while their residual renal function was at 4.8 ± 2.9 ml/min. Discontinuation was decided when the creatinine clearance was stable over 12 ml/min. The mean CAPD period lasted 10.4 ± 5.7 months (4–22 months); 10 patients were treated for more than 6 months, 6 more than 9 months, and 2 more than 1 year. Up to now 8 patients were alive, 6 of them without a dialysis procedure with a mean creatinine clearance of 20 ± 7 ml/min; 2 patients had to return to dialysis 14 and 6 months after discontinuation: one on hemodialysis, one on CAPD. One patient was lost to follow-up after 6 months. Two patients died: one of arteritis and one of a cardiac failure.

Withdrawal of CAPD

One hundred and nine patients, mean age 57 ± 14 years, treated by CAPD during a mean period of 22 ± 18 months had to be transferred to other modes of therapy: 106 to hemodialysis and 6 to intermittent peritoneal dialysis (table 3). Abdominal complications were the most frequent cause of transfer, including 76 patients (70%): peritonitis, recurrent peritonitis or fungal peritonitis in 39 cases, sclerosing encapsulating peritonitis in 11 cases, ultrafiltration failure in 12 cases predominantly in patients treated with acetate buffer dialysates, intestinal perforation of diverticulosis in 8 cases, hernias in 3 cases, tunnel infection in 1 case and abdominal or back pain in 2 cases. Patient's preference was the major reason of transfer in 22 patients: one group of 10 patients with a short experience time of less than 6 months, and one group of 12 patients with a mean experience on CAPD of 30 months – these patients developed weariness to perform 4 exchanges per day every day. Malnutrition and/or cachexia was the reason for the medical team to oblige the transfer of 8 patients to hemodialysis.

All these patients were studied after their transfer: 38 patients are still alive on hemodialysis with a mean time on hemodialysis of 26 ± 18 months. Eleven patients received a kidney transplant after a mean time on hemodialysis of 19 ± 12 months; their major reason for transfer was recurrent peritonitis which entailed repeated temporary withdrawals from the waiting list. After transplantation the outcome was good for all the 11 patients. Fifty of the transferred patients died, 20 of them because of cardiovascular complications in the early period after transfer. Four diabetics died of metabolic complications including hypoglycemia and hyperkalemia. Abdominal complications were responsible for death in 8 cases: 6 with sclerosing peritonitis, 2 with gastrointestinal hemorrhage. Sepsis with predominantly pulmonary infections led 11 patients to death. There were 7 other deaths for various reasons. The mean time between transfer and death for all these patients was relatively short: 12 ± 10 months.

Death on CAPD

One hundred and eight patients died while they were treated by CAPD (table 4). Half of these deaths, 54 patients, were in relation to cardiovascular complications including myocardial infarction in 18 cases, cerebrovascular accident in 14 cases, congestive or other cardiac failures in 8 patients. Fourteen diabetic patients died after lower limb amputations required for gangrene and sepsis. The mean age of these patients with cardiovascular deaths was 65 ± 12 years at the start of CAPD and they all belonged to the high-risk group of patients.

Abdominal complications were responsible for 15 deaths (14%): peritonitis in 9 cases (fungal peritonitis in 4), sclerosing peritonitis in 1 case, calcifying peritonitis in 1, intestinal perforation in 2 cases and necrotizing enteritis in 2 cases. Various malignancies led to death in 10 patients. Cessation of treatment was decided, in agreement with the relatives, for 10 patients (mean age 73 ± 8 years) when facing a situation where multiple complications including dementia led to permanent and definitive hospital-

Table 4. Cause of death in 108 CAPD patients

Cardiovascular disease	54
Myocardial infarction	18
Cerebrovascular accident	14
Lower limb amputation and sepsis	14
Various cardiac failure	8
Abdominal complication	15
Peritonitis	9
Sclerosing peritonitis	1
Calcifying peritonitis	1
Intestinal perforation	2
Necrotizing enteritis	2
Malignancy	10
Cessation of treatment	10
Sepsis	4
Various reasons	7
Unknown reasons	8

ization; the mean duration of CAPD in these patients was 32 ± 14 months. Sepsis and specifically pulmonary infections were responsible for 4 deaths, various known reasons for 7 and unknown reasons including some sudden deaths without any obvious laboratory abnormalities for 8 deaths.

Discussion

Since its introduction in our department, CAPD-CCPD has had a considerable impact on the management of ESRD patients: during the same follow-up period approximatively 800 patients were beginning an hemodialysis program; that is to say that the proportion of patients trained on CAPD-CCPD was around 38% of the entire ESRD population seen at the Hôpital de la Pitié during the last decade [12]. Our policy during the first part of our study (1978–1985) was to select for CAPD patients who presented some contraindications to hemodialysis or even to any form of dialysis: diabetics, elderly patients, patients with cardiac disease. With experience and with the decrease in the peritonitis rate seen with the new disconnectable systems [13–15] a positive indication for CAPD was decided for young patients awaiting a kidney transplant [16]. In some groups such as diabetics [17] or elderly patients [18], the results obtained on CAPD compare favorably with those obtained on hemodialysis. The data from other centers such as Toronto Western Hospital clearly indicate that age, diabetes and preexisting cardio-vascular disease have an adverse effect on the outcome of the treatment [19]. The survival rate of young patients without any systemic or cardiovascular disease was 100% at 4 years [19]. But in the American National Registry, exclusion of elderly patients and diabetic population had little effect on outcome [20]. One of the reasons to maintain our patient's recruitment policy until 1985 was the detrimental effect of the failure of the peritoneal membrane observed in our population due to the loss of ultrafiltration secondary to an extensive use of acetate dialysates [8, 21] in about 40 patients treated with those solutions for more than 1 year. It was reversible when the patients were switched to lactate solutions, but participated in the drop-out of the technique in more than 20 patients through direct failure (12 patients), patient's preference (5 patients) or malnutrition (3 patients). This problem was less frequent with the lactate solutions as described in the United States [19] and United Kingdom [4]. Furthermore, 18 CAPD patients, even after transfer to hemodialysis (2 patients) or after transplantation (1 patient) developed progressive sclerosing peritonitis [21] with 8 direct deaths and 5 related deaths. The high incidence of peritonitis observed in our unit during the early phase of our experience (1 episode every 6–10 patient-months) did not encourage us to propose CAPD to every ESRD patient. The good results obtained with the disconnectable systems [14] was one of the reasons for changing our policy.

Two groups of patients were considered as positive drop-outs: patients receiving a kidney transplant and patients having a recovery of renal function. Expansion of CAPD coupled with recent advances in clinical transplantation led to an increasing number of renal allografts recipients with prior CAPD therapy [1]. In Manchester, 25% of the patients receiving a transplant were patients whose only form of dialysis was CAPD [22]. This proportion is less important in our group but reached 20% in 1988. Patient and graft survivals after transplantation for CAPD patients were at least as good as that achieved for ESRD patients receiving prior hemodialysis when identical selection criteria, preparation and immunosuppressive therapy were employed [22]. Active peritonitis is a contraindication to transplanta-tion [23]. Most would agree that transplantation is safe if an episode of peritonitis has been adequately cleared and the patient's treatment com-pleted. In our practice, a period of 4 weeks between therapy and transplantation was probably too high: 10–15 days seems to be reasonable [22]. Peritoneal dialysis could be employed posttransplant but was deemed as associated with too high a risk of peritonitis and was thus never used.

During the follow-up 11 patients (4%) treated by CAPD recovered a renal function allowing a prolonged discontinuation of the procedure [24]. A lower percentage was observed for the patients treated in the hemodialysis unit. Similar results were observed by Cancarini et al. [25]. The reasons for this recovery were not obvious: a slower decline of renal function as pointed out in a study comparing hemodialysis and CAPD patients [26], the correction of hypertension and/or cardiac failure. Such factors as constant high plasma osmolality, stable high plasma urea concentration, absence of acute shifts similar to those observed during the hemodialysis sessions were considered by several authors [25, 26].

The two most important failures on CAPD were withdrawal from the technique mainly in relation to abdominal complications and death mainly related to cardiovascular complications. Each one accounted for 35% of our whole population. Peritonitis was responsible for 35% of all transfers, a proportion similar to that reported by Tranaeus et al. [27] but is higher than in other long-term studies [4, 19]. In addition to peritonitis, the other two major problems described in our unit, loss of ultrafiltration and sclerosing peritonitis, led a total of 62 patients to be transferred to hemodialysis [21]. Ten patients developed intestinal perforation, 2 of them died and 8 were transferred to hemodialysis. These numbers emphasize the role of diverticulosis as a risk factor for development of fecal peritonitis [28]. Patients particularly at risk of diverticulosis, namely those older than 60 years, those with previous history of constipation, those with polycystic kidney disease should have a barium enema before starting CAPD. One should avoid in these patients constipating medicines, aluminum gels and give osmotic laxatives or stool softeners to prevent constipation. Patient's preference was the second major reason of transfer: 22 patients (20%). This percentage is the same that was observed in the American CAPD registry [29]. In these patients 2 groups emerged: one who rejected the technique early after the training period, frequently consecutively to the first peritonitis episode, and another group of mainly elderly patients who developed weariness to perform four exchanges per day after 3–5 years of treatment [30].

Cardiovascular complications accounted for half of the deaths reported in our study. This number is higher than that reported in the European registry [1] or other long-term studies [4, 19, 27] but our high proportion of insulin-dependent diabetic (28%) or elderly patients (one-third over 70 years) and the presence of cardiac risk factors in two-thirds of the patients could explain such a lethality. Despite the fact that hypertension is very often well controlled during CAPD [19], its long adverse effects prior to CAPD may increase the cardiovascular mortality. Abdominal complications leading to death remained too high during the entire follow-up; however, two-thirds of these deaths occurred at the early phase of our program and these causes of mortality should progressively decline or hopefully disappear.

Based on our experience CAPD is now proposed to different types of patients: young patients awaiting a transplant, diabetic patients, and elderly patients in good clinical condition. Preexisting cardiovascular diseases remain the main cause of death. Abdominal complications should progressively disappear as the peritonitis rate decreases, loss of ultrafiltration and sclerosing peritonitis is also becoming much less frequent. This first decade was the pioneering stage for CAPD, the next one will certainly see CAPD taking a truly prominent part in the treatment of ESRD patients.

References

1   Brunner FP, Fassbinder W, Broyer M, et al: Combined report on regular dialysis and transplantation in Europe XVIII 1987. Nephrol Dial Transpl 1989;4:5–32.
2   Rottembourg J, Jacobs C: La dialyse péritonéale continue ambulatoire. Concepts actuels après dix ans d'expérience. Presse Méd 1989;18:1018–1023.
3   Nolph KD, Lindblad AS, Nowak JW: Current concepts. Continuous ambulatory peritoneal dialysis. N Engl J Med 1988;318:1595–1600.
4   Gokal R, Baillod R, Bogle S: Multicentre study on outcome of treatment in patients on continuous ambulatory peritoneal dialysis and hemodialysis. Nephrol Dial Transplant 1987;2:172–178.
5   Diaz Buxo JA: Current status of continuous cyclic peritoneal dialysis. Periton Dial Int 1989;9:9–14.
6   Rottembourg J, Jacq D, Vonlanthen M, et al: Straight or curled Tenckhoff peritoneal catheter for CAPD. Periton Dial Bull 1981;1:123–124.
7   Rottembourg J, Jacq D, Krouri A, et al: La dialyse péritonéale continue ambulatoire. Résultats cliniques. Nouv Presse Méd 1980;9:3158–3163.
8   Rottembourg J, Brouard R, Issad B, et al: Role of acetate in loss of ultrafiltration during CAPD. Contr Nephrol. Basel, Karger, 1987, vol 57, pp 197–206.
9   Balducci A, Slama G, Rottembourg J, et al: Intraperitoneal insulin in uremic diabetics undergoing continuous ambulatory peritoneal dialysis. Br Med J 1981;283:1021–1023.
10   Rottembourg J: Peritoneal dialysis in diabetics; in Nolph KD (ed): Peritoneal Dialysis. Dordrecht, Kluwer Acad Publ, 1989, pp 365–379.
11   Maiorca R, Cancarini G, Manilil, et al: Life table analysis of patient and method survival in continuous ambulatory peritoneal dialysis and hemodialysis after six years experience; in Khanna R, Nolph KD, Prowant B, Twardowski ZJ, Oreopoulos

DG (eds): Advances in Continuous Ambulatory Peritoneal Dialysis, 1986. Toronto, Periton Dial Bull Inc, 1986, pp 27–30.

12 Rottembourg J, Michel C, Verger C, Issad B: La dialyse péritonéale continue ambulatoire en Ile de France; in Chatelain C, Jacobs C (eds): Seminaires d'Uro-Nephrologie. Paris, Masson, 1989, vol 14, pp 177–184.

13 Maiorca R, Cantaluppi A, Cancarini GC, et al: Prospective controlled trial of a Y connector and disinfectant to prevent peritonitis in continuous ambulatory peritoneal dialysis. Lancet 1983;ii:642–644.

14 Rottembourg J, Brouard R, Issad B, et al: Prospective randomized study about Y connectors in CAPD patients; in Khanna R, Nolph KD, Prowant B, Twardowski ZJ, Oreopoulos DG (eds): Advances in Continuous Ambulatory Peritoneal Dialysis, 1987. Toronto, Periton Dial Bull Inc, 1987, pp 107–113.

15 Faller B, Pierre D, Verger C, et al: French multicenter study on drop out and peritonitis rate on CAPD; in Khanna K, Nolph KD, Prowant B, Twardowski ZJ, Oreopoulos DG (eds): Advances in Continuous Ambulatory Peritoneal Dialysis, 1987. Toronto, Periton Dial Bull Inc, 1987, pp 179–182.

16 Fries D, Benarbia S, Brocard JF, et al: Dialyse péritonéale continue ambulatoire et transplantation rénale. Presse Méd 1985;14:819–821.

17 Rottembourg J: Le traitement de l'insuffisance rénale du diabétique. Presse Méd 1987;46:437–440.

18 Dombros NV: CAPD versus hemodialysis in the elderly. Contr Nephrol. Basel, Karger, 1988, vol 57, pp 291–292.

19 Khanna R, Wu G, Vas S, Oreopoulos DG: Mortality and morbidity on continuous ambulatory peritoneal dialysis. ASAIO J 1983;6:197–204.

20 Nolph KD, Pyle K, Hiatt M: Mortality and morbidity in continuous ambulatory peritoneal dialysis. Full and selected registry populations. ASAIO J 1983;6:220–226.

21 Rottembourg J, Gahl GM, Poignet JL: Severe abdominal complications in patients undergoing continuous ambulatory peritoneal dialysis. Proc Eur Dial Transplant Assoc 1983;20:236–242.

22 O'Donoghue DJ, Dyer PA, Gokal PR: Renal transplantation in patients treated with continuous ambulatory peritoneal dialysis; in La Greca G (ed): Peritoneal Dialysis. Milano, Wichtig Editore, 1989, pp 259–264.

23 Ryckelynck JP, Verger C, Pierre D, et al: Early post transplant infections risk in CAPD. Periton Dial Bull 1984;4:40–42.

24 Rottembourg J, Issad B, Allouache M, Jacobs C: Recovery of renal function in patients treated by CAPD; in Khanna R, Nolph KD, Prowant B, Twardowski ZJ, Oreopoulos DG (eds): Advances in Peritoneal Dialysis, 1989. Toronto, Periton Dial Bull Inc, 1989, pp 63–66.

25 Cancarini GC, Brunori G, Camerini C, et al: Renal function recovery and maintenance of residual diuresis in CAPD and hemodialysis. Periton Dial Bull 1986;6:77–79.

26 Rottembourg J, Issad B, Gallego JL, et al: Evolution of residual function in patients undergoing maintenance hemodialysis or CAPD. Proc Eur Dial Transplant Assoc 1982;19:397–409.

27 Tranaeus A, Heimburger O, Lindholm B, Bergstrom J: Six years' experience of CAPD at one centre. A survey of major findings. Periton Dial Int 1988;8:31–41.

28 Wu G, Khanna R, Vas S, Oreopoulos DG: Is extensive diverticulosis of the colon a contraindication to CAPD. Periton Dial Bull 1983;3:180–183.

29 Lindblad AS, Nowak JW, Nolph KD: The USA CAPD registry; in Nolph KD (ed): Peritoneal Dialysis. Dordrecht, Kluwer Acad Publ, 1989, pp 389–413.
30 Delattre S, Sibertin-Blanc D, Montassine MC, Rottembourg J: Autonomie des patients traités par DPCA; in Kuss R, Legrain M (eds): Seminaires d'Uro-Néphrologie. Paris, Masson, 1983, vol 9, pp 117–126.

Prof. J. Rottembourg, MD, Department of Nephrology, Hôpital de la Pitié, 83, Boulevard de l'Hôpital, F–75013 Paris (France)

Different Approaches to Peritoneal Access

La Greca G, Olivares J, Feriani M, Passlick-Deetjen J (eds): CAPD – A Decade
of Experience. Contrib Nephrol. Basel, Karger, 1991, vol 89, pp 28–30

Endoscopic Peritoneal Dialysis Catheter Placement

Ch. Beyerlein-Buchner, F.W. Albert

Medizinische Klinik III, Städtisches Klinikum, Kaiserslautern, BRD

In the last decade, surgical implantation of long-term catheters in
patients undergoing peritoneal dialysis was the therapy of choice [1]. Alternative methods of peritoneal access placement have recently been described [2–
5]: the guide wire controlled insertion, placing the peritoneal catheter after
filling the peritoneal cavity with dialysis solution, the peritoneoscopic insertion using either one access [5] or the 'two trocar' technique which will be
described in this report.

Patients and Methods

From 1.1.1978 to 31.12.1988 the 'two trocar' technique was performed in 95
patients (31 males, 64 females; mean age 59.2, range 10–89; 67% diabetics). Twenty-six
patients underwent CAPD while 69 patients were on IPD. In 61 patients a straight double-
cuff Tenckhoff catheter [6] (from January 1978 to November 1978 and since March 1984)
and in 32 patients a coiled double-cuff Tenckhoff catheter (from December 1978 to
February 1984) were used. In 2 patients a pneumoperitoneum could not be achieved and
endoscopic placement failed.

The anatomical points chosen for the insertion technique are depicted in figure 1. On
Monroe's point the so-called Veress needle is introduced to inflate 2–3 liters of dinitrogen
oxide in order to achieve a pneumoperitoneum. The first trocar is then inserted two
fingers lateral left and cranial from the navel. In the lower abdomen an incision of 5–7 cm
is made and the tissue is prepared down to the preperitoneal fascia. The peritoneal cavity
is first inspected by the upper trocar in order to find a suitable place to introduce the
second trocar in the median line of the lower abdominal wall.

Under direct optical control the catheter is pushed through the second trocar into the
Douglas space. The metal cannula is carefully removed and the internal cuff is fixed
waterproof in the abdominal fascia with late absorbable thread. The external end of the
catheter is pulled by a redon pike through the subcutaneous tissue and leaves the skin at
3–5 cm cranial off the navel right beside the midline, depending on the length of the
subcutaneous tunnel to prevent cuff protrusion. According to a previous report [7], the

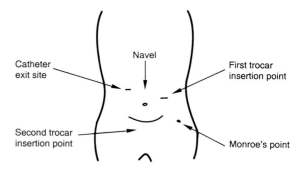

Fig. 1. Anatomical points chosen for the insertion technique.

Table 1. Early complications of endoscopic peritoneal catheter placement (n = 93)

Complication	n
Catheter tip migration (X-ray proved)	7
Catheter obstruction with poor drainage	2
Early peritonitis (first 2 weeks)	2
Leakage	1

direction of the subcutaneous tunnel is made craniocaudal. Finally, the peritoneal catheter adapter is fixed and wounds are closed in layers.

The whole procedure is carried out under local anesthesia in sterile conditions and lasts about 30 min. Immediately afterwards, peritoneal dialysis, usually IPD, is started with small exchange volumes from 500 to 2,000 ml for 4–5 days.

Results and Discussion

In the last 11 years, 12 catheter complications were observed in 9 out of 93 patients (table 1). Eleven complications occurred in 36 implantations between 1978 and 1983, while there has only been one insertion-related complication in 57 implantation procedures since 1984.

All these events were observed within 4 weeks after the first catheter placement. In 8 of these patients, surgical intervention was necessary and in only 1 case of peritonitis conservative management was effective.

Surgical implantation was chosen in hernias of the abdominal wall, in extreme obesity, if extensive intra-abdominal adhesions were expected, if simultaneous surgical treatment of an intestinal disease was indicated or if general anesthesia was wanted. Twenty surgical peritoneal catheter implantations were carried out in the above-mentioned period but, to date, no data are available on late complications.

Our results demonstrate that the 'two trocar' technique is simple, almost risk-free and yields as good results as the surgical implantation [8, 9] because the whole peritoneal cavity can be inspected, the best point of the catheter passage through the abdominal wall can be determined and the catheter can be placed under direct visual control.

References

1   Slingeneyer A, Balmes M, Mion C: Surgical implantation of the Tenckhoff catheter in peritoneal dialysis; in La Greca G, Biasioli S, Ronco C (eds): Peritoneal Dialysis. Milano, Wichtig Editore, 1983, pp 133–136.

2   Gloor HJ, Nichols K, Sorkin MI, et al: Peritoneal access and related complications in CAPD. Am J Med 1983;74:593–598.

3   Rubin J, Adair C, Raju S, et al: The Tenckhoff catheter for peritoneal dialysis – an appraisal. Nephron 1982;32:370–374.

4   Lovinggood J: Peritoneal catheter implantation for CAPD. Periton Dial Bull 1984;4:106–109.

5   Ash S, Handt A, Bloch R: Peritoneoscopic placement of the Tenckhoff catheter: Further clinical experience. Periton Dial Bull 1983;3:8–12.

6   Tenckhoff H, Schechter H: A bacteriologically safe peritoneal access device. Trans Am Soc Artif Intern Organs 1968;14:181–186.

7   Colombi A, Ayer G: Straight Tenckhoff catheter implantation technique; in Augustin R (ed): Peritonitis in CAPD. Contrib Nephrol. Basel, Karger, 1987, vol 57, pp 130–135.

8   Bierman MH, Kasperbauer J, Kusek A, et al: Peritoneal catheter survival and complications in ESRD. Periton Dial Bull 1985;5:229–233.

9   Khanna R, Twardowski ZJ: Peritoneal dialysis access; in Nolph KD (ed): Peritoneal Dialysis. Dordrecht, Kluwer, 1989, pp 319–342.

Dr. Ch. Beyerlein-Buchner, Medizinische Klinik III, Städtisches Klinikum, Friedrich-Engels-Strasse 25, D–W–6750 Kaiserslautern (FRG)

La Greca G, Olivares J, Feriani M, Passlick-Deetjen J (eds): CAPD – A Decade
of Experience. Contrib Nephrol. Basel, Karger, 1991, vol 89, pp 31–34

The Straight Tenckhoff Catheter

A. Colombi[a], *G. Ayer*[b], *G. Burri*[b]

Renal Unit of the Departments of [a]Medicine and [b]Surgery,
Kantonsspital, Lucerne, Switzerland

In contrast to the genealogy of mankind, the *Homo erectus* of peritoneal
catheters has survived all his descendants (fig. 1). The straight Tenckhoff
catheter is still the most widely used catheter for CAPD. At the first CAPD
congress held in Paris in 1979, we presented a new technique of implantation
using the so-called strictly craniocaudal method [1]. Later on, we explained
the philosophy of this implantation technique [2]. We stressed that the
catheter tip should be placed properly in the Douglas pouch, and that the
tunnel should be straight for the shape memory of the silastic catheter.
Finally, the fascial suture should be waterproof over the inner cuff and the
outer cuff should be at a safe distance from the skin exit site. Moreover, we
asked for constant care and dressing at this site.

Since 1978, a total of 90 Tenckhoff catheters have been implanted in 84
patients with end-stage renal failure. Total experience time was 1,934
patient-months. The mean technique survival time was 21.4 ± 16 months.
Only 9 catheters failed, 6 of which were replaced. The main reason for
catheter failure was obstruction (5 cases) followed by peritonitis (2 cases).
While infection or irritation at the exit site was frequently observed, the
peritoneal catheter had to be removed in only 1 case because of tunnel
infection. This was in an elderly diabetic male. The ninth catheter removal
was due to cuff extrusion, a situation which, later on, was no longer regarded
as an indication for catheter removal.

Since 1983, when 3-year catheter survival was 74%, this percentage has
increased steadily. At present 3- and 4-year survival is 91% (fig. 2). Simultaneously, the number of catheters at risk increased from 3 to 19 at 3 years.
After 1979, only every second year a catheter had to be removed because of
catheter failure. The annual experience being constant at between 150 and
220 patient-months (fig. 3). Of course, there is also some correlation between

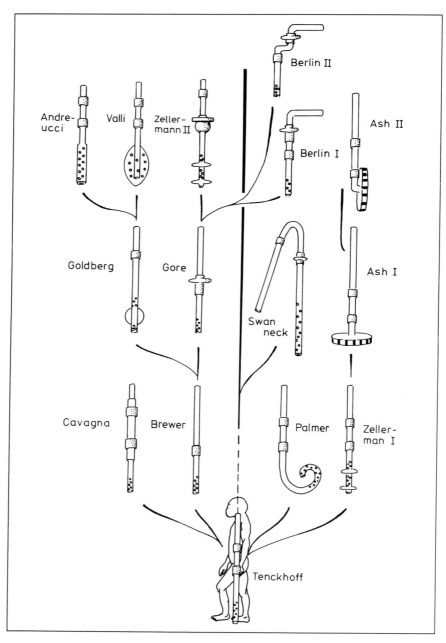

Fig. 1. 'Pedigree' of peritoneal catheters for CAPD.

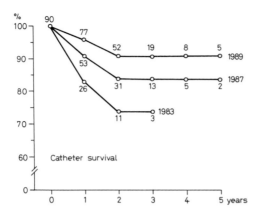

Fig. 2. Catheter survival 1983, 1987 and 1989. Number of catheters at risk is shown above the line.

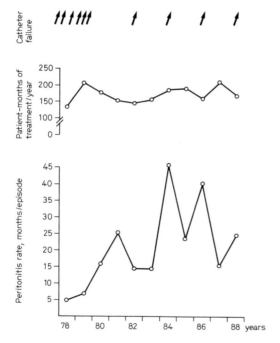

Fig. 3. Catheter failure, patient-months of treatment per year, and peritonitis rate between 1978 and 1989. Lucerne experience.

peritonitis rate and frequency of catheter malfunction. Mean peritonitis rate during this period was 24.4. ± 11.7 months/episode ranging from 14.2 to 46.3 months/episode per year.

Our results indicate that with the correct implantation technique of the straight Tenckhoff catheter and with adequate care of the peritoneal access, a long catheter survival time can be expected. No further development of such catheters is really mandatory.

References

1   Colombi A, Gianella C: Straight implantation of the Tenckhoff catheter for CAPD; in Legrain M (ed): Continuous Ambulatory Peritoneal Dialysis. Proc Int Symp. Amsterdam, Excerpta Medica, 1980, pp 69–72.
2   Colombi A, Ayer G: Straight Tenckhoff catheter implantation technique; in Augustin R (ed): Peritonitis in CAPD. Contr Nephrol. Basel, Karger, 1987, vol 57, pp 130–135.

A. Colombi, MD, Renal Unit of Department of Medicine,
Kantonsspital, CH–6000 Lucerne (Switzerland)

La Greca G, Olivares J, Feriani M, Passlick-Deetjen J (eds): CAPD – A Decade of Experience. Contrib Nephrol. Basel, Karger, 1991, vol 89, pp 35–39

Peritoneoscopic Implantation of Catheters for Peritoneal Dialysis: Effect on Functional Survival and Incidence of Tunnel Infection

Cosme Cruz, Mark D. Faber

Henry Ford Hospital, Detroit, Mich., USA

The creation of a safe and durable access to the peritoneal cavity remains one of the most formidable challenges in chronic peritoneal dialysis [1]. Catheter failure, caused by migration, outflow obstruction, leakage and tunnel infection leads to substantial morbidity and is a major cause of the high attrition rate seen in patients on continuous ambulatory peritoneal dialysis (CAPD) worldwide. These catheter problems are often the consequence of limitations in catheter design and implantation methodology.

This study analyzes the effect of the peritoneoscopic method of catheter implantation on the functional survival and the incidence of catheter-related complications in a CAPD program.

Materials and Methods

The outcome of 150 double-cuffed Tenckhoff catheters implanted peritoneoscopically [2] between June 1986 and December 1989 was compared retrospectively to that of 118 catheters implanted using a standard surgical method between March 1980 and May 1986.

The peritoneoscopic method involved a small (average 5 cm) paramedial incision following local anesthesia. Parietal peritoneum was punctured with a 2.6 mm trocar (Y-Tec^{TM}; Medigroup, North Aurora, Ill.) through the rectus abdominis muscle. Direct visualization of the peritoneal space was accomplished with needle peritoneoscope inserted through the trocar. After catheter insertion through a plastic sheath wrapped around the trocar, the distal cuff was placed within the body of the rectus muscle, and an exit orifice created inferior and lateral to the primary incision. The catheters implanted peritoneoscopically were by and large available for use after implantation without a 'break-in' period. Routine care for this group of patients consisted of daily washing with

Table 1. Patient demographic data and incidence of catheter failure according to the implantation method used

	Surgical method (n = 118)	Peritoneoscopic method (n = 150)	
Males/females	65/53	91/59	
Mean age, years	47 ± 21	53 ± 17	
Follow-up, days (±SD)	398 ± 341	360 ± 221	
Tunnel infection	26	1	p = 0.001
Inadequate function or leakage	22	3	p = 0.005

soap and water and thorough blow-drying when wet. Gauze dressing was not used routinely. In contrast, the surgical method involved light general anesthesia and a midline approach. Parietal peritoneum was incised by scalpel under direct visualization and the exit orifice was created cephalad to the primary incision.

Differences in the functional survival according to placement technique were assessed using the Kaplan-Meier actuarial method. The incidences of catheter failure caused by leakage, obstruction and tunnel infection were analyzed by the log rank test.

Results

Table 1 summarizes the patient demographic data and incidence of catheter failure according to the method of implantation used. The incidences of tunnel infection and catheter malfunction were markedly lower during the period of peritoneoscopic implantation. Only 2 patients (both among the first 24 cases done) experienced early failure caused by outflow obstruction. One patient experienced transient leakage which resolved with the discontinuation of dialysis for 2 weeks, after which dialysis using 1-liter exchanges was resumed. Figure 1 illustrates the significant difference in Kaplan-Meier survival rates for surgically (30% at 2 years) and peritoneo-scopically (84% at 2 years) implanted catheters.

Figure 2 shows the typical appearance of a catheter and exit orifice 2 years after peritoneoscopic implantation. There is a complete absence of inflammatory signs at the catheter-skin junction despite its proximity to the groin area.

Figure 3 demonstrates a patient with scars from multiple previous abdominal surgeries including two surgically implanted catheters that failed

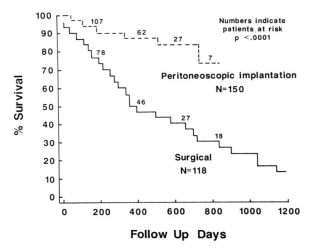

Fig. 1. Kaplan-Meier survival estimates for surgically and peritoneoscopically implanted catheters.

because of tunnel infections and two transplant nephrectomies. This catheter implanted peritoneoscopically remains functional 32 months after implantation.

Figure 4 shows an ileostomy patient 14 months after the peritoneoscopic implantation of a catheter. She remains peritonitis-free after 3 years on CAPD.

Figure 5 shows another patient 22 months after the peritoneoscopic implantation of a peritoneal dialysis catheter and a healthy exit orifice.

Discussion

This relatively new refinement in catheter implantation methodology offers a clear advantage, as these results indicate. The advantages of both the open surgical and blind trocar techniques are combined in that the proper location of the catheter is assured by direct visualization, while the risk of catheter leakage and patient discomfort are greatly reduced by eliminating incision of the parietal peritoneum. Because the procedure is well tolerated with local anesthesia, it can be carried out outside the standard operating room, offering additional advantages in terms of low cost and convenience.

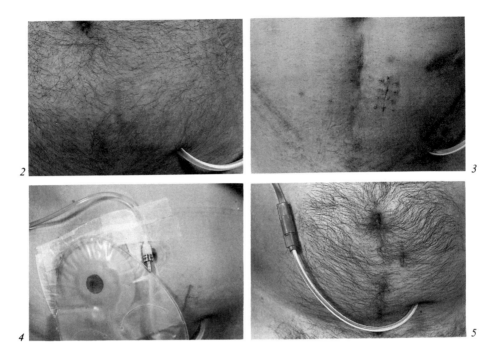

Fig. 2. Catheter and exit orifice 2 years after peritoneoscopic implantation.
Fig. 3. Patient with multiple previous abdominal surgeries.
Fig. 4. Peritoneoscopically implanted catheter in a patient with an ileostomy.
Fig. 5. Peritoneoscopically implanted catheter 22 months after implantation.

The marked difference in the incidence of tunnel infections seen in these two groups of patients may reflect the role that the orientation of the catheter tunnel and exit orifice play in the pathogenesis of this complication. It is now generally believed that a caudally oriented exit orifice away from interference by garment belts is less likely to become encumbered by sweat and debris, as well as being easier to conceal under standard garments. Another possible advantage the patients on the peritoneoscopic method group may have had was the catheter care routine [3]. This regimen has resulted in the preservation of pericatheter skin integrity and the virtual elimination of exit orifice inflammation.

In summary, the peritoneoscopic method of catheter implantation is associated with better functional survival and a lower incidence of tunnel infection.

References

1   Lindblad AS, Hamilton RW, Nolph KD: Special Reports 1987: Complications of peritoneal catheters; in Lindblad A, Novak JW, Nolph KD (eds): Continuous Ambulatory Peritoneal Dialysis in the USA – Final Report of the National CAPD Registry 1981–1988. Dordrecht, Kluwer, 1989, pp 157–166.
2   Ash SR, Wolf GC, Bloch R: Placement of the Tenckhoff peritoneal dialysis catheter under peritoneoscopic visualization. Dial Transplant 1981;10:383–386.
3   Cruz C, Faber MD: Peritoneal catheter and exit site practices. Periton Dial Int 1988;8:57–58.

C. Cruz, MD, Division of Nephrology and Hypertension,
Henry Ford Hospital, 2799 W. Grand Blvd, Detroit, MI 48202 (USA)

La Greca G, Olivares J, Feriani M, Passlick-Deetjen J (eds): CAPD – A Decade of Experience. Contrib Nephrol. Basel, Karger, 1991, vol 89, pp 40–42

Need for Vascular Access in CAPD Patients in Brazil

J.C. Divino Filho[a], *F.P. Almeida*[a], *E. Lobo*[a], *N. Boccato*[b],
J. Moron[c], *F. Linardi*[c], *J.A. Costa*[c]

[a]Nephrology, [b]General Surgery and [c]Vascular Surgery Sections,
Hospital Saõ Severino, Sorocaba, Brazil

Repeated episodes of peritonitis and tunnel infections are still the most frequent complications in CAPD patients. These complications often require temporary discontinuation of CAPD and a vascular access. Thus, many CAPD units have recommended that an arteriovenous fistula (AVF) should be established before the patient is admitted to CAPD to make hemodialysis (HD) available whenever it is needed.

This study presents our experience in this field.

Patients and Methods

From January 1984 to June 1988, 66 patients were treated with CAPD, 35 of them had some type of vascular access before or during CAPD. They were divided into 4 groups: (1) 16 patients who already had an AVF when transferred from HD to CAPD; (2) 7 patients in whom an AVF was established before starting CAPD; (3) 8 patients who did not have any vascular access during CAPD but, in acute situations, needed one; (4) 4 patients who were transferred from HD to CAPD because of inadequate vascular access. There were no significant differences in age, sex or etiology among the groups.

During the same period 115 double-cuff Tenckhoff catheters were implanted as peritoneal access for CAPD in our hospital. All the catheters were inserted by the same surgeon who, routinely, performed a mini-laparotomy under local anesthesia. The catheters were inserted in the midline (28%) or through the rectus muscle sheath (72%).

Intermittent peritoneal dialysis was the dialysis modality used during the 2-week break-in period.

All the costs for HD, CAPD and IPD are paid by the National Institute for Medical Assistance (INAMPS), while the acute vascular access materials (femoral, subclavian and jugular catheters) are imported and cost up to three times more than the retail prices in the USA or Europe.

Results

At the end of the observation period, in group 1 (16 patients) 12 AVF were still functioning (mean survival period 19 months) and 10 of 16 AVF were mainly used during peritonitis episodes (7 patients).

In group 2 (7 patients), there were 5 AVF still functioning (mean survival period 21 months) and 2 of 7 AVF needed to be used (both cases due to peritonitis).

In group 3 (8 patients) different forms of vascular access were used (femoral, 5; jugular, 2; A-V shunt, 1) and in all cases the indication was peritonitis.

In group 4 none of the 4 patients needed acute vascular access and the mean CAPD period was 38 months.

The most frequent early catheter complications were in/outflow obstruction (9 cases), while the most frequent late complications of CAPD were peritonitis episodes resistant to antibiotic therapy (26 cases), exit site tunnel infection (9 cases) and hernias (11 cases).

Discussion

Both vascular and peritoneal access implantation techniques are easy to perform by any general or vascular surgeon. The adequate performance of the operation is a basic condition for the viability of the dialysis treatment. In our hospital the catheter implantation was always performed by the same surgeon and the AVF by 3 vascular surgeons. Their interest and experience played an important role in the success of our dialysis program.

The advent of CAPD created not only a new dialysis alternative for patients with chronic renal failure but also a new opportunity for life in patients in whom AVF or transplantation could not be performed.

Shaldon et al. [1] already showed in 1964 that the use of a large bore vein for vascular access provided reasonable access in acute situations. Along with the technological development, new types of acute vascular access – subclavian [2] or jugular [3] catheters – became available, allowing patients to be kept on HD for a long time.

In Brazil, on the other hand, the costs of acute vascular access materials are not reimbursed by INAMPS, thereby making them unavailable for the majority of the dialysis population.

Thus, in Brazil, an AVF in CAPD patients can be important for both patient and staff as the need for acute HD could emerge. In our experience peritonitis was the main reason to use a vascular access in CAPD patients. Any severe medical complications due to AVF have never been observed in our study and the long survival rate of AVF supports its indication in CAPD patients whenever possible.

In contrast with other reports [4], the costs and complications of the acute vascular access [5] reinforce our policy to establish a primary distal AVF in every new nondiabetic CAPD patient. If the first AVF does not work, we create a new AVF or graft when HD is needed.

The main reason for such a policy is the economic aspect linked to the use of an acute vascular access.

The Tenckhoff catheter in our experience provides a very reliable peritoneal access for CAPD and IPD and its survival can be further improved if the peritonitis incidence, the treatment of complicated peritonitis episodes (*S. aureus*, gram-negative, fungi) and exit site infections could be improved.

In fact, these complications are the most important reasons for catheter removal as well as for the use of vascular access in our CAPD population.

References

1   Shaldon S, Silva H, Pomeroy J, Rae AI, Rosen SM: Percutaneous femoral venous catheterization and reusable dialysers in the treatment of acute renal failure. Trans Am Soc Artif Intern Organs 1964;10:133–135.

2   Uldall PR, Dyck RF, Woods F, Merchant N, Martin GS, Cardella C, Sutton DMC, de Veber GA: A subclavian cannula for temporary vascular access for hemodialysis or plasmapheresis. Dial Transplant 1979;8:963–968.

3   Cimochowski GE, Rutherford WE, Blondin J, Harter H, Worley E, Sartan JA: Experience with 100 consecutives internal jugular catheters for temporary access. Kidney Int 1988;33:218.

4   Joffe P, Skov R, Olsen F: Do patients on continuous ambulatory peritoneal dialysis need arterio-venous fistula? Periton Dial Bull 1986;6:193–195.

5   Stalter KA, Stevens GF, Sterling WA Jr: Late stenosis of the subclavian vein after hemodialysis catheter injury. Surgery 1986;100:924–927.

Dr. J.C. Divino Filho, Hospital São Severino, Av. Roberto Simonsen, 987, 18090 Sorocaba-São Paulo (Brazil)

La Greca G, Olivares J, Feriani M, Passlick-Deetjen J (eds): CAPD – A Decade of Experience. Contrib Nephrol. Basel, Karger, 1991, vol 89, pp 43–46

Experimental CAPD: A Rat Model

N. Gretz[a], J.J. Lasserre[a], P. Drescher[a], K. Mall[b], M. Strauch[a, 1]

[a]Clinic of Nephrology, University of Heidelberg, Klinikum Mannheim;
[b]Department of Nephrology, University of Heidelberg, FRG

The rat is a suitable animal model for the induction of chronic renal failure by performing a 5/6 nephrectomy. Thus, a simulated replacement therapy of renal function could be performed in this animal, as the dog does not seem to be suitable for the purpose [1]. The peritoneal access is the major problem to be solved when CAPD treatment is applied to a rat model. In a previous study [2] on the effect of a bicarbonate-containing CAPD solution, we injected the solution daily into the peritoneal cavity of Sprague-Dawley rats. However, this approach only partly simulates real CAPD conditions since the lack of a peritoneal catheter does not allow overcoming the rat's natural resistance to infection.

For the study of percutaneous access devices in CAPD, the mini-pig has recently been proposed as an animal model [3]. Comparable models for rabbits, mini-pigs, dogs, sheep and, in part, for rats have already been described [4–11]. However, it can be noted that the rats tend to pull out and damage any external catheter. In this study a normal catheter was inserted; the exit site was tunnelled under the neck, capped and left under the skin of the rat.

Materials and Methods

Sixty male Sprague-Dawley rats, with body weights ranging from 300 to 400 g, were studied. The animals received a Ketanest®-Valium® anesthesia for the catheter insertion. The skin of the abdomen and neck was then shaved and the abdomen disinfected. All further steps were performed under antiseptic, but not aseptic precautions. A transverse incision (<1 cm) was made roughly in the middle of the abdomen, the peritoneal cavity

[1] The authors are indebted to Mrs. S. Meisinger, Mrs. I. Sellger and Mrs. A. Helbig for their excellent technical assistance when performing the animal experiments. We appreciate the skilful help of Mrs. S. Redies in preparing the manuscript.

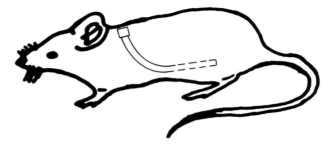

Fig. 1. Schematic drawing of the placement of the catheter as currently used in our model.

was opened in the midline and the catheter was inserted. The catheter was the usual Tenckhoff catheter (Fresenius, Bad Homburg, FRG) for adults. The intra-abdominal part had been reduced to 3 cm, whereas the extraperitoneal part was reduced to a length of approximately 7 cm. The peritoneal cavity was then closed and the cuff placed directly on the insertion site. After that the animal was turned round and the skin of the neck was disinfected. A transverse incision of about 1 cm was made. Then a tunnel was prepared with a forceps and the catheter was pulled through to the neck. A plastic cap with a rubber part for injection was fixed on the catheter by a thread. The tunnel was then extended towards the head of the animal so that the cap could be put into the tunnel proximal to the incision. Thereafter, the whole tunnel was rinsed with Braunol® and the skin was closed.

In another set of animals the skin of the neck was not opened but the catheter was directly tunnelled to the neck of the animal with a forceps. In these animals the tunnel was also rinsed with Braunol®. A schematic drawing of the catheter placement is shown in figure 1.

Results

A wound dehiscence due to early infection occurred in 12 animals. Also, the catheter was often pulled out by the rats and had to be surgically removed. In addition, abscess formation also occurred. After removing the cuff and opening the abscess, a new catheter was inserted some days later.

Eight of the 60 animals died of peritonitis or bowel obstruction. After 2 weeks no further deaths or catheter problems were recorded. In 2 out of the 60 rats the catheter could not be used for the CAPD solution injection because the device had been damaged by the injection needle. In only 50% of all animals could small amounts of the solution be drawn from the catheter. However, these amounts were not sufficient for a biochemical analysis; probably a sufficient amount of drained fluid could be collected by a reduction of the catheter diameter.

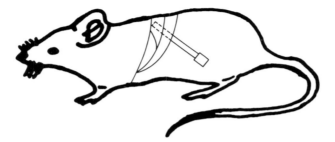

Fig. 2. Proposed catheter placement in the rat. Again, all parts of the catheter remain under the skin.

In the other animals, despite an easy injection of dialysate due to one-way obstruction, no drainage took place.

Discussion

Our data clearly show that peritonitis occurs in rats despite the common belief that these animals are fairly resistant to any type of infection. Probably in the future the peritoneal catheter insertion should be performed under strict aseptic conditions. Antiseptic conditions are not sufficient.

Our results demonstrate that rats are also suitable for trials on peritonitis treatment modalities. However, it should be pointed out that a catheter insertion is mandatory for such a study. In order to obtain a sufficient drainage volume we recommend reducing the total length of the catheter to less than 5 cm. Furthermore, it should be considered to implant the catheter not in the midline but laterally and perhaps to use a Swan-Ganz catheter in order to keep the gut and the omentum away from the catheter. A malfunction might thus be prevented. This type of lateral catheter placement has been used successfully in infants and small children [12]. Buntain [12] pointed out that by means of the lateral placement the catheter is located between liver, lateral abdominal wall and diaphragm, which has been advantageous since this area is completely free of omentum. Our proposed method of catheter placement is depicted in figure 2. In this approach the catheter also remains under the skin.

Furthermore, the injection volume should be reconsidered. A volume of at least 7–12% of body weight is likely to be needed in order to obtain a reasonable drainage volume.

References

1   Bovée, K.C.; Kronfeld, D.S.; Ramberg, C.; Goldschmidt, M.: Long-term measurement of renal function in partially nephrectomized dogs fed 56, 27, or 19% protein. Invest. Urol. *16:* 378–384 (1979).

2   Gretz, N.; Kraft, K.; Meisinger, E.; Lasserre, J.J.; Strauch, M.: Calcium deposits due to bicarbonate-containing CAPD solutions? Adv. CAPD *4:* 220–223 (1988).

3   Cardona, P.R.; Freed, P.S.; Rios, C.E.; Keller, D.M.; Vaughan, F.L.; Bernstein, I.S.; Bernstam, L.; Kantrowitz, A.: An animal model for study of percutaneous access devices in CAPD. Adv. CAPD *4:* 240–244 (1988).

4   Eschbach, J.W.; Adamson, J.W.; Dennis, M.B.: Physiologic studies in normal and uremic sheep. I. The experimental model. Kidney int. *18:* 725–731 (1980).

5   Landsberg, M.; Gnoinski, H.: Recherches sur la diffusion de l'urée dans le peritoine sur le vivant. Comp. Rend. Soc. Biol. *93:* 787–788 (1925).

6   Lankisch, P.G.; Koop, H.; Winckler, K.: Peritoneal dialysis in small laboratory animals. Experientia *33:* 743–745 (1977).

7   Levin, T.N.; Rigden, L.B.; Nielsen, K.H.; Moore, H.L.; Twardowski, Z.J.; Khanna, R.; Nolph, K.D.: Maximum ultrafiltration rates during peritoneal dialysis in rats. Kidney int. *31:* 731–735 (1987).

8   Moulin, G.C.; Lynch, S.E.; Hedley-Whyte, J.; Broitman, S.A.: Detection of gram-negative bacteremia by limulus amebocyte lysate assay: Evaluation in the rat model of peritonitis. J. infect. Dis. *151:* 148–152 (1985).

9   Rubin, J.; Jones, Q.; Quillen, E.: A model of long-term peritoneal dialysis in the dog. Nephron *35:* 259–263 (1983).

10 Webster, S.K.; Salit, M.; Burhop, K.E.; Borgia, J.F.: Peritoneal white blood cells during chronic peritoneal catheterization in micropigs. Adv. CAPD *4:* 309–311 (1988).

11 Wells, I.C.; Durr, M.P.; Grabner, B.J.; Holladay, F.P.; Campbell, A.S.; Zielinski, C.M.; Hammeke, M.D.; Egan, J.D.: Experimental study of chronic ambulatory peritoneal dialysis. I. Inhibition of protein and amino acid losses by single amino acids. Clin. Physiol. Biochem. *3:* 8–15 (1985).

12 Buntain, W.L.: A new technique for the placement of continuous ambulatory peritoneal dialysis catheters in infants and small children. Surgery Gynaec. Obstet. *160:* 362–364 (1985).

Dr. N. Gretz, Clinic of Nephrology, Klinikum Mannheim,
D–W–6800 Mannheim 1 (FRG)

La Greca G, Olivares J, Feriani M, Passlick-Deetjen J (eds): CAPD – A Decade of Experience. Contrib Nephrol. Basel, Karger, 1991, vol 89, pp 47–52

The Oreopoulos-Zellermann Catheter

P.R. Verreet[a], J. Passlick-Deetjen[b], B. Grabensee[b]

Departments of [a]Surgery A (Head: Prof. Dr. *H.-D. Röher*) and [b]Nephrology (Head: Prof. Dr. *B. Grabensee*), Heinrich-Heine University, Düsseldorf, FRG

A low risk access to the abdominal cavity via an implanted catheter is the key to successful peritoneal dialysis. Since Palmer et al. [1] designed the first silicone catheter for the purpose of peritoneal dialysis, many different catheter models [2] were produced showing that the procedure has not so far been optimized. Up to now, there is still a high rate of catheter-dependent complications implicating the reevaluation of the whole concept of catheter designs.

One of the main shortcomings in traditional catheter construction is the choice of materials used. Silicone is one of the materials that has found widespread acceptance and has eventually been used as a basic substance for all varieties of catheters [2–4]. It is characterized by an acceptable degree of elasticity and has proved to be almost biologically inert (table 1).

The catheter model most commonly used is probably the Toronto Western Hospital Catheter according to Oreopoulos-Zellermann made of silicone (fig. 1) [2, 3]. It has certain advantages compared to other models. The course through the abdominal wall is secured by two Dacron felt cuffs, but the pass point through the peritoneum is supplied with a silicone ball which is faced to a Dacron plate to prevent leakage. Two silicone plates attached to the intraabdominal part of the catheter will prevent dislocation. The catheter shows perforations over almost the whole intraabdominal segment. The plates protecting the transrectal implanted catheter against dislocation come to lie approximately to the Douglas pouch. The point of passing through the peritoneal layer is sealed with a Dacron-disc faced to the silicone ball and the catheter itself describes a soft curved way through the muscle and the subcutaneous layer.

The implantation technique practiced at the Heinrich-Heine University of Düsseldorf since 1983 [5] is carried out under general anesthesia. The

Table 1. Comparison of different materials used as permanent implants

	Elasticity	Workability	Biocompatibility	Price
Polyethylene	–	0/–	0	+
Polyvinylchloride	0/–	+	–	+
Silicone	+	–	+	0
Polyurethane	+	+	+	0

– = Bad; 0 = acceptable; + = good.

main advantage is the relaxation of the abdominal wall which enables a primary watertight closure of the abdomen. The left lower abdomen is chosen as the site of implantation for placing the intraabdominal course of the catheter at the left side of the mesenterial axis up to the Douglas pouch so that any dislocation of the implant's end out of the Douglas pouch by movements of the intestine is prevented. The transrectal approach is a well-vascularized covering of the catheter's course in the abdominal wall. The craniocaudal incision is approximately 5 cm long. After opening and inspection of the abdominal cavity the tip of the catheter is advanced ventrally to the promontory to the Douglas pouch under visual control. Again adequate exposure is only possible on the condition of relaxation in general anesthesia. The closure of the abdomen begins with a continuous watertight peritoneal suture which includes the given catheter segment in the distal wound angle. The catheter itself has to be fastened tightly with a monophile resorbable suture (PDS/3-0).

After a tight peritoneal closure the external end of the catheter is pulled through a separate stab incision far away from the implantation wound. Therefore, the catheter is armed with a guide pin. The stab incision is carried out in such a way that the catheter comes to lie in a wide curve without acute angle. The catheter is furthermore placed through the rectus muscle as a well-vascularized and flexible covering. The incision size is created so that the skin encloses the implant firmly but without tension.

As soon as the catheter is moved into its final position, the external opening is connected to the system and a first flow trial and test of water-tightness can be performed. After closing the wound in layers the peritoneal dialysis has thus already started with a reduced volume of 500 ml of dialysis fluid. It is worth mentioning that the Oreopoulos-Zellermann catheter is

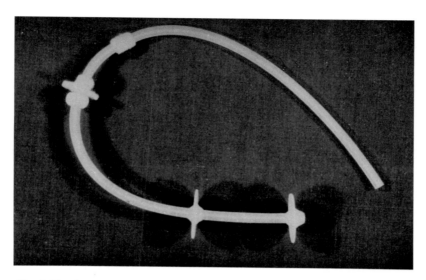

Fig. 1. The Oreopoulos-Zellermann catheter.

radiopaqued to identify any misplacement radiologically by an abdominal X-ray.

Before 1983 the implantation technique had not been standardized in our unit. The number of primary implantations performed at the Department of Surgery at the University of Düsseldorf amount to 32 from 1979 to 1983 and to 102 from 1983 to 1989. The continual increase of implantations might show that this procedure has gained a certain popularity in the Federal Republic of Germany, but so far only 4.3% of all patients with terminal renal insufficiency are treated with CAPD, while in the USA, Canada, Italy and Spain the proportion of peritoneal dialysis is considerably higher [6]. The first period to June 1983 covers the time when different catheter models with different techniques were implanted. In July 1983 the technique was standardized with the introduction of the Oreopoulos-Zellermann catheter. It was followed by a decrease of methodical complications [5–9]. Catheter dislocation has completely disappeared in our study, which is probably due to the antidislocation features of the Oreopoulos-Zellermann catheter's intraabdominal part. Furthermore, no more cases of leakage with fistula formation at the site where the catheter passes through the peritoneum were observed. This may be explained by a modified suture technique under general anesthesia with a relaxed abdominal wall. The intraoperative test for watertightness seems also quite important to be able to suture pos-sible leaking sites.

The major remaining complications are, on the one hand, the so-called 'tunnel' infection and, on the other hand, peritonitis [10]. The aim of implantation is to place the intraabdominal catheter tip exactly in the Douglas pouch to drain the dialysis fluid almost completely. The course of the catheter at the abdominal wall should be without any tension to the surrounding tissue to avoid any cellular reaction – a so-called 'bland tunnel'. This can only be achieved when the stiffness of the catheter permits a sufficient curvature and flexibility without impairment of the lumen, which is mainly dependent on the elasticity of the material.

In actually used silicone catheters elasticity is not sufficiently given to prevent certain pressure areas in the tunnel. Even correct implantation may not prevent a so-called 'tunnel decubitus' which will show up in the subcuta-neous course at any pressurized site a cellular demarcation of the catheter's course. This histological finding causes the necessity for new implants without any spring back force as in common silicone catheters.

Tunnel decubitus presents a primarily aseptic inflammatory reaction of the surrounding tissue. Macroscopically, a fine film of fluid is filling out the tunnel which again may possibly be colonized and ultimately develops a full-blown tunnel infection with associated tissue reaction. Those mostly staphy-lococcal infections might reach the Dacron felt cuff in the subcutaneous tunnel region. It is understandable that –once this area has been infected – this may spread along the tunnel into the abdomen and cause a generalized peritonitis by the periluminal route (fig. 2).

The problems previously mentioned are mainly caused by material- and surface-dependent properties of the long-term implant itself and by the implantation technique. The Oreopoulos-Zellermann catheter – as well as other silicone implants – is blamed for a low elasticity and workability resulting in a not acceptable rigidity leading to tunnel decubitus and in a too compact surface but with a certain roughness, which makes smooth tissue invasion impossible.

Regarding different alternative materials, the lack of elasticity excluded polyethylene for continuous use in peritoneal lavage catheters. The same applies for PVC which proved to be too hard a substance to be permanently implanted in the abdominal wall.

In contrast, in laminated polyurethane the elasticity of the material can be varied to a high degree by adding soft or hard segment substrates in variable proportions. Moreover, when medically used, it has proven to be

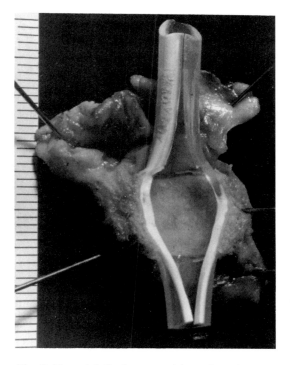

Fig. 2. Tunnel infection – position of an Oreopoulos-Zellermann catheter surrounded by a chronic 'tunnel decubitus' and an insufficiently sealing Dacron cuff.

absolutely inert. Another advantage besides the variability of elasticity is the fact that, for example, catheter perforations can be added as smooth as the rest of the catheter surface, so polyurethane has been modified according to detailed conceptions with regard to the production of a permanent peritoneal catheter. In addition, a test quantifying the growth inhibition of fibroblasts demonstrated that silicone and polyurethane provoke only a minimal reduction in fibroblast activity [11].

A final evaluation of all substances with regard to elasticity, workability, biocompatibility and, last but not least, costs shows polyurethane to be the material with most technical advantages but with a higher price. The main disadvantage of silicone remains that the workability of this material is limited (table 1).

Refraining from criticizing all different varieties of catheters by pointing out the chemical and physical features of the materials used, it is easy to remark that advantageous material properties of commonly used implants have not yet been sufficiently utilized. This applies to surface properties, elastic behavior, biostability, and biocompatibility.

Therefore, based on the Oreopoulos-Zellermann catheter's advantages, the superiority of a new implant made of laminated polyurethane in a special sandwich technique showing only 35% of the silicone catheter's stiffness retaining its initial shape was worked out and should encourage long-term results in animal tests. The first clinical results of a prospective randomized trial of the Oreopoulos-Zellermann catheter and the new so-called 'Braun-Verreet catheter' [11] will in future be reported after a 1-year follow-up and will hopefully be an advantageous alternative.

References

1　Palmer RA, Quinton WE, Gray JF: Prolonged peritoneal dialysis for chronic renal failure. Lancet 1964;i:700–702.
2　Oreopoulos DG, Baird-Helfrich G, Khanna R, Lum GM, Matthews R, Paulsen K, Twardowski ZJ, Vas SI: Peritoneal catheters and exit-site practices: Current recommendations. Periton Dial Bull 1987;7:130–137.
3　Oreopoulos DG, Robson M, Izatt S, Clayton S, De Veber GA: A simple and safe technique for continuous ambulatory peritoneal dialysis. Trans Am Soc Artif Intern Organs 1978;24:484–489.
4　Tenckhoff H, Schechter H: A bacteriologically safe peritoneal access device. Trans Am Soc Artif Intern Organs 1968;14:181–186.
5　Verreet PR, Rötzscher V, Ulrich B: Implantationstechnik des Oreopoulos-Zellermann-Katheters zur Peritonealdialyse. Chirurg 1983;54:609–612.
6　Verreet PR, Grabensee B, Röher H-D.: Chirurgie und Peritonealdialyse. Dtsch Med Wochenschr 1991, in press.
7　Verreet PR, Passlick J, Haacke C: Die Chirurgie der Peritonealdialyse. Langenbecks Arch/Kongressband. 104. Kongr Dtsch Ges Chir, 1987, p 341.
8　Verreet PR: Implantation, Konzept und Nachsorge eines dauerhaften Peritonealdialysesystems. Acta Chir Austr 1988;137:152–153.
9　Verreet PR, Fakir C, Ohmann C, Röher H-D: Preventing recurrent postoperative adhesions: An experimental study in rats. Eur Surg Res 1989;21:267–273.
10　Passlick J, Chlebowski H, Thomas L, Risler T, Peters U, Rosin H, Grabensee B: Klinik und Verlauf der Peritonitis bei Patienten mit kontinuierlich ambulanter Peritonealdialyse. Med Welt 1982;33:1797–1799.
11　Verreet PR: The Braun-Verreet-Catheter for CAPD, a new well functioning approach; in Bengmark S (ed): Peritoneum and Peritoneal Access. Tranberg, 1987, p 102.

Dr. med. P.R. Verreet, Department of Surgery A, Heinrich-Heine-University, Moorenstrasse 5, D–W–4000 Düsseldorf (FRG)

La Greca G, Olivares J, Feriani M, Passlick-Deetjen J (eds): CAPD – A Decade of Experience. Contrib Nephrol. Basel, Karger, 1991, vol 89, pp 53–58

Peritonitis Prevention by Eliminating the Risk Factor Disconnection

F.U.W. Jethon, I. Weber-Fürsicht, V. Steudle, R. Güleke, U. Kirschner

Intensive Medicine and Infection Control, Research and Development Department, Fresenius AG, Bad Homburg, FRG

The use of CAPD in a larger number of patients with chronic renal insufficiency is partly limited by peritonitis episodes, which are mostly caused by germs entering the peritoneal cavity primarily via the catheter lumen (transluminal, intraluminal) [1, 2] and more seldom via the catheter tunnel in the abdominal wall (periluminal) or the wall of the inner organs (transmural) [3, 4].

Each connection and disconnection is a potential risk step for the contamination of the CAPD system, resulting in peritonitis episodes.

The introduction of disconnect flush systems (reusable Y or O systems, single-use Y systems and integrated double bag systems) [5–10] or assist devices, e.g. the Thermoclav® [11, 12], could considerably reduce the incidence of peritonitis. However, even with disconnect systems a potential risk of contamination remains. The flush effect has been demonstrated to be effective only after a fresh contamination, but not after a prolonged dwell time [13–15]. Therefore, the most severe risk step is disconnecting. Recently, the ANDY® system (A non-disconnect Y system, Fresenius AG, Bad Homburg, FRG) was made available for CAPD. With this system the most severe risk steps are eliminated as no disconnection takes place after the exchange of dialysate; instead, the transfer set is sealed by a clamp and cut off distal to the clamp (fig. 1).

The objective of our study was to investigate bacterial growth in fresh CAPD solution and in native peritoneal dialysis effluent, in test tubes as well as in catheters, in order to evaluate whether the used dialysate could influence the flush effect. Furthermore, we examined whether the sealed tube is bacteria-proof over a prolonged period of time.

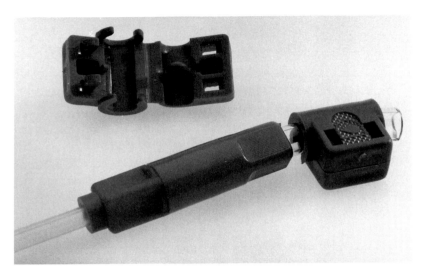

Fig. 1. ANDY clamp. In the upper part the clamp is open, in the lower part the clamp is closed and the transfer set cut off distal to the clamp.

Material and Methods

Test Strains. *Pseudomonas diminuta* (ATCC 19146), an extremely small germ usually chosen to test sterile filters, was used to examine the imperviousness of the ANDY set to germs.

Pseudomonas aeruginosa (ATCC 15442), *Staphylococcus epidermidis* (ATCC 12228), *Staphylococcus aureus* (ATCC 6538) and *Candida albicans* (ATCC 10231), which are frequently found in CAPD peritonits [16, 17], were used for the investigation of the growth of germs in the dialysate.

Cultivation of Overnight Cultures. This was performed in Tryptone soy broth (TSB Oxoid). Germs from stock cultures on Tryptone soy agar (TSA Oxoid) plates were inoculated into 40 ml TSB and incubated at 37 °C for 16 h (fungus 20 h).

Experimental Design. For growth experiments in CAPD solutions overnight cultures were diluted in 0.9% NaCl solution and then added to 50 ml fresh CAPD solution (CAPD 2, 1.5% glucose, pH 5.5, Fresenius AG) or native dialysis effluent from patients free from peritonitis and not on antibiotic therapy (initial inoculum: 100–300 CFU/ml). These mixtures were incubated under slight shaking at 37 °C in a water bath. Samples were taken every 2 h, diluted, plated with 20 ml TSA and incubated at 37 °C for 24–72 h. Control experiments were carried out in TSB.

In order to investigate the growth *of P. aeruginosa* and *S. epidermidis* in catheters, 12 fragments of Tenckhoff catheters (Fresenius AG) with an approximate length of 20 cm were filled with fresh CAPD solution or native dialysis effluent, adding 0.1 ml of

Table 1. Growth of different germs in fresh CAPD solution and in native dialysis effluent after 0, 12 and 24 h in CFU/ml

	Growth medium						
	CAPD fresh			CAPD effluent			control TSB
	0 h	12 h	24 h	0 h	12 h	24 h	24 h
S. epidermidis	210	0	0	221	110	22	5×10^8
S. aureus	327	108	14	291	153	18	1×10^9
P. aeruginosa	274	886	1.7×10^4	261	4,000	4×10^5	5×10^9
C. albicans	110	21	0	112	485	1,104	1×10^7

prediluted overnight culture (initial inoculum per catheter: 850 CFU of *P. aeruginosa* and 300 CFU of *S. epidermidis*). The catheter fragments were locked, loaded with a weight of 1 kg and slowly rotated on a shaking device at 37 °C for 12 h. After this they were flushed with 100 ml CAPD solution. The solution was completely filtered through a membrane filter (Sartorius) with a pore size of 0.45 μm. The filter was placed on a TSA pad (Sartorius) and then incubated for 24–72 h at 37 °C.

Three independent experiments with 10 clamps each were carried out to investigate whether the sealed tube is bacteria-proof. Fragments of tubes were clamped in the middle, the lower part was filled with 2 ml 0.9% NaCl solution and then welded. The upper part was filled with 1 ml overnight culture of *P. diminuta* (5×10^8 CFU/ml) and closed. These tube fragments were kept upright at 37 °C for 24 h. Thereafter, the NaCl solution was plated with 20 ml TSA and incubated for 72 h at 37 °C.

Results

Growth of Germs in CAPD Solution. In table 1 the results of germ growth in fresh dialysis fluid and in native peritoneal dialysis effluent in test tubes are given. The marked reduction of staphylococci in fresh dialysis solution as well as in native dialysis effluent could not be observed with *P. aeruginosa*, the CFU of which increased exponentially in both media. In spite of the low titers of CFU of staphylococci, there was an evident turbidity of the solution. With *C. albicans* a decrease in CFU was observed in fresh solution, whereas CFU increased in native dialysis effluent.

Growth of Germs in Catheters. With fresh dialysis solution a complete elimination of *S. epidermidis* was noticed, whereas with *P. aeruginosa* a

Table 2. Growth of germs in catheters filled with fresh CAPD solution or with native dialysis effluent

Growth medium	S. epidermidis		P. aeruginosa	
	number of positive sets	CFU/ catheter	number of positive sets	CFU/ catheter
CAPD fresh	0/0%	0	12/100%	$>2.5 \times 10^3$
CAPD effluent	3/25%	50	12/100%	$>1.0 \times 10^4$

The number of catheters with positive proof of germs after 12 h (total/%) as well as the number of CFU per catheter are given (initial inoculum per catheter: 850 CFU for *P. aeruginosa* and 300 CFU for *S. epidermidis*).

dramatic increase could be observed. In contrast, with native PD effluent, *S. epidermis* was only markedly reduced, while CFU of *P. aeruginosa* increased even more compared to fresh dialysis solution (table 2).

Safety of the ANDY Clamp. No germs could be detected in the NaCl solution in the noncontaminated part of the tube (table 3).

Discussion

Since the flush is not effective after a prolonged dwell time [13–15], it was proposed to fill reusable systems with disinfectants between the exchanges in order to increase the flush effect [13]. Yet, even this involves a considerable risk for the patient [18] and recent studies could not prove the effectiveness of in-line disinfectants [9, 19]. Our study indicates that fresh dialysis solution alone has an inhibitory effect on microbial growth, although our results revealed a remarkable difference among different species.

The significant reduction of germs (with the exception of *P. aeruginosa*) in fresh dialysis solution was also observed by other authors [20]. However, the total disappearance of *S. epidermidis* and *C. albicans* after 24 h in our study could not be explained sufficiently. This inhibitory effect might partially be due to the low pH of the solution. The exponential growth of *P. aeruginosa* not only in fresh dialysis fluid, but also in native PD effluent, might explain the ineffectiveness of a flush after a prolonged dwell time and stresses the need for new devices which provide sufficient protection from contamination.

Table 3. Safety of the tube clamp of the ANDY set

Test series	Clamp No.	Number of positive sets
I	1–10	0
II	11–20	0
III	21–30	0

Three series with 10 tube fragments cut off from ANDY sets separated with the clamp in the middle, were contaminated with 5×10^8 CFU of *P. diminuta* on one side. CFU in the noncontaminated tube segment were examined.

This is even more stressed by our findings in the catheter experiments, where *P. aeruginosa* increased to the same extent as in the test tubes. Again, with *S. epidermidis* in fresh dialysis solution, no germs could be detected.

With the ANDY system the most severe risk step in the exchange procedure, the disconnection, during which a further contamination may take place, is avoided. Our findings indicate that under the above conditions no germ could pass the closed clamp. Thus, no contamination of the system can occur while the clamp is closed. After the dwell time the remainder of the system is disconnected and immediately afterwards the new transfer set is connected and an effective flush started.

Therefore, the ANDY system meets two requirements of a CAPD system, which hitherto seemed to exclude each other – minimum risk of contamination combined with maximum comfort and maximum freedom of movement for the patient.

References

1   Augustin R, Kuhlmann U, Schmid E, et al: Bacterial peritonitis in CAPD: Pathogenesis, symptoms, therapy and progress; in Augustin R (ed): Peritonitis in CAPD. Contrib Nephrol. Basel, Karger, 1987, vol 57, pp. 10–22.
2   Oreopoulos DG, Vas S, Khanna R: Prevention of peritonitis during continuous ambulatory peritoneal dialysis. Periton Dial Bull 1983;3:518–520.
3   Gokal R: Peritonitis in continuous ambulatory peritoneal dialysis. J Antimicrob Chemother 1982;9:417–422.
4   Vas SI, Low DE, Layne S, et al: Microbiological diagnostic approach to peritonitis in CAPD patients; in Atkins RC (ed): Peritoneal Dialysis. Edinburgh, Churchill-Livingstone, 1981, pp 264–271.

5 Bazzato G, Coli U, Landini S, et al: Six years experience of CAPD with double bag system. Periton Dial Bull 1984;4:S4.

6 Buonchristiani U, Cozzari M, Quintaliani G, et al: Abatement of exogenous peritonitis risk using the Perugia CAPD system. Dial Transplant 1983;12:14–24.

7 Cantaluppi A, Scalamogna A, Castelnovo L, et al: Peritonitis prevention in CAPD: Efficacy of a Y-connector and disinfectant. Periton Dial Bull 1986;6:58–61.

8 Maiorca R, Cancarini GC, Colombrita D, et al: Further experience with Y system in continuous ambulatory peritoneal dialysis; in Khanna R, Nolph KD, Prowant BF, Twardowski ZJ, Oreopoulos DG (eds): Advances in Continuous Ambulatory Peritoneal Dialysis, 1986. Toronto, Peritoneal Dialysis Bulletin Inc, 1986, pp 172–175.

9 Ryckelynck JP, Verger C, Cam G, et al: Importance of the flush effect in disconnect systems; in Khanna R, Nolph KD, Prowant BF, Twardowski ZJ, Oreopoulos DG (eds): Advances in Continuous Ambulatory Peritoneal Dialysis. Toronto, Peritoneal Dialysis Bulletin Inc, 1986, pp 282–284.

10 Vas SI: Can advances in connector technology reduce peritonitis in CAPD? Periton Dial Bull 1985;5:5–6.

11 Martinez V, García Caballero J, Munoz I, et al: Heat sterilization of Safe·Lock connectors using Thermoclav® in experimental conditions. Contrib Nephrol. Basel, Karger, 1991, vol 89, pp 59–61.

12 Thomae U: Heat sterilisation of Safe·Lock connectors using the Thermoclav; in Augustin R (ed): Peritonitis in CAPD. Contrib Nephrol. Basel, Karger, 1987, vol 57, pp 172–177.

13 Luzar MA, Slingeneyer A, Cantaluppi A, et al: In vitro study of the flush effect in two reusable continuous ambulatory peritoneal dialysis (CAPD) disconnect systems. Periton Dial Int 1989;9:169–173.

14 Schmid E, Augustin R, Kuhlmann U, et al: Quantitative in vitro contamination and recovery studies: the flush principle in CAPD; in Augustin R (ed): Peritonitis in CAPD. Contrib Nephrol. Basel, Karger, 1987, vol 57, pp 185–190.

15 Verger C, Luzar MA: In vitro study of the CAPD Y line systems; in Khanna R, Nolph KD, Prowant BF, Twardowski ZJ, Oreopoulos DG (eds): Advances in Continuous Ambulatory Peritoneal Dialysis, 1986. Toronto, Peritoneal Dialysis Bulletin Inc, 1986, pp 160–164.

16 Michael J, Adu D, Gruer LD, et al: Bacteriological spectrum of CAPD peritonitis; in Augustin R (ed): Peritonitis in CAPD. Contrib Nephrol. Basel, Karger, 1987, vol 57, pp 41–44.

17 Rodriguez-Pérez JC: Fungal peritonitis in CAPD – Which treatment is best? in Augustin R (ed): Peritonitis in CAPD. Contrib Nephrol. Basel, Karger, 1987, vol 57, pp 41–44.

18 Junor BJR, Briggs JD, Forwell MA, et al: Sclerosing peritonitis. The contribution of chlorhexidine in alcohol. Periton Dial Bull 1985;5:101–104.

19 Werner HP: Efficacy of 'disinfectants' frequently used in dialysis; in Augustin R (ed): Peritonitis in CAPD. Contrib Nephrol. Basel, Karger, 1987, vol 57, pp 147–157.

20 Verbrugh HA, Keane WF, Conroy WE, et al: Bacterial growth and killing in chronic ambulatory peritoneal dialysis fluids. J Clin Microbiol 1984;20:199–203.

Dr. U. Kirschner, Intensive Medicine and Infection Control, Research and Development, Fresenius AG, POBox, D–W–6380 Bad Homburg (FRG)

La Greca G, Olivares J, Feriani M, Passlick-Deetjen J (eds): CAPD – A Decade
of Experience. Contrib Nephrol. Basel, Karger, 1991, vol 89, pp 59–61

Heat Sterilization of Safe·Lock Connectors Using Thermoclav® in Experimental Conditions

*V. Martinez, J. García Caballero, I. Muñoz, O. Celadilla,
B. Miranda, R. Selgas*

Hospital La Paz, Madrid, Spain

Exogenous peritonitis is one of the most frequent complications in
CAPD [1, 2]. It is usually caused by inappropriate handling of the CAPD bag
connectors. Disconnect systems with flush before fill and an ultraviolet
germicide chamber have recently been introduced to prevent these types of
infections. Different results have been reported following the use of these
devices [3–5]. However, complete sterilization of the touched zones cannot
be achieved with these systems. A new assist device, the Thermoclav®
(Fresenius AG, Bad Homburg), has been proposed for germ eradication [6].
Actually, the autoclave method should provide a complete sterilization of the
accidentally touched zones during the exchange procedures. The aim of this
paper is to study this device under experimental contamination conditions to
confirm its usefulness and security in vivo.

Material and Methods

Six double experiments were performed. The Safe·Lock connector (Fresenius AG,
Bad Homburg) was contaminated prior to the passage of dialysate and before breaking the
breaking cone. A simultaneous inoculum of 10 µl (10,000 colony forming units, cfu) of
Escherichia coli (ATCC 1376), *Staphylococcus aureus* (ATCC 2554), and a spore strip of
Bacillus subtilis and *Bacillus stearothermophilus* (Lab. Pergut) was placed in the male part
of the connector. In a different setting, a contaminated gauze swab (only *E. coli* and
S. aureus) was placed into the connector lumen. Thereafter, the Thermoclav device was
switched on. At the end of the process, after 8 minutes, samples for microbiological
analysis, taken from the dialysate collected downstream from the connector and from the
swab in the lumen, were cultured.

In a second experiment every procedure was repeated in the same way except that the
Thermoclav was not completely closed. 24–48 h after incubation at 37 °C microbiological

Table 1. Experiment performed under optimal and appropriate conditions

Microorganism	Inoculum, cfu	Results
E. coli, ATCC 1376	10,000	negative
S. aureus, ATCC 2554	10,000	negative
B. subtilis (spore strip)	10,000	negative
B. stearothermophilus (spore strip)	10,000	negative

Table 2. Experiment performed by incomplete closure of the Thermoclav device

Microorganism	Inoculum, cfu	Results
E. coli, ATCC 1376	10,000	positive
S. aureus, ATCC 2554	10,000	positive
B. subtilis (spore strip)	10,000	positive
B. stearothermophilus (spore strip)	10,000	positive

growth was assessed by usual methods. Positive and negative bacteriological controls were also studied. During the procedure usual bag exchange conditions for the Safe·Lock system were exactly reproduced.

Results

Positive and negative culture controls resulted in appropriate positive and negative bacterial growth. No microbiological growth was detected after the Thermoclav exposure in any of the six double experiments. Therefore, neither *S. aureus* nor *E. coli* nor *Bacillus* spores survived the heating procedure (table 1). However, when the working conditions of the Thermoclav device were altered by not completely closing it, germs were not eradicated at all (table 2).

Discussion

In CAPD patients, the exogenous peritonitis rate has progressively decreased since the introduction of new technology [3–6]. However, in some patients the new assist devices were unsuccessful in completely preventing exogenous peritonitis.

In addition, disconnect systems with chlorhexidine in line as disinfectant, expose patients to a risk of an accidental disinfectant introduction into the abdomen, whereas disconnect systems without chlorhexidine are not proved effective in eradicating *P. aeruginosa* and *S. aureus* with the flush before fill effect [7].

The interest in developing new and effective devices for preventing CAPD peritonitis should be permanent. The results obtained in the present study performed under experimental contamination conditions are unequivocal concerning the capacity of eradicating all forms of germs by the Thermoclav device. Only when the process of sterilization was altered by hindering the complete closure of the device was this assist device unsuccessful in sterilizing contaminated connectors. Probably, the incomplete closure did not allow the achievement of the correct temperature.

We conclude that under experimental conditions the Thermoclav device eradicates any germs introduced into the CAPD connection zone, including the spore forms.

References

1   Mion C, Slingeneyer A, Canaud C: Peritonitis; Gokal R (ed): Continuous Ambulatory Peritoneal Dialysis. Edinburgh, Churchill Livingstone, 1986, pp 163–217.
2   Vas SI: Peritonitis; in Nolph KD (ed): Peritoneal Dialysis. Boston, Martinus Nijhoff, 1985, pp 411–440.
3   Nolph KD; Prowant B, Serker KD, et al: A randomized multicenter clinical trial to evaluate the effects of an ultraviolet germicidal system on peritonitis rate in CAPD. Periton Dial Bull 1985;5:19–24.
4   Cantaluppi A, Scalamogna A, Castelnovo C, Graziani G: Long-term efficacy of a Y-connector and disinfectant to prevent peritonitis in CAPD; in Khanna R, Nolph KD, Prowant B, Advances in Continuous Ambulatory Peritoneal Dialysis 1986. Toronto, Peritoneal Dialysis Bulletin, Inc., 1986, pp 182–185.
5   Burkar J, Hylander B, Durnell T: Comparison of peritonitis rates during long-term use the standard spike vs. the Y set in CAPD. Periton Dial Int 1989;9 (suppl 1): abstr 21.
6   Thomae U: Heat sterilization of Safe·Lock connectors using the Thermoclav; in Augustin R (ed): Peritonitis in CAPD. Contr Nephrol. Basel, Karger, 1987, vol 57, pp 172–177.
7   Verger C, Luzar MA: In vitro study of CAPD-Y line systems; in Khanna R, Nolph KD, Prowant B (eds): Advances in Continuous Ambulatory Peritoneal Dialysis, 1986. Toronto. Peritoneal Dialysis Bulletin, Inc., 1986, pp 160–164.

Rafael Selgas, MD, Servicio de Nefrologia, Hospital La Paz,
Castellana 261, E–28046 Madrid (Spain)

La Greca G, Olivares J, Feriani M, Passlick-Deetjen J (eds): CAPD – A Decade of Experience. Contrib Nephrol. Basel, Karger, 1991, vol 89, pp 62–67

Reduction of the Incidence of Peritonitis in CAPD: Effectiveness of Heat Sterilization of Safe·Lock Connectors

E. Olivas, C. Jiménez, A. López, E. Andres, L. Sánchez Tárraga

Nephrology Service, General Hospital, Albacete, Spain

Bacterial peritonitis is the most frequent complication of CAPD patients and greatly affects morbidity, mortality and dropout of these patients [1–3]. The germs reach the peritoneal cavity by several routes: intraluminal (through the lumen of the catheter), periluminal (around the catheter), transmural (from the bowel) and ascending (from the vagina). Though in some studies [4] the intraluminal route only accounted for 30–35% of the overall peritonitis, this route is still considered the most common way of infection by most of the authors [5]. Consequently, the development of new systems aims at eradicating this important route of peritoneal infection. Heat sterilization of the Safe·Lock connectors using the Thermoclav® device is one of these systems. The connector placed in this device is heated up in a few minutes to sterilize the connection [6].

In this study we assess our recent experience with this system, comparing the incidence of peritonitis with that of other systems.

Patients and Methods

The high incidence of peritonitis has been a consistent and worrying factor since the beginning of our CAPD program in 1985 (table 1).

In 1987, 32 episodes of exogenous peritonitis were detected in 50% of the 24 CAPD patients (1 episode/6.6 patient-months). The spike connector, Safe·Lock connector and UV-XD germicide chamber were used during that year.

In March 1988, the heat sterilization system for the Safe·Lock connectors was utilized in patients starting the CAPD program. During 1988, 35 patients were treated with CAPD: 12 of these with the Thermoclav device, the others with the previously used systems (8 spike connector and 17 UV-XD device). Twenty-six episodes of peritonitis

Table 1. Incidence of peritonitis 1985–1988

Year	Patients n	Patient- months	Peritonitis		Incidence episodes/ patient-months
			n	% of patients	
1985	11	45	3	27	1/15
1986	19	142	10	26	1/14.2
1987	24	211	32	50	1/6.6
1988	35	286	26	45	1/11

Table 2. Incidence of peritonitis according to the system used in 1988

System	Patients n	Patient- months	Peritonitis		Incidence episodes/ patient-months
			n	% of patients	
Spike	8	76	8	75	1/9.5
UV-XD	17[1]	157	16	53	1/9.8
Thermoclav	12	53	2	16	1/26.5
Thermoclav[2]	12	53	1	8	1/53.0

[1] Two patients transferred from spike connector to UV-XD.
[2] Without periluminal peritonitis, $p < 0.001$.

were detected. Two of these occurred in patients using the Thermoclav system, one in connection with an exit site infection and the other the day after a session in which the use of the Thermoclav device was not possible because of a power problem. If the peritonitis episodes associated with a prior and simultaneous tunnel infection are excluded, the incidence of infection with this system was 1 episode/53 patient-months, significantly less than that obtained with the other two systems (table 2).

From March 1988 to April 1989, 38 patients were treated with CAPD: the Thermo-clav device was used in 17 patients (group A), while the remaining 21 patients (group B) utilized the spike connector (7 patients) and UV-XD chamber (14 patients). During this period, 2 patients using the spike connector were transferred to the UV-XD device.

The mean age and the percentage of diabetic patients were similar in both groups (table 3). A double-cuff Tenckhoff catheter, using a titanium connector in group B and a Safe · Lock connector in group A, was chosen as peritoneal access in all patients.

Four exchanges per day with 2-liter bags were performed in all patients. Only 1 diabetic patient in group B used intraperitoneal insulin. In the other diabetic patients of both groups, subcutaneous insulin for the management of their diabetes was administered. The transfer system was changed at the patient's home every 8 weeks. The

Table 3. Patient population and causes of end-stage renal failure (% values)

Group A: n = 17, mean age 55.8 ± 13.2		Group B: n = 21, mean age 56.1 ± 11.6	
Diabetes	41	Diabetes	38
Nephroangiosclerosis	12	Chronic pyelonephritis	10
Adult polycystic disease	12	Amyloidosis	9
Chronic glomerulonephritis	7	Chronic glomerulonephritis	9
Unknown	28	Unknown	34

Table 4. Incidence of peritonitis according to the system used (March 88 to April 89)

	Patients n	Patient-months	Peritonitis		Incidence episodes/ patient-month	
			n	% of patients		
Group A	17	113	3 (1)[1]	17 (6)[1]	37.6 (113)[1]	p < 0.01
Group B	21	264	24 (23)[1]	66 (62)[1]	11 (11.5)	
Group B						
Spike	7	77	1	86	8.5	NS
UV-XD	16	187	14	44	13.3	

[1] Without periluminal peritonitis.

diagnosis of peritonitis was based on leukocyte count ($>100/mm^3$) in the cloudy peritoneal effluent, abdominal pain, fever and leukocytosis.

The comparative data for both groups were analyzed by the χ^2 test with Yates' correction and the analysis of the actuarial risk curve was calculated by Kaplan-Meier's method.

Results

During the trial period, in group A (with a cumulative period of 113 patient-months), 3 peritonitis episodes were detected in 3 patients (17%) with an incidence of 1 episode/37.6 patient-months) (table 4). As already mentioned, one of these events occurred for technical reasons, and the other two episodes occurred in 2 patients immediately after the catheter insertion and before starting CAPD. Both cases were associated with subcutaneous

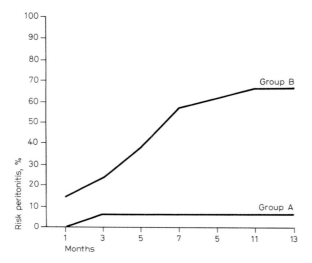

Fig. 1. Actuarial risk curves of the two groups (p < 0.001).

tunnel infection. The same bacteria *(Staphylococcus aureus)* were identified both in the tunnel exudate and in the peritoneal effluent culture.

In group B (with a cumulative period of 264 patient-months), 24 peritonitis episodes were recorded in 14 patients (66%) with an incidence of 1 episode/11 patient-months (table 4). Only 1 of these patients suffered from subcutaneous tunnel infection at the same time; immediately after the surgical insertion of the catheter the same germ was detected in the tunnel exudate and in the peritoneal effluent. The incidence of peritonitis was statistically different in the two groups (p < 0.01). If only the intraluminal peritonitis episodes were taken into account, this difference is even more evident (1 episode/113 patient-months in group A and 1 episode/11.5 patient-months in group B). No significant difference between the patients using spike connector and those using the UV-XD chamber were recorded (table 4). The actuarial risk curves for the two groups are depicted in figure 1.

Discussion

One of the most interesting aspects of a CAPD program is the development of new alternative methods and systems to reduce the possible contamination routes, thus reducing the incidence of peritonitis.

In October 1985, heat sterilization of the Safe · Lock connectors using the Thermoclav device was introduced in clinical practice [6]. Using this method, three phases (heating, sterilization and cooling) take place over a period of about 8 min. In theory, during this period the connection between the catheter and the dialysate bag is sterilized, thus neutralizing intraluminal contamination, which is perhaps the most frequent cause of peritonitis in CAPD patients [4].

In 70% of CAPD patients at least one episode of peritonitis occurs during the first 12 months of treatment [7], 9 months being the average period till the first peritonitis incident [8].

In our study lasting 13 months a highly significant reduction of the peritonitis incidence was observed with the Thermoclav device in comparison with the other systems used (spike connector and UV-XD chamber). However, the short observation period does not allow, at the moment, drawing general conclusions about the effectiveness of this system in preventing peritonitis of intraluminal origin in CAPD patients. The incidence of peritonitis related to an exit site infection (periluminal) has been reported to be 0.6–0.7 episodes/patient-year [9]. It is generally very difficult to eradicate and is a major cause of catheter replacement [10]. In 70% of these cases the causative bacteria was *S. aureus* [11].

Inadequate exit site management, poor biocompatibility of the materials used [12], humoral and cellular immune response disturbances [3] and metabolic derangements (diabetes) [13] are the etiologic predisposing factors mainly involved in this type of infection. Obviously the Thermoclav system cannot prevent the periluminal peritonitis. However, despite the short observation period, this system was highly effective in preventing peritonitis caused by contamination in our patients.

References

1 Slingeneyer A, Mion C, Beraud JJ, Oules R, Branger B, Balmes M: Peritonitis, a frequently lethal complication of intermittent and continuous ambulatory peritoneal dialysis. Proc Eur Dial Transplant Assoc 1981;18:212.

2 Mion C, Slingeneyer A, Elie M, Canaud B, Morad G, Flavier LJ, Oules R, Branger B, Florence P: Transfers from maintenance peritoneal dialysis to hemodialysis: causes and outcome; in La Greca G, Chiaramonte S, Fabris A, Feriani M, Ronco C (eds): Peritoneal Dialysis. Milano, Wichtig, 1988, pp 223–232.

3 Wing AJ, Broyer M, Brunner FB: Combined report on regular dialysis and transplantation in Europe. Proc Eur Dial Transplant Assoc 1983;20:5.

4   Oreopoulos DG, Vas S, Khanna R: Prevention of peritonitis during continuous ambulatory peritoneal dialysis. Periton Dial Bull 1983;3:518–520.
5   Nolph KD: A multicenter study group. A randomized multicenter clinical trial to evaluate the effects of an ultraviolet germicidal system on peritonitis rate in continuous ambulatory peritoneal dialysis. Periton Dial Bull 1985;5:19–24.
6   Thomas U: Heat sterilization of Safe·Lock connectors using the Thermoclav; in Augustin R (ed): Peritonitis in CAPD. Contrib Nephrol. Basel, Karger, 1987, vol 57, pp 172–177.
7   Strippoli P, Coviello F, Martella AS, Misserini A, Scatizzi A: Prevention of *Staphylococcus aureus* in CAPD patients: a stimulating experience; in Khanna R, Nolph KD, Prowant B, Twardowski ZJ, Oreopoulos DG (eds): Advances in Continuous Ambulatory Peritoneal Dialysis. Toronto, Peritoneal Dialysis Bulletin, Inc, 1986, pp 114–117.
8   Nolph KD: CAPD, CCPD overview; final NIH CAPD Registry Reports and summaries of special studies. 9th Annual Conference on Peritoneal Dialysis, Dallas, Tex 1989.
9   Nolph KD, Cutler SJ, Steinberg SM: Continuous ambulatory peritoneal dialysis in the United States: a three-year study. Kidney Int 1985;28:198–205.
10 Hamilton RW, Ingriam J: An assessment of peritoneal catheters; in Khanna R, Nolph KD, Prowant B, Twardowski ZJ, Oreopoulos DG (eds): Advances in Continuous Peritoneal Ambulatory Dialysis. Toronto, Peritoneal Dialysis Bulletin, Inc, 1986, pp 151–154.
11 Augustin R, Kuhlmann U, Schmid E, Wisser H: Bacterial peritonitis in CAPD: Pathogenesis, symptoms, therapy and progress; in Augustin R (ed): Peritonitis in CAPD. Contrib Nephrol. Basel, Karger, 1987, vol 57, pp 10–22.
12 Twardowski ZJ, Nolph KD, Khanna R, Prowant BF, Ryant LP, Nicholls WK: The need for a 'swan neck' permanently bent, arcuate peritoneal dialysis catheter. Periton Dial Bull 1985;5:219–223.
13 Rottembourg J, Shahat Y, Agrafiotis A, Thuilliers Y, De Groo F, Jacobs C, Legrain M: Continuous ambulatory peritoneal dialysis in insulin-dependent diabetic patients: 40-months' experience. Kidney Int 1983;23:40–45.

Emilio Olivas, MD, Servicio de Nefrologia, Hospital General,
c/Hermanos Falco s/n, E–02006 Albacete (Spain)

La Greca G, Olivares J, Feriani M, Passlick-Deetjen J (eds): CAPD – A Decade
of Experience. Contrib Nephrol. Basel, Karger, 1991, vol 89, pp 68–73

Influence of the Preservative Sorbic Acid on Human and Bacterial Cells [1]

H.A. Verbrugh[a], M. Hazenberg[a], V. Steudle[b]

[a]Laboratory of Microbiology, University of Utrecht Medical School, Utrecht,
The Netherlands; [b]Science Department, Fresenius AG, Oberursel/Taunus, FRG

Fresh peritoneal dialysis solutions do not well support the growth of
bacterial species. The bacteriostatic nature of dialysis fluids changes rapidly,
however, during the dwell time in the peritoneal cavity of peritoneal dialysis
patients [1]. Thus, effluents obtained from CAPD patients allow microorganisms to multiply and, thereby, cause infection. It would theoretically be
beneficial if dialysis solutions retained their bacteriostatic activity throughout the dwell period in patients. Except for the use of antibiotics, other agents
that may limit the growth of bacteria in dialysis solutions have not been
tested.

Preservatives are classes of agents that are added to foodstuffs, cosmetics
and drug formulations to inhibit the growth of bacteria and, especially, fungi.
Taken with these products, preservatives are relatively innocuous for the
consumers. Organic acids are used extensively as preservatives. Sorbic acid is
one of the most thoroughly investigated organic acid preservatives and was
found to be harmless in numerous acute, subchronic and chronic toxicity
tests [2]. We studied the effects of sorbic acid on human and bacterial cells
that are relevant to the setting of CAPD. Sorbic acid was found to inhibit the
growth of bacterial cells in a concentration- and pH-dependent manner.
However, the function of human phagocytic and peritoneal mesothelial cells
was also affected by the presence of sorbic acid.

[1] This study was supported in part by a research grant from the Fresenius Foundation, Bad Homburg, FRG.

Inhibition of Bacterial Growth

At pH 5.3, sorbic acid (Hoechst AG, Frankfurt/M, FRG) inhibited the growth of *Escherichia coli* strain ON-2 in tissue culture medium M199 [1]. The minimal inhibitory concentration of sorbic acid under these conditions was 1 g/l. Multiplication of *E. coli* could not be detected over a 6-hour incubation. However, sorbic acid did not reduce the number of colony-forming units and was thus not bactericidal for *E. coli* at concentrations up to 2 g/l. Higher concentrations of sorbic acid were not used since its solubility in water is limited [2]. At 0.5 g/l sorbic acid was not bacteriostatic for *E. coli* but did reduce the rate of bacterial multiplication by approximately 50%.

At pH 6.3 sorbic acid was not bacteriostatic. However, the rate of bacterial multiplication was reduced by half in the presence of 1–2 g/l sorbic acid. At pH 7.3 the addition of sorbic acid to the medium had no detectable influence on the growth of *E. coli*.

Influence on Phagocytosis

The uptake and intracellular killing of radiolabeled *E. coli* by human polymorphonuclear leukocytes (PMN), monocytes (MN) and peritoneal macrophages (PMP) were measured using previously described techniques [3]. All assays were performed in medium M199 with or without sorbic acid. At pH 5.3, sorbic acid did not inhibit the uptake of *E. coli* by PMN. In contrast, 2 g/l sorbic acid in medium set at pH 7.3 was slightly inhibitory on the phagocytic activity of PMN. The phagocytosis by MN and PMP was similarly affected under these conditions (table 1). However, the reduced rate of uptake by MN did not reach statistically significant levels. Lower concentrations of sorbic acid were not inhibitory.

Likewise, the rate of intracellular killing of *E. coli* was not affected by the extracellular presence of sorbic acid at pH 7.3. At pH 5.3, however, the intracellular killing of *E. coli* by PMN was progressively reduced by increasing concentrations of sorbic acid (table 2).

Influence on Oxygen Metabolism

The uptake of molecular oxygen and its subsequent conversion to toxic oxygen species by phagocytic cells contribute significantly to the capacity of

Table 1. Inhibitory effect of sorbic acid on the uptake of E. coli by human phagocytes in M199 at pH 7.3

Cell type	Time min	% uptake of E. coli in	
		M199	M199 + 0.2% sorbic acid
Polymorphonuclear	2	50 ± 4	32 ± 4*
leukocytes	6	57 ± 5	46 ± 6
	12	67 ± 4	47 ± 1
	30	71 ± 5	43 ± 8*
Monocytes	2	30 ± 5	26 ± 4
	6	45 ± 3	34 ± 6
	12	69 ± 3	49 ± 8
	30	79 ± 5	64 ± 8
Peritoneal	2	29 ± 3	25 ± 4
macrophages	6	34 ± 1	26 ± 1
	12	40 ± 2	29 ± 3
	30	46 ± 5	31 ± 5*

Mean ± SEM, based on at least three separate experiments performed in duplicate.
* $p < 0.05$ compared to M199 without sorbic acid.

Table 2. pH-dependent inhibitory effect of sorbic acid on the intracellular killing of E. coli by human PMN

Sorbic acid g/l	% killing of E. coli by PMN at	
	pH 5.3	pH 7.3
0 (control)	96 ± 1	98 ± 1
0.5	88 ± 3	99 ± 1
1.0	65 ± 3*	97 ± 1
1.5	63 ± 7*	97 ± 1
2.0	60 ± 10*	96 ± 1

Mean ± SEM, based on three experiments performed in duplicate.
* $p < 0.05$ compared to control medium without sorbic acid.

these cells to kill bacteria [4]. We therefore studied the uptake of O_2, the production and release of superoxide anions (O_2^-), and the chemilumines-cence of PMN in the presence of sorbic acid. In all experiments PMN were stimulated with phorbol-myristate-actate (PMA) and the chemiluminescence was enhanced by the addition of luminol to the medium [3]. At pH 5.3, sorbic

Table 3. pH-dependent effect of sorbic acid on the consumption of oxygen by human PMN

M199 at pH	Stimulus	O_2 consumption by PMN in	
		M199	M199 + 0.2% sorbic acid
5.3	none (resting PMN)	7.2 ± 1.1	0.2 ± 0.1
	phorbol-myristate-actate	16.6 ± 4.4	0.9 ± 0.5
7.3	none (resting PMN)	0.6 ± 0.1	24.6 ± 3.3
	phorbol-myristate–actate	29.5 ± 1.5	35.4 ± 2.1

Mean $\pm$ SEM nmol/4 $\times$ 10^6 PMN/10 min, based on three separate experiments performed in duplicate.

acid completely blocked the uptake of oxygen by PMN; consequently, superoxide anions and chemiluminescence were not detected. In contrast, the uptake of oxygen by PMN was stimulated by sorbic acid when the tests were performed at pH 7.3 (table 3). However, the increased uptake of oxygen by PMN was not followed by a comparable increase in the amount of superoxide or of chemiluminescence released by the PMN (data not shown). Surprisingly, the chemiluminescent response of PMN was even reduced by 60–70% in the presence of sorbic acid at pH 7.3.

Influence on Mesothelial Cells

Mesothelial cells form a mononolayer covering the inner wall of the abdominal cavity. Quantitatively, the mesothelial cells are the most important cells exposed to the intraperitoneal milieu. We have previously described the isolation and culture of human mesothelial cells from pieces of omentum [5]. The rate of mesothelial cell growth was observed over a 5-day period in culture medium with increasing concentrations of sorbic acid. The pH of the medium (M199) was 7.3. The growth of mesothelial cells was reduced in the presence of concentrations of sorbic acid exceeding 1 g/l. At 2 g/l, sorbic acid completely inhibited mesothelial cell proliferation. However, concentrations of sorbic acid ≤ 1 g/l had little influence on the ability of mesothelial cells to multiply. Acute toxicity studies using standard ^{51}Cr-release assays showed sorbic acid to be nontoxic at pH 7.3. In contrast,

Table 4. Summary of sorbic acid effects

Cell system	Inhibitory at	
	pH	concentration, g/l
Bacterial cells		
Growth of *E. coli*	≤ 6.5	≥ 0.5
Human phagocytes		
Uptake of *E. coli*	7.3	≥ 2.0
Killing of *E. coli*	5.3	≥ 1.0
O_2 consumption	5.3	≥ 2.0
	(7.3 stimulatory!	≥ 2.0)
O_2^- production	7.3	≥ 2.0
Chemiluminescence	5.3–7.3	≥ 1.0
Mesothelial cells		
Growth rate	7.3	≥ 1.0
Membrane integrity (^{51}Cr-release)	5.3	≥ 1.0

sorbic acid at concentrations ≥ 1 g/l induced mesothelial cell lysis when the assays were run at pH 5.3.

Summary and Discussion

Sorbic acid is a straight-chain α,β-unsaturated monocarboxylic acid. Sorbic acid is widely used to preserve foods, cosmetics and pharmaceutical products. Given orally, sorbic acid has been shown to be virtually harmless. Like other fatty acids, sorbic acid is degraded in animals and in humans to CO_2 and water through β-oxidation [6, 7]. Typical use levels of sorbic acid in foods range from 0.2 g/l in wine to 3 g/l in some cheeses [2]. With sorbic acid and other organic acids it is the undissociated molecule that provides antimicrobial activity [8]. The antimicrobial activity of sorbic acid increases as the pH approaches its dissociation constant, which is 4.75. We also showed the activity of sorbic acid on bacterial as well as on human cells to be highly pH dependent. The upper pH limit of its antimicrobial activity was 6.0–6.5, as has been shown by previous investigators [9]. However, the mechanisms of the antimicrobial activity of sorbic acid are not clearly defined. Most likely, several mechanisms are involved, including the inhibition of various enzyme systems, the inhibition of respiration and the inhibition of substrate transport into the cell; the inhibition is, thus, relatively nonspecific [2]. We found sorbic acid to have inhibitory as well as stimulatory effects on human phagocytic and mesothelial cells, usually in a pH-dependent fashion. Our results are summarized in table 4. The mechanisms of sorbic acid inhibition of human cell function remain to be further investigated; clearly, enzyme systems such as the membrane NADPH-oxidase that converts O_2 into O_2^- may be involved [10]. The critical level of sorbic acid would seem to be 1.0 g/l; concentrations above this level may be inhibitory on several human cell functions. Further study is needed with sorbic acid and other preservatives to fully explore their potential as antimicrobial additives for peritoneal dialysis solutions.

References

1   Verbrugh HA, Keane WF, Conroy WE, Peterson PK: Bacterial growth and killing in chronic peritoneal dialysis fluids. J Clin Microbiol 1984;20:199–203.
2   Liewen MB, Marth EH: Growth and inhibition of microorganisms in the presence of sorbic acid: A review. J Food Protect 1985;48:364–375.
3   Verbrugh HA, Keane WF, Hoidal JR, Freiberg MR, Elliott GR, Peterson PK: Peritoneal macrophages and opsonins: antibacterial defense in patients undergoing chronic peritoneal dialysis. J Infect Dis 1983;147:103–111.
4   Klebanoff SJ: Antimicrobial mechanisms in neutrophilic polymorphonuclear leukocytes. Semin Hematol 1975;12:117–142.
5   van Bronswijk H, Verbrugh HA, Bos HJ, et al: Cytotoxic effects of commercial CAPD fluids and bacterial exoproducts on human mesothelial cells in vitro. Periton Dial Int 1989;9:197–202.
6   Deuel HJ, Alfin-Slater R, Weil CS, et al: Sorbic acid as a fungistatic agent for foods. I. Harmlessness of sorbic acid as a dietary component. Food Res 1954;19:1–12.
7   Deuel HJ, Calbert CE, Anisfeld L, et al: Sorbic acid as a fungistatic agent for foods. II. Metabolism of α,β-unsaturated fatty acids with emphasis on sorbic acid. Food Res 1954;19:13–19.
8   Cowles PB: The germicidal action of the hydrogen ion and of the lower fatty acids. Yale J Biol Med 1941;13:571–578.
9   Park HS, Marth EH: Inactivation of *Salmonella typhimurium* by sorbic acid. J Milk Food Technol 1972;35:535–539.
10 Babior BM: Oxygen-dependent microbial killing by phagocytes. N Engl J Med 1978; 298:659–668, 721–725.

H.A. Verbrugh, MD, Laboratory of Medical Microbiology, Diakonessenhuis, Bosboomstraat 1, NL–3582 KE, Utrecht (The Netherlands)

La Greca G, Olivares J, Feriani M, Passlick-Deetjen J (eds): CAPD – A Decade
of Experience. Contrib Nephrol. Basel, Karger, 1991, vol 89, pp 74–78

Assist Devices Used in the Prevention of Peritonitis in the USA

J.F. Winchester, C. Rotellar, T.A. Rakowski, W.P. Argy, G.E. Schreiner

Georgetown University Medical Center, Washington, D.C., USA

The frequency of peritonitis has stimulated the search for devices which
would prevent bacterial contamination during a dialysis exchange in continuous ambulatory peritoneal dialysis (CAPD). The simple early devices have
evolved into sophisticated and attractive machinery to protect the connections, in most cases, without bacterial contamination. Numerically, the most
important devices used in the US are the UV-XD, the O-Set, the Ultraset,
and the Mechanical Assist Device (all Baxter Healthcare Corporation).
Several other devices are also marketed in the US: the Abbott Optima
system, the Dupont SCD devices and the McGaw Bagless Connection device
and also the Fresenius Safe·Lock connector. The largest numbers of patients
have been treated with the Baxter devices which allow for a more in-depth
analysis of results.

Peritonitis Rates

The latest and final report from the NIH CAPD Registry [1] reports an
unchanged incidence in class 1A patients (i.e. no previous experience with
dialysis) of 1.3 episodes of peritonitis per year from 1981 through 1987. In
class 1B patients (previous alternative forms of ESRD replacement therapy),
however, the incidence rate of peritonitis has actually risen from 1.3 to 1.6
episodes of peritonitis per year. In contrast, however, is the single center
experience with peritonitis which in most centers not using assist devices is
around one episode of peritonitis per patient year [2–4]. The NIH CAPD
Registry has analyzed data from a very large number of patients; in 1987

Table 1. Peritonitis rates per patient-year with different assist devices [1, 6]

	Manual	In-line filter	Sterile weld	Ultra-violet	Other
Number of patients	3,178	50	38	1,046	226
Peritonitis rate/ patient-year	1.26	1.47	1.07	1.12	1.35

approximately 3,000 were analyzed. Peritonitis still continues to be the major cause of dropout from CAPD from relapsing peritonitis, recurrent peritonitis, exit site and tunnel infections and catheter replacement. A recent editorial has highlighted the fact that assist devices may well have been responsible for a global reduction in peritonitis in the CAPD population at large [5]. This has also been stressed in the 1987 NIH CAPD Registry Report [6].

Assist Devices

The 1987 CAPD Registry Report and the 1988 NIH CAPD Registry Report [1, 6] analyzed a subset of approximately 4,000 patients in whom devices were used for assist of CAPD exchanges in a group of approximately 1,500. Numerically, the ultraviolet device (UV-XD) was used in 1,000, the sterile weld device (Dupont SCD) was used in 38, the in-line filter (Peridex, Millipore Corporation, Bedford, Mass.) was used in 50, and other devices were used in 226. As shown in table 1, the devices did reduce the peritonitis rate, particularly with the sterile weld device, but also highly significantly for the ultraviolet device. The in-line filter, on the other hand, was responsible for a higher rate of peritonitis than the manual rate.

Previous reports have shown that the sterile weld device reduces the incidence of peritonitis appreciably in the high-risk patient population [7, 8] as does the ultraviolet device [9, 10].

Both national cooperative studies of a multicenter nature and single center studies have shown that the ultraviolet device reduces the incidence of peritonitis in high-risk populations as well as in global populations on a large scale. A recent introduction of the 'flash' UV-XD device is too recent for analysis of data, but the device is supposed to deliver a higher energy ultraviolet charge than the earlier model.

The largest impact, however, on peritonitis and acceptability to patients has been the introduction of the 'flush before fill' concept and in-line sterilization with antiseptics (hypochlorite solution) in various modifications of the original 'Y'-set (namely the O-set, the Ultraset and other disconnect devices) [11–13]. Introduction of hypochlorite has been shown to kill adherent bacteria (pseudomonas), while other bacteria would be flushed out without requiring the use of hypochlorite, as shown by Vas [14]. The Italian experience [11, 12] has been confirmed [13]. Flush before fill with in-line sterilization has now become widely accepted in the US giving a frequency of peritonitis of approximately 1 in 2 years.

All assist devices benefit the high-risk patient significantly, in that in-line sterilization with disconnect has been shown to considerably reduce the overall frequency of peritonitis.

Discussion

Despite initially very encouraging results with both the in-line [15] filter and the sterile weld device [7], they are no longer being widely used in the US. Reasons for their nonuse are not well defined, but in the former the in-line filtration device was bulky and did not find wide patient acceptance, as well as requiring changing every 2 weeks, with increased cost for doing so (approximately 160 dollars per month) and, in the latter, the high cost of the heat sealing exchange blade was also felt to be too costly.

The two systems which have found most widespread acceptance are both relatively inexpensive, although the UV-XD device is fairly costly. The simplicity of the Y-set and its modifications has found widespread patient acceptance, although the costs of complete disconnect without reuse of the lines will inevitably raise the price of CAPD maintenance higher than previously. The advantages of disconnect, however, with the patient remaining bagless and free to perform normal daytime activities, largely offsets this particular disadvantage.

While the incidence of peritonitis has been generally reduced with assist devices, it has become clearly apparent that peritonitis is not totally abolished with the use of these devices. This has heightened the awareness of noncontamination as a source of peritonitis in the CAPD patient. Sources of bacteria from bowel, from skin, with transfer of bacteria alongside the catheter have all been demonstrated and have led to the search for a more compatible catheter design as well as catheter materials. The challenge to

CAPD in the future is the development of a completely biocompatible catheter with prevention of exit site and tunnel infections which are now felt to be responsible for approximately 30% of all peritonitis infection [2]. A smaller proportion of blood-borne or bowel wall transfer of bacteria to cause infection of the peritoneum remains a further challenge.

References

1 Lindblad A, Novak JW, Nolph KD (eds): Continuous Ambulatory Peritoneal Dialysis in the USA – Final Report of the National CAPD Registry 1981–1988. Dordrecht, Kluwer, 1989.
2 Vas SI: Peritonitis; in Nolph KD (ed): Peritoneal Dialysis. Dordrecht, Kluwer, 1988, pp 261–288.
3 Winchester JF, Rakowski TA, Barnard WF, Gelfand MC, Argy WP, Schreiner GE: Clinical experience with CAPD; in Paul JP, Gaylor JDS, Courtney JM, Gilchrist T (eds): Biomaterials in Artifical Organs. London, Macmillan Press, 1984, pp 17–27.
4 Pierratos A, Amair P, Corey P, Vas SI, Khanna R, Oreopoulos DG: Statistical analysis of the incidence of peritonitis on continuous ambulatory peritoneal dialysis. Periton Dial Bull 1982;2:32–36.
5 Schreiber MJ: The impact of assist devices in the prevention of peritonitis. Periton Dial Int 1988;8:7–9.
6 Lindblad AS, Novak JW, Stablein DM, Cutler SJ, Nolph KD: Report of the National CAPD Registry, 1987.
7 Hamilton W, Charyton C, Kurtz S, Ogden D, Rakowski T, Schreiber M, Sorkin M, Suki W, Winchester J, Adams P, Caruana R, Burkart J, Vidt D, Piraino B, Silver M, Argy W: Reduction in peritonitis frequency by the DuPont sterile connection device. Trans Am Soc Artif Intern Organs 1985;31:651–654.
8 Winchester JF: CAPD systems and solutions; in Gokal R (ed): Continuous Ambulatory Peritoneal Dialysis. Edinburgh, Churchill-Livingstone, 1986, pp 94–109.
9 Nolph KD, Prowant B, Serkes KD, Morgan LM, Pyle WR, Hiatt MP, Grant JE: A randomized multicentric clinical trial to evaluate the effects of an ultraviolet germicidal system on peritonitis rate in continuous ambulatory peritoneal dialysis. Periton Dial Bull 1985;5:19–24.
10 Popovich R, Moncrief JW, Sorrels-Akar AJ, Mullins CV, Pyle K: The ultraviolet germicidal system: the elimination of distal contamination in CAPD; in Maher JF, Winchester JF (eds): Frontiers in Peritoneal Dialysis. New York, Field Rich, 1986, pp 169–175.
11 Maiorca R, Cantaluppi A, Cancarini GC, Scalamogna A, Broccoli R, Raziana Brasa S, Ponticelli C: Prospective controlled trial of a Y-connector and disinfectant to prevent peritonitis in continuous ambulatory peritoneal dialysis. Lancet 1983;ii:642–644.
12 Cantaluppi A, Scalamogna A, Guerra L, Castelnovo C, Graziani G, Ponticelli C: Peritonitis prevention in CAPD: Efficacy of a Y-connector and disinfectants; in Maher JF, Winchester JF (eds): Frontiers in Peritoneal Dialysis. New York, Field Rich, 1986, pp 198–202.

13   Lempert K, Kolb J, Swartz R, Campese V, Golper TA, Winchester JF, Nolph KD, Husserl FE, Zimmerman SW, Kurtz SB: A multicenter trial to evaluate the use of the CAPD 'O'-set. Trans Am Soc Artif Intern Organs 1986;32:557–559.

14   Vas SI: The role of bacterial adherence in infections; in La Greca G, Chiaramonte S, Fabris A, Feriani M, Ronco C (eds): Peritoneal Dialysis. Milano, Wichtig, 1988, pp 69–72.

15   Rotellar C, Winchester JF, Ash SR, Rakowski TA, Barnard WF, Heeter E: Long-term use of unidirectional bacteriologic filters to reduce peritonitis frequency in CAPD; in Maher JF, Winchester JF (eds): Frontiers in Peritoneal Dialysis. New York, Field Rich, 1986, pp 203–206.

J.F. Winchester, MD, Georgetown University,
3800 Reservoir Road NW, Washington, DC 20007 (USA)

Therapy of Peritonitis

La Greca G, Olivares J, Feriani M, Passlick-Deetjen J (eds): CAPD – A Decade of Experience. Contrib Nephrol. Basel, Karger, 1991, vol 89, pp 79–86

Tuberculous Peritonitis in Patients on CAPD

F. Ahijado[a], *J. Luño*[a], *I. Soto*[a], *E. Gallego*[a], *E. Junco*[a], *J.R. Polo*[b], *A. Galan*[a], *F. Valderrabano*[a]

[a]Nephrology and [b]General Surgery Services,
Hospital General Gregorio Marañon, Madrid, Spain

CAPD has been recognized as an effective method of treatment of chronic renal failure. Unfortunately, peritonitis continues to be the most frequent and serious complication of peritoneal dialysis [1, 2]. The most common causes of peritonitis are gram-positive cocci *(Staphylococcus epidermidis, Staphylococcus aureus)* and less frequently gram-negative bacteria (Enterobacteriacae, Pseudomonas sp., Acinetobacter sp.). Fungal and anaerobe peritonitis are more rarely seen. Peritonitis due to *Mycobacterium tuberculosis* has been reported only occasionally in the literature [3–14]. Difficulties in diagnosis may have been responsible for its low incidence.

Pulmonary and extrapulmonary tuberculosis occur with higher frequency in end-stage renal failure patients than in the general population [13–18], but peritoneal localization seems to be restricted to those uremic patients undergoing peritoneal dialysis. High mortality rates have characterized tuberculous peritonitis among the previously reported cases. A low index of suspicion added to the poor sensitivity of the skin test and the Ziehl-Neelsen stain in peritoneal fluid could explain a delayed diagnosis with a subsequent fatal outcome.

In this paper we present 4 CAPD patients with tuberculous peritonitis and we would like to emphasize the need to consider this diagnosis in chronic peritoneal dialysis patients who have nonresponsive or relapsing peritonitis with a progressive loss of ultrafiltration.

Patients and Methods

In the last 7 years 43 uremic patients underwent CAPD in our unit. Peritonitis was the most common complication with a rate of 1 episode per patient every 10.8 months.

Table 1. Tuberculous peritonitis: patients' data

Patient No.	Age	Sex	Etiology	Months on CAPD	Previous peritonitis episodes
1	34	M	diabetes	42	4
2	52	M	CGN	13	4
3	55	M	diabetes	7	2
4	63	F	diabetes	38	5

CGN = Chronic glomerulonephritis.

In each episode of peritonitis, specimens of peritoneal fluid (40–50 ml) were collected for cell count, gram stain and specific stain for acid-alcohol fast bacteria (AAFB) by means of the Ziehl-Neelsen technique. Fluid cultures for the most usual bacteria (blood-agar and thioglycolate broth), fungi (Sabouraud medium) and mycobacteria (Löwenstein-Jensen medium) were performed, If mycobacteria were isolated, they were then characterized following the criteria of the Center for Disease Control [19].

During the last 2 years we have also included in our CAPD program the Peritoneal Equilibrium Test (PET) to periodically evaluate the dialysis efficiency following the procedure described by Twardowski [20]. Thus, possible effects due to tuberculosis on ultrafiltration and solute transport properties of the peritoneum could also be evaluated in tuberculous patients before and after the disease was diagnosed.

Results

Four of 43 patients (9%) developed tuberculous peritonitis. In all cases tuberculous peritonitis was associated with bacterial peritonitis episodes and *M. tuberculosis* was demonstrated by smear of culture from the cloudy peritoneal fluid.

Age, sex, time on CAPD, and original disease for end-stage renal failure in tuberculous patients are shown in table 1. Three of them were diabetics. The time on peritoneal dialysis ranged from 7 to 42 months. No one had shown a history of pulmonary or extrapulmonary tuberculosis and only in 1 patient was other coexisting extraperitoneal localization (urinary tract) demonstrated. Two or more episodes of peritonitis preceded tuberculous diagnosis (table 1) in all cases. Peritonitis incidence in the tuberculous peritonitis patients was higher than in the rest of the CAPD patients: 1 episode/patient/4.9 months vs. 1 episode/patient/12.4 months. In both

Table 2. Tuberculous peritonitis: clinical findings (n = 4)

Abdominal tenderness	3/4
Astenia	3/4
Anorexia	3/4
Fever	2/4
Nausea/vomiting	4/4
Inadequate ultrafiltration	4/4
Coincident bacterial peritonitis	4/4
Cloudy effluent	4/4

groups relapsing or refractory simultaneous peritonitis due to other than *M. tuberculosis* was always documented.

Anorexia, malaise, abdominal tenderness and cloudy dialysate were the most common clinical findings at presentation of the patient to the unit. Fever was not uniformly observed (2 of 4 patients) (table 2). Failure in peritoneal ultrafiltration for at least 2 months before diagnosis was an invariable feature in all 4 cases, associated with a nonsignificant increase in peritoneal solute transport rate for glucose and creatinine (table 3).

Laboratory data and culture results are also shown in table 3. WBC count in blood was always normal or minimally increased. Cell counts in peritoneal fluid disclosed 2,200–5,900 leukocytes/μl. Only 1 patient had positive acid-fast bacteria smears of the peritoneal effluent, but *M. tuberculosis* grew in dialysate cultures in all cases 1 month later. Extraperitoneal bacteria were isolated only in 1 patient (No. 3) in a urine sample. Skin test was positive in only 2 patients.

Catheters were removed from all our patients because of relapsing or nonresponsive bacterial peritonitis. When diagnosis of tuberculosis was made, treatment with two or three drugs (isoniazid, rifampin with or without etambutol) had already been started in 3 patients (table 4). One of them (No. 3) refused to continue on CAPD and was switched to hemodialysis. The other 2 patients (Nos. 1, 4) were again treated with CAPD, after the catheter had been replaced 1 month later. However, only in patient No. 1 was a notable improvement in ultrafiltration overt (table 3). He received a kidney allograft 6 months after diagnosis and no tuberculous reactivation has appeared until now. In contrast to this, 1 patient (No. 4) still maintained loss of peritoneal ultrafiltration despite 5 months of therapy. This was probably due to a sclerosing process which had developed.

Table 3. Laboratory data and PET results

Patient No.	Laboratory findings				
	peritoneal fluid				blood
	WBC	RBC	AAFB	culture	WBC
1	2,400	1,200	–	*M. tuberculosis* Pseudomonas sp.	11,000
2	3,700	–	–	*M. tuberculosis/ S. aureus/* Candida sp.	10,000
3	5,900	8,500	–	*M. tuberculosis/ S. aureus*	10,500
4	2,200	11,000	+	*M. tuberculosis/ S. epidermidis/* Corynebacteria	11,300

WBC = White blood cell count; RBC = red blood cell count; AAFB = acid-alcohol fast bacteria.

The unique patient who was not treated early (patient 2) died before diagnosis of tuberculosis was made. He suffered from a protracted course of *S. aureus* peritonitis when fungi (Candida sp.) were isolated in the peritoneal fluid. Catheter removal, i.v. amphotericin B plus vancomycin and hemodialysis were required, but despite all these measures, symptoms of peritonitis continued. Ten days after his admission, he committed suicide. Three weeks later growth of *M. tuberculosis* was detected in the dialysate culture.

Discussion

Since Khanna et al. [3] described the first case, 21 new patients on CAPD with tuberculous peritonitis have been reported (excluding the 4 mentioned here). Therefore, *M. tuberculosis* is a rare but not exceptional germ causing peritonitis in CAPD patients. The experience accumulated at this time has merely permitted the unmasking of the clinical picture.

PET results before/after diagnosis
(values given at the end of a 4-hour dwell time)

months	D_t/D_o glucose	D/P creatinine	ultrafiltration rate ml/min
−2/+1	0.30/0.32	0.77/0.83	1.04/1.66
−/−	−/−	−/−	−/−
−1.5/−	0.27/−	0.74/−	0.20/−
−2.2/+1.5	0.31/0.30	0.79/0.81	0.62/0.4

Table 4. Treatment and clinical course

Patient No.	Treatment	Catheter	Clinical course
1	I+R+E	removed	continued on CAPD; renal transplant 6 months later
2	−	removed	death (suicide)
3	I+R+E	removed	chronic hemodialysis
4	I+R	removed	continues on CAPD

I = Isoniazid; R = rifampicin; E = ethambutol.

Peritoneal tuberculosis no doubt requires a high index of suspicion nowadays, since incidence of the disease has declined in all the developed countries. But in recent years there has been a recrudescence with pulmonary and most frequently extrapulmonary localization among a new target population group constituted of immunosuppressed patients who clearly include uremic patients because of the well-known impairment in cellular and humoral-mediated immunity associated with uremia [21]. Diabetes mellitus in this setting might be an additional immunosuppressive factor predisposing to infection by *M. tuberculosis*. Three of our patients presented here were diabetics, which represents a rate of incidence of over 19% of all our diabetic CAPD patients. Also, previous steroid therapy has been reported by some authors [3, 4, 6, 14] as an additional predisposiong factor for *M. tuberculosis* peritonitis. Thus, all this suggests that tuberculous peritonitis in patients on CAPD is a consequence of the reactivation of a latent genital or peritoneal focus rather than a primary infection through the catheter.

Tuberculous peritonitis in CAPD patients usually shows no specific clinical data and seldom a history of tuberculosis or simultaneous extraperitoneal localization of *M. tuberculosis* is found (3 of 21 cases described). Typical clinical symptoms most commonly referred to as fever and abdominal pain are also observed in other bacterial peritonitis episodes. In fact, many patients had had a previous or simultaneous peritonitis due to microorganisms other than *M. tuberculosis*. Findings related to peritoneal fluid include nonremarkable leukocytosis with polymorphonuclear predominance and a variable amount of proteins. Red blood cell presence in effluent, although not a common feature as reported previously, was noted in 3 of our patients and it could be a distinctive clue in differential diagnosis.

According to other authors and also confirmed in our experience, alcohol-acid fast bacteria stains seem to be not sensitive (1/4), the effluent culture being the more effective method for diagnosis (positive in all of our cases). Notwithstanding, *M. tuberculosis* growth in specific culture is not always reliable [5–7, 12], therefore serial cultures could be advisable when tuberculosis is suspected. In contrast, peritoneal biopsy had always been definite when performed in cases reported in the literature, so that if the culture continues to be negative, a histological examination of the peritoneum can provide the diagnosis.

The 4 patients mentioned in this paper developed ultrafiltration failure. This is a remarkable event only previously observed in 4 other patients with tuberculous peritonitis [12, 13]. We noted loss of ultrafiltration at least 2 months before tuberculosis diagnosis was made. Indeed, in our CAPD unit the tuberculous patients have suffered more episodes of previous peritonitis than nontuberculous patients which, together with the damage ascribed to the granulomatous disease on the peritoneal membrane, could explain the ultrafiltration failure. However, as in patient 1, this situation appears to be reversible after treatment in some patients [13] but not in others, perhaps reflecting the appearance of a sclerosing process as a consequence of multiple episodes of previous peritonitis or a delayed diagnosis of tuberculous disease.

Therapy guidelines for patients on CAPD have not yet been well-established in tuberculous peritonitis but regimens with a combination of two or three drugs seem to be sufficiently effective over 9–12 months. Catheter removal also appears not to be mandatory in all cases provided that prompt diagnosis and chemotherapy are carried out. Thus, peritoneal dialysis does not need to be interrupted while clinical improvement is being achieved, as other authors have observed [12–16]. However, this conservative management is not always possible since, as mentioned earlier, tuberculous peritonitis is usually preceded by a protracted culture-negative peritonitis or by a relapsing/nonresponsive peritonitis due to other bacteria. These conditions make catheter removal necessary before *M. tuberculosis* growth in culture is found. Notwithstanding, successful CAPD after catheter replacement appears to be feasible without additional problems in many patients.

Despite the high mortality rate in CAPD patients with peritoneal tuberculosis reported to the present time (8/21), 3 of our patients survived. An early diagnosis seems to be crucial in this setting.

In summary, tuberculous peritonitis must be suspected in CAPD patients with frequent episodes of peritonitis. It follows a prolonged and protracted course with progressive loss of ultrafiltration. Diabetes mellitus is thought to be an additional risk factor in our experience. This group of patients at risk must be considered overall for prophylaxis with isoniazid if they are living in an area of high tuberculosis incidence.

References

1   Nolph KD, Prowant B, Sorkin MI, Gloor H: The incidence and characteristics of peritonitis in the fourth year of a continuous ambulatory peritoneal dialysis program. Periton Dial Bull 1981;1:50–53.
2   Gokal R, King J, Bogle S, et al: Outcome in patients on continuous ambulatory peritoneal dialysis and hemodialysis: 4 years analysis of a prospective multicenter study. Lancet 1987;ii:1105–1109.
3   Khanna R, Fenton SS, Cattran DC, Thompson D, Deitel M, Oreopoulos DG: Tuberculous peritonitis in patients undergoing continuous ambulatory peritoneal dialysis (CAPD). Periton Dial Bull 1980;1:10–12.
4   O'Connor J, MacCormich M: Tuberculous peritonitis in patients on CAPD. The importance of lymphocytosis in the peritoneal fluid. Periton Dial Bull 1981; 1:106.

5   Holley HP, Tucker CT, Moffat TL, Dodds KA, Dodds HM: Tuberculous peritonitis in patients undergoing chronic home peritoneal dialysis. Am J Kidney Dis 1982;1:222–226.

6   McKerrow KJ, Neale TJ: Tuberculous peritonitis in chronic renal failure managed by continuous ambulatory peritoneal dialysis. Aust NZ J Med 1983;13:343–347.

7   Kluge GH: Tuberculous peritonitis in a patient undergoing chronic ambulatory peritoneal dialysis (CAPD). Periton Dial Bull 1983;3:189–190.

8   Morford DW: High index of suspicion for tuberculous peritonitis in CAPD patients. Periton Dial Bull 1982;2:189–190.

9   Cuss FMC, Carmichael DJS, Linington A, et al: Tuberculosis in renal failure: A high incidence in patients born in the third world. Clin Nephrol 1986;25:129–133.

10 Ludlam H, Jayne D, Phillips J: Mycobacterium tuberculosis as a cause of peritonitis in a patient undergoing continuous ambulatory peritoneal dialysis. J Infect 1986;12: 75–77.

11 Tranaeus A, Petrini B: Early diagnosis of tuberculosis should be the aim in peritonitis associated with peritoneal dialysis (in Swedish). Läkartidningen 1987;84: 2125–2126.

12 Mallat SG, Brensilver JM: Tuberculous peritonitis in a CAPD patient cured without catheter removal: Case report, review of the literature and guidelines for treatment and diagnosis. Am J Kidney Dis 1989;2:154–157.

13 Cheng IKP, Chang PCK, Chan MK: Tuberculous peritonitis complicating long-term peritoneal dialysis. Am J Nephrol 1989;9:155–161.

14 Baumgartner DD, Arterbery VE, Hale AJ et al: Peritoneal dialysis-associated tuberculous peritonitis in an intravenous drug user with acquired immunodeficiency syndrome. Am J Kid Dis 1989;14:154–157.

15 Amedia C, Oettinger CW: Unusual presentation of tuberculosis in chronic hemodialysis patients. Clin Nephrol 1977;8:363–366.

16 Rotsky EA, Rostand SG: Mycobacteriosis in patients with chronic renal failure. Arch Intern Med 1980;140:57–61.

17 Andrew OT, Schoenfeld PY, Hopewell PC, et al: Tuberculosis in patients with end-stage renal disease. Am J Med 1980;68:59–65.

18 Mion CM, Slingeneyer A, Canaud B: Peritonitis; in Gokal R (ed): Continuous Ambulatory Peritoneal Dialysis. New York, Churchill Livingstone, 1986, pp 163–217.

19 Procedures for the Isolation and Identification of Mycobacteria. Washington, Center for Disease Control, 1976, DHEW Publ No (CDC) 76:8230.

20 Twardowski ZJ, Nolph KD, Khanna R, et al: Peritoneal equilibration test. Periton Dial Bull 1987;7:138–147.

21 Wilson WEC, Kirpatrick CH, Talmage DW: Suppression of immunologic responsiveness in uremia. Ann Intern Med 1965;62:1–14.

J. Luño, MD, Hospital General Gregorio Marañon, Servicio de Nefrologia,
Dr. Esquerdo 46, E–28007 Madrid (Spain)

La Greca G, Olivares J, Feriani M, Passlick-Deetjen J (eds): CAPD – A Decade of Experience. Contrib Nephrol. Basel, Karger, 1991, vol 89, pp 87–95

Changing Antimicrobial Resistance in CAPD Peritonitis?[1]

*E.W. Boeschoten[a, b], P.J.G.M. Rietra[b], D.G. Struijk[a],
R.T. Krediet[c], L. Arisz[c, 2]*

[a]Foundation for Home Dialysis Midden-West Nederland, Amsterdam;
[b]Department of Microbiology and [c]Medicine (Renal Unit),
Academic Medical Centre, Amsterdam, The Netherlands

Peritonitis is still considered to be an important complication of CAPD [1, 2]. In most centers, the incidence of peritonitis is between 0.5 and 2 episodes per patient per year [3]. From the beginning of the CAPD era concern was expressed about the possibility of shifts in causative microorganisms and increasing antibiotic resistance [4, 5]. To analyze the magnitude of these possible problems during long-term CAPD treatment, we studied all peritonitis episodes occurring during a 6-year period.

Materials and Methods

The patient group studied consisted of 79 adult patients (40 male; mean age at the start of CAPD 47 years, range 16–75 years) trained for CAPD during a 5-year period. The study was completed 1 year later, giving a patient follow-up of at least 1 year. The total experience during the studied period was 131 patient years.

Peritonitis was diagnosed when two of the following criteria were present: (a) cloudy fluid due to a raised white cell count (more than 100 cells/µl); (b) presence of microorganisms in gram stain or culture of peritoneal dialysate; (c) clinical symptoms of peritoneal inflammation. When peritonitis was caused by one or more gram-positive bacteria the episode was called gram-positive. When one or more gram-negative bacteria were cultured, the episode was called gram-negative, even in the presence of gram-positive bacteria. When fungi were cultured the episode was classified fungal.

[1] This study was supported by the Praeventiefonds (grants: 28–649, 28–649–1, 28–1228) and by Baxter Nederland BV.

[2] Mrs. M.J. Visser is acknowledged for her accurate microbiologic assistance. Mrs. A. de Jong is acknowledged for the preparation of the manuscript.

All dialysate samples for microbiological examination were taken from the dialysate bag in the laboratory of medical microbiology under standardized aseptic conditions. Five ml of the dialysate was added to Brewer's thioglycollate containing 0.5% Tween-80. Two hundred ml dialysate was centrifuged for 30 min at 10,000 g. The sediment was used for gram's stain and was inoculated on blood-agar both under aerobic and anaerobic conditions, chocolate-agar, serum-agar containing 0.5% Tween-80, CLED medium and Brewer's thioglycollate with 0.5% Tween-80. Incubations were carried out for 7 days at 35 °C. When no causative microorganisms were obtained, the preserved sediment of the dialysate was cultured at lower temperatures (28 °C) on a medium for lipophilic yeasts (pepton-agar with glucose and yeast extract and olive oil), on blood-agar under Campylobacter conditions and, when tuberculosis was suspected, cultured on special media for mycobacteria. Uncentrifuged dialysate was used for total cell count (Bürker method) and differential cell count (Giemsa stain).

To demonstrate resistance to antibiotics a disc-diffusion technique with Isosensitest-agar (Oxoid) and Neo-sensitabs was used at 37 °C. Sensitivity to methicillin was tested at 30 °C using a heavy inoculum. Blood-agar was used to demonstrate patterns of sensitivity of alpha-hemolytic streptococci. Incubations were performed for 48 h. The size of the zones of inhibition were related to the MIC break-points recommended by the 'Reference Group for Antibiotics' in Sweden (SIR system) [6].

Results

During the 6-year period a total of 280 episodes of peritonitis occurred in 69 of the 79 patients. According to the culture results 207 were classified gram-positive, 42 gram-negative, 10 fungal and one was caused by *Mycobacterium tuberculosis*. In 20 episodes no positive cultures were obtained. Ten of these culture-negative episodes occurred within 1 week after implantation of the peritoneal dialysis catheter. The Giemsa stain showed a predominance of mononuclear cells in 9 and predominance of eosinophilic cells in 1 of these episodes. Four culture-negative episodes occurred in patients who used the Braun® CAPD system. For reasons not yet classified, the incidence of 'sterile peritonitis' with this system was unusually high. In one case of culture-negative peritonitis the patient had started antibiotic treatment before dialysate was taken to the hospital for microbiological examination. The remaining culture-negative episodes were unexplained. These five truly 'sterile' episodes accounted for 1.8% of all 280 peritonitis episodes.

The 309 microorganisms which were cultured in the 260 culture-positive peritonitis episodes are shown in table 1. The majority of the peritonitis episodes were caused by coagulase-negative Staphylococci, 158 of these 164 strains being *Staphylococcus epidermidis*.

Table 1. Microorganisms cultured during 260 culture-positive peritonitis episodes

Gram-positive		
Staphylococcus coagulase-negative	164	
Staphylococcus aureus	25	
Micrococcus spp.	9	
Streptococcus spp. (not enterococcus)	27	
Enterococcus	7	
Corynebacterium spp.	10	
Propionibacterium acnes	4	
Bacillus sp.	1	
Nocardia sp.	1	
Gram-negative		
Neisseria spp.	2	
Moraxella sp.	1	
Campylobacter sp.	1	
Escherichia coli	9	
Citrobacter sp.	1	
Klebsiella pneumoniae	2	
Enterobacter spp.	6	
Proteus spp.	4	
Pseudomonas aeruginosa	2	
Pseudomonas spp.	4	
Acinetobacter spp.	13	
Flavobacterium sp.	1	
V e-strain	1	
Bacteroides spp.	2	
Alcaligenes faecalis	1	
Mycobacteriae		
Mycobacterium tuberculosis	1	
Fungi		
Candida spp.	7	
Ulocladium	1	
Malassezia furfur	1	
Rhodotorula rubra	1	
Total	309	

Figure 1 shows that the relative proportion of gram-positive, gram-negative, fungal and culture-negative peritonitis episodes was not markedly different in each of the 6 years of CAPD. Also, when successive episodes of peritonitis were analyzed, no change was observed in the relative incidence of the various causative microorganisms (fig. 2).

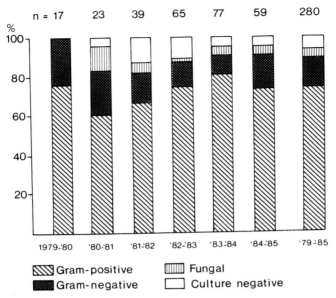

Fig. 1. The relative proportion of gram-positive, gram-negative, fungal and culture-negative peritonitis episodes in each of the 6 years of CAPD. n = Number of peritonitis episodes in each year.

To analyze whether antimicrobial resistance changed during CAPD the patterns of sensitivity to antibiotics were studied of all 158 *S. epidermidis* strains. In all strains analysis of sensitivity was performed for: penicillin, methicillin/cephalosporin, tetracycline, gentamicin, sulphonamide, trimethoprim, erythromycin and fusidic acid. Eighty-two strains were tested for vancomycin and rifampicin. Of the 158 strains 40 (25%) were sensitive to all antibiotics. In 28 (18%) resistance to only one antibiotic was present, whereas 90 (57%) of the strains were resistant to two or more antibiotics and classified as multiresistant. Table 2 shows that only a small portion of these 90 strains was truly multiresistant. Nineteen of the 28 monoresistant *S. epidermidis* strains were resistant to penicillin. The proportional distribution of antibiotic resistance in the 90 multiresistant strains is shown in figure 3.

In the 6 years of the study period no shift in patterns of sensitivity of the *S. epidermidis* strains could be established. Despite the consequent use of cephradine as antibiotic of first choice, the percentage of *S. epidermidis* resistant to methicillin/cephalosporin did not change in the successive years.

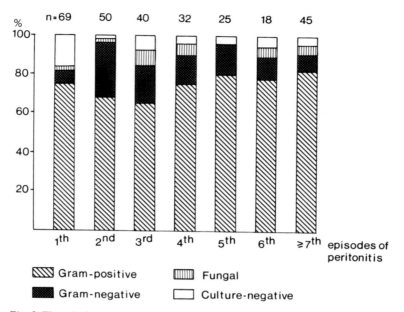

Fig. 2. The relative proportion of gram-positive, gram-negative, fungal and culture-negative episodes in succeeding episodes of peritonitis. n = Number of peritonitis episodes involved.

Table 2. Resistance to antibiotics of 90 multiresistant strains of *S. epidermidis*

Resistant to	Number of strains	Percentage
2 antibiotics	27	30
3 antibiotics	18	20
4 antibiotics	19	21
5 antibiotics	13	14
6 antibiotics	7	8
7 antibiotics	5	6
9 antibiotics	1	1

In figure 4, the percentage of methicillin/cephalosporin strains is compared with resistance to sulphonamides and/or trimethoprim. Figure 5 shows that the relative proportion of nonresistant, monoresistant and multiresistant *S. epidermidis* strains did not change during the 6-year period. The percentage of multiresistant *S. epidermidis* strains in successive episodes of perito-

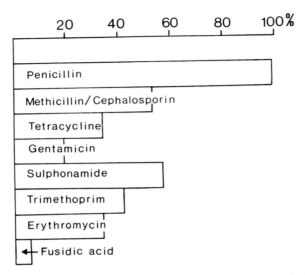

Fig. 3. Proportional distribution of antibiotic resistance in 90 multiresistant *S. epidermidis* strains.

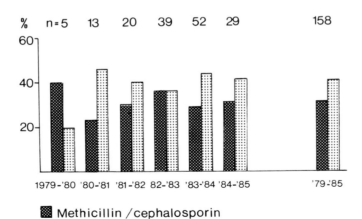

Fig. 4. Proportional resistance of *S. epidermidis* to methicillin/cephalosporin and to sulphonamides and/or trimethoprim in 6 years of CAPD. n = Number of *S. epidermidis* strains cultured in each year.

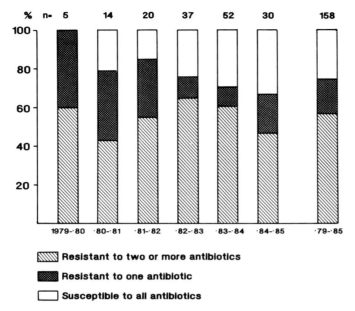

Fig. 5. Relative proportion of nonresistant, monoresistant and multiresistant *S. epidermidis* strains in each of the 6 years of CAPD. n = Number of *S. epidermidis* strains involved.

nitis in which *S. epidermidis* was involved is shown in figure 6. The differences between the successive episodes were not significant.

Discussion

In this study, gram-positive bacteria were by far the most frequent causative microorganisms of peritonitis. This is also the experience of almost all other CAPD centers [3]. Half of all culture-negative episodes were found shortly after the implantation of the peritoneal dialysis catheter, a situation in which dialysate leucocytosis is not uncommon [7]. In this series only 1.8% of all peritonitis episodes were culture-negative. During the 6 years of the study no shift in the distribution of causative microorganisms was observed. Furthermore, no preference for specific microorganisms was observed in a patient's first, second or subsequent episode of peritonitis. The risk of contracting peritonitis caused by gram-positive bacteria remained un-

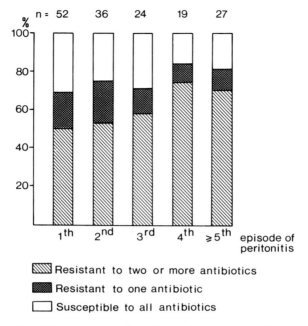

Fig. 6. Relative proportion of nonresistant, monoresistant and multiresistant *S. epidermidis* strains in successive episodes of peritonitis in which *S. epidermidis* was involved. n = Number of *S. epidermidis* strains involved.

changed. Similar observations were reported by others [8, 9]. They disprove the early findings of Nolph et al. [4], who found a significant increase of infections caused by gram-negative bacteria from 1979 to 1980.

Antibiotic resistance of *S. epidermidis* strains involved in CAPD peritonitis did not change during the studied period. The percentage of *S. epidermidis* strains resistant to methicillin/cephalosporin was 30–40%. A similar percentage has been reported by others [5, 10, 11]. Despite repeated treatment with cephradine as the antibiotic of first choice [12], this percentage did not change during the 6 years of the study. The percentage of *S. epidermidis* strains resistant to methicillin/cephalosporin remained comparable to the percentage of strains resistant to sulphonamides and/or trimethoprim, antibiotics rarely used in our patients. After a peritonitis episode with a methicillin/cephalosporin-resistant *S. epidermidis,* the chance of finding a resistant *S. epidermidis* as causative microorganism in the next episode was only 50%. We conclude that there is no indication for increasing antimicrobial resistance in CAPD peritonitis.

References

1 Tranaeus A, Heimbürger O, Lindholm B: Peritonitis during continuous ambulatory peritoneal dialysis (CAPD): Risk factors, clinical severity and pathogenetic aspects. Periton Dial Int 1988;8:253–263.

2 Vas SI: Peritonitis; in Nolph KD (ed): Peritoneal Dialysis. Dordrecht, Kluwer Academic Publishers, 1989, pp 261–288.

3 Boeschoten EW: Continuous ambulatory peritoneal dialysis; thesis, University of Amsterdam, 1988, pp 116–152.

4 Nolph KD, Prowant B, Sorkin MI, et al: The incidence and characteristics of peritonitis in the fourth year of a continuous ambulatory peritoneal dialysis program. Periton Dial Bull 1981;1:50–53.

5 Atkins RC, Humphery T, Thomson N, et al. Efficacy of treatment in CAPD-peritonitis – the problem of staphylococcal antibiotic resistance; in Atkins RC, Thomson NM, Farrell PC (eds): Peritoneal Dialysis. Edinburgh, Churchill-Livingstone, 1981, pp 337–339.

6 The Swedish Reference Group for Antibiotics: A revised system for antibiotic sensitivity testing. Scand J Infect Dis 1981;13:148–152.

7 Fijen JW, Struijk DG, Krediet RT, et al: Dialysate leucocytosis in CAPD patients without clinical infection. Neth J Med 1988;33:270–280.

8 Prowant B, Ryan L, Nolph KD: Six years experience with peritonitis in a CAPD program. Periton Dial Bull 1983;3:199–201.

9 Swartz RD: Chronic peritoneal dialysis: Mechanical and infectious complications. Nephron 1985;40:29–37.

10 Chan MK, Baillod RA, Chuah P, et al: Three years' experience of continuous ambulatory peritoneal dialysis. Lancet 1981;i:1409–1412.

11 Gruer LD, Barlett R, Aylitte GAJ: Species identification and antibiotic sensitivity of coagulase negative staphylococci from CAPD peritonitis. J Antimicrob Chemother 1984;13:577–583.

12 Boeschoten EW, Rietra PJGM, Krediet RT, et al.: CAPD peritonitis: A prospective randomized trial of oral versus intraperitoneal treatment with cephradine. J Antimicrob Chemother 1985;16:789–797.

E.W. Boeschoten, MD, Renal Unit, F4-215, Academic Medical Centre,
Meibergdreef 9, NL-1105 AZ Amsterdam (The Netherlands)

La Greca G, Olivares J, Feriani M, Passlick-Deetjen J (eds): CAPD – A Decade
of Experience. Contrib Nephrol. Basel, Karger, 1991, vol 89, pp 96–107

Pharmacokinetic Considerations for Treatment of Bacterial Peritonitis during Continuous Ambulatory Peritoneal Dialysis

*J.-L. Bouchet[a], M. Aparicio[b], G. Vinçon[c], F. Demotes-Mainard[c],
Cl. Quentin[d], J.P. Bourdenx[a], J. Dupoux[a], L. Potaux[b]*

[a]CTMR Saint-Augustin, Departments of [b]Nephrology, [c]Clinical Pharmacology,
and [d]Bacteriology, Hôpital Pellegrin, Bordeaux, France

Continuous ambulatory peritoneal dialysis (CAPD) is now considered as a good alternative to hemodialysis (HD) for patients with end-stage renal disease (ESRD). The introduction of new connection systems [1, 2] was recently followed by a net decrease in the rate of peritonitis episodes. However, the development of bacterial peritonitis remains a major complication during CAPD. The choice of antimicrobial agents is based on two important criteria: first, the efficacy against the isolated species responsible for the peritonitis, and second, the lack of side effects when the total plasma clearance of the drug is reduced by renal failure. This second criterium can be evaluated by pharmacokinetic studies measuring several parameters, i.e. the elimination half-life ($t_{1/2}$), the volume of distribution and peritoneal, renal and total plasma clearances. These parameters are all important and helpful in determining the best route for drug administration and dosing guidelines. Staphylococci and some gram-negative enterobacteria are the principal species found during peritonitis episodes in subjects undergoing CAPD [3].

The aim of this study was to examine the behavior of fosfomycin, a unique antimicrobial agent, cefotaxime, a third-generation cephalosporin and latamoxef, a synthetic oxa-β-lactam antibiotic, after intravenous (IV) and intraperitoneal (IP) administration in CAPD patients who were free of infection.

Table 1. Clinical characteristics of subjects undergoing CAPD

Study	Subject No.	Age years	Sex	Body weight kg	Primary diagnosis	Creatinine clearance ml/min	Duration of CAPD months
Fosfomycin	1	46	F	60	hypertensive nephrosclerosis	0	13
	2	46	F	75	renal atrophy	7.5	6
	3	64	F	52	hypertensive nephrosclerosis	6	4
	4	57	M	57	hypertensive nephrosclerosis	0	24
	5	59	F	54	polycystic kidneys	0	5
	6	58	M	63	renal atrophy	0	6
Cefotaxime	7	26	F	39	chronic glomerulonephritis	3	5
	8	31	M	65	polycystic kidneys	0	11
	9	55	F	87	polycystic kidneys	0	9
	10	51	M	60	chronic glomerulonephritis	4	11
	11	72	M	63	interstitial nephritis	5	3
	12	24	M	64	diabetic nephropathy	6	1
	13	54	M	58	hypertensive nephrosclerosis	0	3
	14	63	M	55	hypertensive nephrosclerosis	0	12
Latamoxef	15	24	F	51	chronic glomerulonephritis	1.2	13
	16	25	F	56	interstitial nephritis	0	14
	17	36	F	60	interstitial nephritis	5.8	10
	18	50	F	50	hypertensive nephrosclerosis	3.9	4
	19	51	F	78	polycystic kidneys	0.5	12
	20	62	F	60	renal tuberculosis	0.5	4
	21	73	F	40	undetermined etiology	1.2	4
	22	49	M	66	chronic glomerulonephritis	10	9
	23	58	M	65	hypertensive nephrosclerosis	0	1
	24	80	M	72	undetermined etiology	1	1
Mean ±SD		50.58 ±15.9		60.41 ±10.8		2.56 ±3.10	1 ±5.44

Material and Methods

Patients. Our subjects were 24 voluntary patients (11 male and 13 female) with ESRD who had all given their informed consent and had undergone CAPD for 1–24 months. The clinical characteristics of these patients are summarized in table 1. Mean age was 51 ± 16 years (range 24–73 years). The subjects were clinically stable and without evidence of peritonitis (white blood cell count in peritoneal fluid <100/ml). None had ever presented signs or symptoms of liver disease. CAPD was carried out with a Tenckoff catheter and with a 1.36% dextrose solution for peritoneal dialysis. During the study, patients were hospitalized and CAPD was performed with four 4-hour exchanges and one overnight 8-hour exchange. A randomized cross-over design was used whereby patients received both an IV and IP dose of 1 g of fosfomycin (6 patients), cefotaxime (8 patients) or latamoxef (10 patients) with 1 week washout between the different doses.

Fosfomycin Study (6 Patients) and Latamoxef Study (10 Patients). During IV studies, fosfomycin or latamoxef (1 g) were injected into a forearm vein over 3 min just after IP infusion of the dialysate. Blood samples (5 ml) were collected from an indwelling venous catheter in the other arm at 0, 0.05, 0.08, 0.17, 0.33, 0.50, 0.75, 1, 1.5, 2, 3, 4, 5, 6, 7, 8, 9, 10, 12, 16, 24, 28, 32, 36, 40, 48, 52, 56, 60, 64 and 72 h after drug injection. A 5-ml dialysate sample was also collected at corresponding intervals for drug assay. Urine samples were collected before injection and at intervals of 0–4, 4–8, 8–12, 12–16, 16–24, 24–36, 36–48, 48–60 and 60–72 h after administration. For the IP study a single dose of 1 g of fosfomycin was mixed with 1.5 liters of dialysis fluid and was infused into the peritoneal cavity by gravity over 15 min; blood samples were collected at 0, 0.25, 0.50, 0.75, 1, 1.5, 2, 3, 4, 5, 6, 7, 8, 9, 10, 12, 16, 24, 36, 48, 60 and 72 h after fosfomycin administration. Urine samples were collected as described after IV dosing.

Cefotaxime Study (8 Patients). The protocol of IV and IP administration of a dose of 1 g of cefotaxime was the same as described for fosfomycin and latamoxef. Blood, urine and dialysate samples were also collected as previously reported. After IV administration, blood samples (5 ml) were drawn at 0, 0.08, 0.16, 0.25, 0.33, 0.5, 0.75, 1, 1.5, 2, 3, 4, 5, 6, 8, 10 and 12 h. Urine samples were collected before injection and at intervals of 0–2, 2–4, 4–6, 6–8, 8–10, 10–12, and 12–24 h after dosing. At each change of the dialysis bag the collected volume was determined and an aliquot was kept frozen. During IP dosing, the drug was diluted in 2 liters of dialysate before instillation; blood samples were collected at 0, 0.25, 0.5, 0.75, 1, 1.5, 2, 3, 4, 5, 6, 8, 10 and 12 h after cefotaxime dosing. Urine samples were collected as described above.

Antibiotic Assays. During these three studies, blood samples were immediately centrifuged and plasma was frozen at $-20\,^{\circ}C$ (fosfomycin and cefotaxime) or $-80\,^{\circ}C$ (latamoxef) until assayed. Urine and dialysate aliquots were also frozen. Fosfomycin was assayed by a microbiological diffusion technique [4]. Details of the method are reported elsewhere [5]. Cefotaxime and latamoxef were assayed by HPLC, using an already published technique [6, 7].

Pharmacokinetic Analysis. The pharmacokinetics were analyzed by an interactive graphic program [8]. The concentration-time data points were fit to a biexponential model by a Gauss-Newton interactive procedure. The terminal plasma $t_{1/2}\beta$ was calculated by the equation $t_{1/2}\beta = 0.693/\beta$ in which β is the terminal-phase rate constant. The AUCs (area under the curve) were calculated by the trapezoidal rule with extrapolation to infinity by the terminal slope of the fit curve. Total plasma clearance (Cl) was calculated by the formula: $Cl = D/AUC_{0-\infty}$. The apparent volume of distribution (Vd_{area}) was calculated by the formula: $Vd_{area} = Cl/\beta$. Peritoneal (Cl_P) and renal (Cl_R) clearances were calculated: $Cl = Q/AUC_{0-\infty}$ where Q is the amount of drug removed by peritoneal dialysis or by the kidneys during 72 h [9]. The fraction of fosfomycin systemically absorbed after IP instillation (f_{IP}) was calculated as the ratio of AUC after IP and IV dosing with the assumption that Cl remained constant from one part of the study to the next. The percent of fosfomycin absorbed from the peritoneum was also calculated for each patient from the

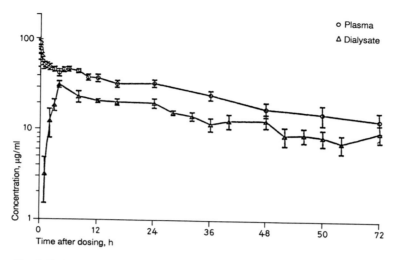

Fig. 1. Relationship between mean plasma and dialysate levels of fosfomycin and time after IV administration.

following equation: $f_{IP} = [(amount\ injected - amount\ recovered)/amount\ injected] \times 100$. After IP instillation, maximum plasma concentration (C_{max}) and time to peak (t_{max}) were determined directly from the data.

Results

Fosfomycin Study

Mean plasma and dialysate concentrations after IV administration of fosfomycin are given in table 2 and figure 1. The maximum mean plasma concentration (measured at the first sampling 3 min after the dose was given) was $94.1 \pm 10.3\ \mu g/ml$. The mean plasma fosfomycin concentrations were $53.3 \pm 3.8\ \mu g/ml$ at 1 h, $38.4 \pm 3.6\ \mu g/ml$ at 12 h, $34.5 \pm 3.2\ \mu g/ml$ at 24 h and $17.9 \pm 3.4\ \mu g/ml$ at 48 h. Fosfomycin was still detected in the plasma 72 h after the dose was administered (mean $13.3 \pm 3.4\ \mu g/ml$). The average concentration of fosfomycin in the peritoneal dialysis fluid reached a maximum value of $32.2 \pm 2.8\ \mu g/ml$ at 4 h postinjection. Although dialysis fluid was exchanged 5 times a day, fosfomycin was detectable in dialysate samples for up to 72 h postdosing (mean $9.9 \pm 2.2\ \mu g/ml$). Mean plasma and dialysate concentrations of fosfomycin after IP instillation are given in table 3 and figure 2. At the end of instillation, the mean plasma fosfomycin concentra-

Table 2. Fosfomycin, cefotaxime and latamoxef kinetics after a single 1 g IV injection in CAPD patients

	Fosfomycin	Cefotaxime	Latamoxef
$t_{1/2}\beta$, h	38.4 ± 8.7	2.31 ± 0.20	17.9 ± 4.2
β, h^{-1}	0.024 ± 0.006	0.318 ± 0.030	0.041 ± 0.011
$AUC_{0-\infty}$, µg/ml/h	$2,892 \pm 556$	153.8 ± 20.1	$1,709 \pm 608$
Vd_{area}	0.32 ± 0.03	0.38 ± 0.05	0.29 ± 0.13
V_{ss}, l/kg	0.20 ± 0.02	0.35 ± 0.04	0.27 ± 0.11
Cl, ml/min	7.0 ± 1.4	118.8 ± 12.3	12.8 ± 7.7
Cl_P, ml/min	3.2 ± 0.2	6.7 ± 1.3	2.1 ± 0.5
Cl_R, ml/min	4.7 ± 1.8	4.9 ± 1.6	1.7 ± 2.5
Urinary excretion, %	ND	3.9 ± 0.1	11.1 ± 13.3
Peritoneal excretion, %	ND	4.9 ± 0.7	20.2 ± 8.3

ND = Not determined; $t_{1/2}\beta$ = elimination half-life; β = terminal phase rate constant; $AUC_{0-\infty}$ = area under the curve; Vd_{area} = distribution volume; V_{ss} = distribution volume steady state; Cl = total plasma clearance; Cl_P = peritoneal clearance; Cl_R = renal clearance.

Table 3. Fosfomycin, cefotaxime and latamoxef kinetics after a single 1 g IP instillation in CAPD patients

	Fosfomycin	Cefotaxime	Latamoxef
$AUC_{0-\infty}$, µg/ml/h	$1,908 \pm 348$	90.5 ± 12.4	762 ± 234
C_{max}, µg/ml	34.7 ± 2.3	15.0 ± 1.5	34.1 ± 8.5
t_{max}, h	5.0 ± 0.6	2.0 ± 0.3	4.3 ± 0.7
k_e, h^{-1}	0.053 ± 0.030	0.334 ± 0.039	0.049 ± 0.017
$t_{1/2}\beta$, h	39.9 ± 8.6	2.3 ± 0.3	15.4 ± 4.1
k_a, h^{-1}	0.580 ± 0.039	0.656 ± 0.121	0.544 ± 0.165
$t_{1/2}\alpha$, h	1.22 ± 0.09	1.3 ± 0.2	1.4 ± 0.5
Absorption, %	68.4 ± 6.0	58.7 ± 6.4	57 ± 16

$AUC_{0-\infty}$ = Area under the curve; C_{max} = peak concentration; t_{max} = time of peak concentration; k_e = elimination rate constant; k_a = absorption rate constant; $t_{1/2}\beta$ = elimination half-life; $t_{1/2}\alpha$ = absorption half-life.

tion was 5.2 ± 1.2 µg/ml. At the end of the first dialysis cycle, the mean peak plasma fosfomycin concentration was 36.2 ± 2.8 µg/ml. At 72 h postdosing, the mean plasma concentration was 8.4 ± 2.4 µg/ml. The fosfomycin plasma concentration-time curves after IV administration of fosfomycin were biphasic in 4 patients, suggesting an open, two-compartment kinetic model. In

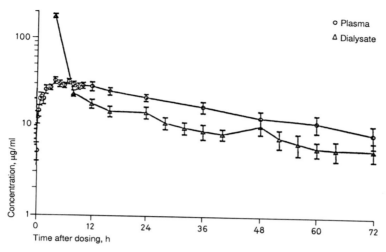

Fig. 2. Relationship between mean plasma and dialysate levels of fosfomycin and time after IP administration.

2 patients, a one-compartment model was used for kinetic analysis. Pharmacokinetic parameters for each patient after IV dosing are listed in table 2. The mean plasma $t_{1/2}$ of fosfomycin during peritoneal dialysis was 38.4 ± 8.7 h (range 12.7–77 h). Mean plasma clearance was 7.0 ± 1.4 ml/min (range 3.2–13 ml/min) and mean volume of distribution was 0.32 ± 0.03 l/kg (range 0.19–0.43 l/kg). The extent of elimination of fosfomycin was reflected by the mean urinary recovery, 37% of the dose (4 patients were functionally anephric without diuresis), and mean dialysate recovery, $37.2 \pm 3.6\%$ of the dose. The mean peritoneal clearance was 3.2 ± 0.2 ml/min (range 2.7–3.9 ml/min). Pharmacokinetic parameters for each patient after IP administration of fosfomycin are listed in table 3. The absorption rate (k_a) was 0.580 ± 0.039 h^{-1} and the time to peak was 5.0 ± 0.6 h. Based on the ratio of plasma AUC after an IP dose to plasma AUC after an IV dose, the mean bioavailability to the systemic circulation was $68.4 \pm 6.0\%$. Based on the IP dose and the amount of unabsorbed fosfomycin drained from the peritoneal cavity, the mean bioavailability was $67.2 \pm 5.3\%$.

Cefotaxime Study

The mean plasma concentrations of cefotaxime after IV injection are shown in figure 3. Data points from all subjects after the IV dose suggest an

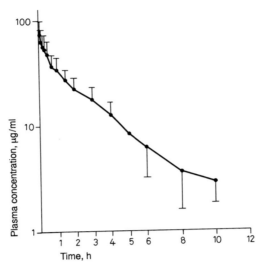

Fig. 3. Mean (± SD) plasma concentrations of cefotaxime/desacetyl-cefotaxime after IV injection of 1 g (n = 8).

early distribution phase of < 30 min, followed by linear elimination kinetics. The mean plasma cefotaxime concentrations were 72.2 ± 8.7 µg/ml 0.08 h and 3.2 ± 1.2 µg/ml 12 h after dosing. Kinetic parameters are listed in table 2. The mean plasma $t_{1/2}$ of cefotaxime during peritoneal dialysis was 2.31 ± 0.20 h. The total amount of drug eliminated through the peritoneal membrane over a single 4-hour dwell time was 28.6 ± 3.4 mg. Peritoneal excretion was low: only 4.9 ± 0.7% of cefotaxime is removed by this route in 24 h. The mean peritoneal clearance was 6.7 ± 1.3 ml/min (range 2.7–12.2 ml/min). Renal excretion of cefotaxime was also low (3.9 ± 0.1% of the dose over 24 h), but there were wide interindividual variations. The mean renal clearance was 4.9 ± 1.6 ml/min (range 0.09–11.4 ml/min). The mean plasma concentrations of cefotaxime after IP administration are shown in figure 4. Serum concentrations of cefotaxime rose rapidly in 5 subjects after peritoneal instillation. At the end of perfusion the mean plasma cefotaxime concentration was 5.3 ± 1.3 µg/ml. For all subjects, mean plasma cefotaxime concentrations were 6.5 ± 1.2 µg/ml 15 min after the end of instillation and 3.1 ± 0.06 µg/ml after 8 h. Because two distinct exponential phases could not be discerned, a one-compartment model was used for the calcula-

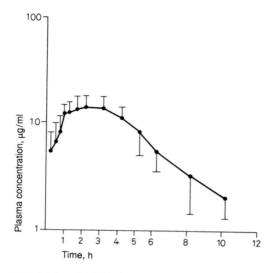

Fig. 4. Mean (± SD) plasma concentrations of cefotaxime/desacetyl-cefotaxime after IP injection of 1 g (n = 8).

tion of kinetic parameters (table 3). The mean plasma cefotaxime $t_{1/2}$ value was 2.29 ± 0.30 h. Cefotaxime absorption kinetics from the peritoneal compartment were calculated by standard equations for estimating oral drug absorption. Because the drug is absorbed into the systemic circulation, plasma drug concentrations would be determined by the absorption and elimination rate constants k_a and k_e. The apparent calculated k_a was found to be 0.656 ± 0.121 h^{-1} by regression analysis and in our subjects the absorption $t_{1/2}$ was 1.3 ± 0.2 h. The total amount of cefotaxime remaining at the end of the first 4-hour dwell time was 371 ± 59 mg (37 ± 6%), and the percent absorption of cefotaxime from the peritoneal space was 58.7 ± 6.4%.

Latamoxef Study

The mean plasma concentrations of latamoxef after the IV and IP injections are shown in figure 5. After IV administration, the mean plasma latamoxef concentrations were 171 ± 62, 19 ± 8.4, 9.4 ± 4.7 and 4.5 ± 2.4 µg/ml after 0.08, 24, 48 and 72 h, respectively. At the end of peritoneal instillation, the mean plasma latamoxef concentration was

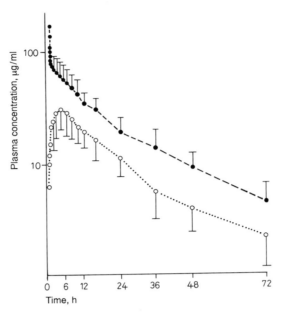

Fig. 5. Mean plasma levels of latamoxef after IV injection (●) and IP instillation (○) of 1 g.

3.5 ± 2.8 µg/ml. Mean plasma latamoxef concentrations were 11.2 ± 2.7 µg/ml after 24 h, 3.9 ± 1.7 µg/ml after 48 h and 2.2 ± 1.6 µg/ml 72 h after dosing. Kinetic parameters after IV injection are listed in table 2. The mean plasma $t_{1/2}$ was 17.9 ± 4.2 h (range 11.7–23.6 h). The mean renal clearance (1.7 ml/min) and mean renal excretion (11% of the dose) were very low. There was wide interindividual variation in the renal elimination of latamoxef, because residual urine flow differed greatly in the patients. Peritoneal excretion was poor; 20.2 ± 8.3% of the dose was removed by this route in 48 h. The mean peritoneal clearance was 2.1 ± 0.5 ml/min (range 1.5–2.8). Kinetic parameters after IP administration are listed in table 3. When latamoxef was placed in the peritoneal fluid, 57 ± 16% of the dose was absorbed, with an absorption $t_{1/2}$ of 1.4 ± 0.5 h. The total amount of latamoxef remaining in the peritoneal fluid at the end of the first 4-hour dwell time was 333 ± 46 mg (33 ± 7%). The mean plasma latamoxef $t_{1/2}$ was 15.4 ± 4.1 h, which was the same as after intravenous injection.

Discussion

The high incidence of adverse drug reactions in uremic patients is generally recognized and may be due to several factors [10]. Drugs are absorbed to various extents, distributed to body tissues where pharmacologic actions and toxic reactions take place, and eliminated by one or more processes at various rates. Abnormalities in any of these factors may occur in uremia and be affected by hemodialysis or CAPD [10].

Bacterial peritonitis remains the major complication during CAPD [11], although the more frequent use of new transfer systems (Y system, double bag systems) has recently been followed by a real decrease in the rate of bacterial peritonitis.

The principal bacteria found during peritonitis episodes are *Staphylococcus aureus, Staphylococcus epidermidis* and some enterobacteria [3, 11]. Fosfomycin, a unique antibiotic extracted from streptomyces, cefotaxime, a third-generation cephalosporin, and latamoxef, a synthetic oxa-β-lactam antibiotic, all have a broad spectrum activity against gram-negative and some gram-positive species and can be used for treatment of bacterial peritonitis.

The purpose of this study was to determine the exchange kinetics of these three antibiotics through the peritoneal membrane after IV and IP administration in patients undergoing CAPD. Details of pharmacokinetics of these antibiotics have previously been reported [5, 12–15]. Fosfomycin and latamoxef are eliminated by the kidneys [16, 17]. After IV administration the mean elimination $t_{1/2}$ and total plasma clearance are 38.4 ± 8.7 h and 7 ± 1.4 ml/min respectively for fosfomycin and 17.9 ± 4.2 h and 12.8 ± 7.7 ml/min for latamoxef.

These results clearly indicate that little fosfomycin or latamoxef is removed from the plasma during CAPD. This is not surprising. Maher [10] previously demonstrated that peritoneal clearance is necessarily less than dialysis flow rate which under the conditions of our experiments was maximally 7 ml/min.

It is noteworthy that the plasma clearances of fosfomycin and latamoxef are influenced by the degree of renal failure [5, 14]. After IV administration, the cefotaxime serum kinetic parameters were as follows: elimination $t_{1/2}$ 2.31 ± 0.20 h, total plasma clearance 118.8 ± 12.3 ml/min and peritoneal clearance 6.7 ± 1.3 ml/min. These data demonstrate that if the peritoneal clearance is low, $t_{1/2}$ and total plasma clearance are poorly affected. It is noteworthy that dialysate concentrations of cefotaxime rose rapidly after IV administration, but only 5% of the dose was eliminated by the peritoneal route.

When given intraperitoneally, fosfomycin, latamoxef and cefotaxime were rapidly absorbed into the vascular compartment. The absorption $t_{1/2}$ and percent of absorption from the peritoneal space were respectively 1.22 ± 0.09 h and 68% for fosfomycin, 1.4 ± 0.5 h and 57% for latamoxef, and 1.3 ± 0.2 h and 58.7% for cefotaxime. Our data show a bidirectional exchange of fosfomycin, latamoxef and cefotaxime between the blood and peritoneal compartments; however, these antibiotics appear to transfer well from the peritoneal to the plasma side of the peritoneal filtration barrier but poorly in the opposite direction. The reasons for these transfer characteristics are not known but similar results have been found with gentamycin, tobramycin, cefazolin, ceftizoxime and vancomycin [15].

Many factors such as concentration gradient, protein binding, molecular size, lipid solubility and drug ionization may influence the rate and extent of the peritoneal excretion of antibiotics. Therefore it appears important to note that effective peritoneal and serum levels of fosfomycin, latamoxef and cefotaxime were achieved by intraperitoneal administration of the drugs. However, during peritonitis the transport of antibiotics, such as cephalosporins across the peritoneal membrane, is enhanced, presumably because of hyperemia of the inflamed membrane [18].

In conclusion, pharmacokinetic studies demonstrate that therapeutic serum concentrations can be produced by administering antibiotics intraperitoneally. Although it is relatively easy to predict the peritoneal clearance of an antibiotic, kinetic studies remain of great interest in the determination of several parameters such as elimination $t_{1/2}$, distribution volume, and total plasma clearance. These pharmacokinetic parameters are helpful for suggesting preliminary dosing guidelines for treatment of bacterial peritonitis: 1 g every 24–36 h for fosfomycin and latamoxef and 1 g every day for cefotaxime.

References

1   Maiorca R, Cantaluppi A, Cancarini GC, et al: Prospective controlled trial of Y connector and disinfectant to prevent peritonitis in continuous ambulatory peritoneal dialysis. Lancet 1983;ii:642–644.
2   Rottembourg J, Brouard R, Issad B, et al: Prévention des péritonites au cours de la dialyse péritonéale continue ambulatoire. Intérêt des systèmes déconnectables. Presse Méd 1988;17:1349–1353.

3   Vas SI: Microbiological aspects of chronic ambulatory peritoneal dialysis. Kidney
    Int 1983;23:83–89.
4   Groue DC, Randall WA: Assay Methods of Antibiotics: A Laboratory Manual. New
    York, Medical Encyclopedia, 1955, p 1978.
5   Bouchet JL, Albin H, Quentin Cl, et al: Pharmacokinetics of intravenous and
    intraperitoneal fosfomycin in continuous ambulatory peritoneal dialysis. Clin Ne-
    phrol 1988;29:35–40.
6   Demotes-Mainard F, Vinçon G, Jarry C, et al: A micromethod for determination of
    cefotaxime and desacetyl cefotaxime in plasma and urine by high performance liquid
    chromatography. J Chromatogr 1984;336:438–445.
7   Diven WF, Obermeyer BD, Wolen L, et al: Measurement of serum and tissue
    concentration of latamoxef using high pressure liquid chromatography. Ther Drug
    Monit 1981;3:291–295.
8   Gomeni R: PHARM – An interactive graphic program for individual and population
    pharmacokinetic parameter estimation. Comput Biol Med 1984;14:25–34.
9   Gibson TP, Matusals E, Nelson LD, et al: Artificial kidneys and clearance calcula-
    tions. Clin Pharmacol Ther 1976;20:720–726.
10 Maher JF: Pharmacokinetics in patients with renal failure. Clin Nephrol 1984;21:
    39–43.
11 Vas SI: Peritonitis; in Nolph KD (ed): Peritoneal Dialysis. Boston, Nijhoff, 1986,
    pp 411–440.
12 Bouchet JL, Quentin Cl, Albin H, et al: Pharmacokinetics of fosfomycin in hemo-
    dialyzed patients. Clin Nephrol 1985;23:218–221.
13 Goto M, Sugiyama R, Nakajima S, et al: Fosfomycin kinetics after intravenous and
    oral administration to human volunteers. Antimicrob Agents Chemother 1981;20:
    393–400.
14 Albin H, Ragnaud JM, Demotes-Mainard F, et al: Pharmacokinetics of intravenous
    and intraperitoneal latamoxef in chronic ambulatory peritoneal dialysis. Eur J Clin
    Pharmacol 1986;30:299–302.
15 Albin H, Demotes-Mainard F, Bouchet JL, et al: Pharmacokinetics of intravenous
    and intraperitoneal cefotaxime in chronic ambulatory peritoneal dialysis. Clin
    Pharmacol Ther 1985;38:285–289.
16 Kawasota N, Shiroha Y, Doi S, et al: A study in serum level and urinary excretion of
    fosfomycin in man with special reference to pharmacokinetic analyses. Jpn J
    Antibiot 1978;31:549–555.
17 Carmine AA, Brodgen AN, Heel RC, et al: Latamoxef: a review of its antibacterial
    activity, pharmacokinetic properties and therapeutic use. Drugs 1983;26:279–333.
18 Petersen J, Steward RDM, Catto GRD, et al: Pharmacokinetics of intraperitoneal
    cefotaxime treatment of peritonitis in patients on continuous ambulatory peritoneal
    dialysis. Nephron 1985;40:79–82.

J.-L. Bouchet, MD, CTMR Saint-Augustin, 106, avenue d'Arès,
F–33074 Bordeaux Cedex (France)

La Greca G, Olivares J, Feriani M, Passlick-Deetjen J (eds): CAPD – A Decade of Experience. Contrib Nephrol. Basel, Karger, 1991, vol 89, pp 108–118

Intraperitoneal Cefazolin and Gentamicin in the Management of CAPD-Related Peritonitis[1]

Jochen Weber, Ulrich Kuhlmann

Robert Bosch Hospital, Teaching Hospital of the
Eberhard Karls University of Tübingen, Department of Internal Medicine,
Division of Nephrology, Stuttgart, FRG

Various antibiotic regimes were recommended for the initial treatment of bacterial peritonitis in CAPD but prospective studies that could demonstrate superiority of any one of them are lacking [1, 2]. The most widely used drugs for the initial treatment of peritonitis are cephalosporins as a single agent or in combination with aminoglycosides [2–9] or aminoglycosides plus vancomycin [10].

We began to study prospectively the effect of intraperitoneal cefazolin and gentamicin in patients with CAPD-related peritonitis in 1983, based on the pharmacokinetic [11–15] and microbiologic [16] investigations of these antibiotics in CAPD. We present the outcome and bacteriologic features of 67 episodes of bacterial peritonitis in 43 unselected patients. We evaluated the effectiveness of the monitoring of the daily white blood cell count in the effluent for the determination of the optimal treatment period.

Patients and Methods

Patients

From July 1983 to March 1989, 80 episodes of peritonitis were diagnosed in 43 of 73 patients who were maintained on CAPD, 48.8% were male and 52.2% were female. The age of the patients at the initiation of CAPD therapy ranged from 17 to 83 years (mean 51.5). Diabetes type I was the underlying disease in 32.6% of the patients and diabe-

[1] This work was supported by a research grant from Fresenius AG, Oberursel, FRG.

tes type II in 11.6%. All patients had a surgically implanted straight Tenckhoff catheter and used CAPD supplies (Safe·Lock connector, Y-connector) of Fresenius, Oberursel, FRG.

Sixty-seven episodes were included in the study, 13 patients with peritonitis were excluded for the following reasons: 8 patients were primarily treated with other antibiotics because of a history of allergic side effects to one of the drugs used in the study, 1 patient had tuberculous peritonitis and 1 fungal peritonitis *(Aspergillus flavus)* and 3 patients died of peritonitis-unrelated causes during peritonitis treatment.

Diagnostic Criteria

The diagnostic criteria of peritonitis were the presence of turbid dialysate with a white blood cell count (WBC) $\leq 100/\mu l$ and abdominal pain if present. Tunnel infection was diagnosed by pain, tenderness and inflammation of the subcutaneous part of the Tenckhoff catheter.

Peritonitis occurring later than 4 weeks after a previous successfully treated episode was classified as reinfection. A peritonitis episode with recovery of the same organism within a period of 4 weeks after termination of a previous antibiotic treatment was the criterion for the diagnosis of a relapse.

Microbiological Investigations

For the microbiological investigations dialysate effluent was collected under sterile conditions from the CAPD bag and 2×10 ml of the effluent were incubated aerobically and anaerobically in two blood culture bottles with brain-heart-infusion media (BCB System, Roche). The culture media were kept at 37 °C and daily subcultures on MacConkey agar, blood agar and Sabouraud agar under aerobic and anaerobic conditions were performed until an organism could be demonstrated. Routine antibiotic susceptibility tests were performed with the agar diffusion technique.

Initial Treatment

All patients were hospitalized for the duration of treatment as soon as symptoms of peritonitis occurred. Two rapid dialysate exchanges without dwell-time were done immediately in all patients, with 500 IU heparin/liter dialysate added to these two and the following bags. Patients then proceeded with their regular CAPD regimen, with antibiotics added to the bags. A loading dose of 500 mg cefazolin/liter dialysate and 40 mg gentamicin/liter dialysate was added to the first bag, the following bags contained a maintenance dose of 125 mg cefazolin and 8 mg gentamicin/liter dialysate.

Modification of Treatment

Modification of the initial antibiotic regimen depended on the results of the susceptibility testing. If the cultured organism was cefazolin-sensitive, gentamicin was discontinued. Gentamicin as a single agent was continued, if cefazolin-resistant and gentamicin-susceptible organisms were isolated. Patients with culture-negative peritonitis received cefazolin and gentamicin throughout the treatment.

If no clinical improvement occurred within the first 4–5 days despite appropriate antibiotic therapy (according to the sensitivity results), a new microbiological investigation was done and appropriate drugs were chosen. In patients who did not respond to the modified therapy after an additional 2–4 days the catheter was removed. This policy was also applied to patients with peritonitis caused by tunnel infection. We did not perform an early removal of the catheter in patients with tunnel infections unless clinical impairment evolved under antibiotic therapy or the dialysate cell count increased.

Duration of Antibiotic Treatment

The daily monitoring of the white blood cell count (WBC) of the dialysate effluent of the 'night bag' was used to determine the duration of antibiotic treatment. Antibiotics were discontinued when the WBC was $\leq 100/\mu l$ for 3 consecutive days. The WBC was performed in a Neubauer chamber.

Definition of Treatment Success

Patients with a successful outcome were defined as responders if they were cured with the initial antibiotic regimen alone (responder group). Patients who were cured only after modification of the antibiotic therapy or catheter removal were not considered to be responders to the cefazolin/gentamicin therapy (nonresponders).

Results

Microbiological Results

In 65 of all 67 peritonitis episodes cultures were done. Eleven of these 65 cultures were negative (16.9%) but 2 of the negative cultures were done while patients already received antibiotics for reasons other than peritonitis. Aside from these two negative cultures, organisms could be recovered in 54 of 63 cultures (85.7%).

Gram-positive species accounted for 72.4% and gram-negative organisms for 27.6% of all 58 isolated organisms (table 1), including the isolates of four peritonitis episodes with recovery of two organisms. Tunnel infections were caused in 80% by *Staphylococcus aureus* and in each 10.0% by *Staphylococcus epidermidis* and *Pseudomonas aeruginosa*. The blood cultures in patients with intra-abdominal pathologic findings, i.e. diverticulitis, yielded no organisms. The results of the sensitivity testing for cefazolin and gentamicin are indicated in table 1. *S. epidermidis* was susceptible to both antibiotics in 80.0%. Methicillin (oxacillin)-resistant *S. epidermidis* (MRS) were isolated in 20.0% of the *S. epidermidis* strains. All MRS showed in vitro sensitivity to cefazolin.

Causes of Peritonitis

The etiology of peritonitis remained unknown in 34 episodes (table 2). Eighteen patients had a history of poor technique performance, 10 patients had tunnel infections and two diverticulitis. Three patients with gram-negative peritonitis had diverticulosis but not diverticulitis.

Table 1. Peritonitis-causing organisms and outcome of patients

Causative organisms				Resistance of isolates to		Outcome of patients			
species	total		tunnel infection	cefa-zolin	genta-micin	responder group		non-re-sponder group	
	n	%	n	n	n	n	%	n	%
Gram-positive species									
S. epidermidis	20	34.6	1	0	4	18	90.0	2	10.0
S. aureus	14	24.1	8	0	1	4	28.6	10	71.4
Streptococcus spp.	5*	8.6	0	0	1	3	75.0	1	25.0
Others	3*	5.2	0	0	0	2	100.0	0	0
Gram-negative species									
Escherichia coli	5*	8.6	0	0	0	4	100.0	0	0
Pseudomonas spp.	5	8.6	1	2	0	2	40.0	3	60.0
Others	6*	10.3	0	4	0	3	60.0	2	40.0
Culture negative	11	16.9				11	100.0	0	0
Culture not done	2	2.9				2	100.0	0	0

The rate of species of all causative organisms was calculated from the total number of isolates (n = 58) of all positive cultures (n = 54). The rate of negative cultures was calculated from the total number of cultures done (n = 65). An asterisk (*) indicates that one organism included in this number was isolated as a second species in 4 patients in whom two organisms were recovered. The number of strains resistant to cefazolin and gentamicin is indicated for the different species. The clinical outcome was calculated separately for the different species, the culture-negative episodes and for the patients in whom no culture was done. In peritonitis episodes with multiple organisms (*) the species-related outcome was calculated for only one of the isolates.

In 37 patients peritonitis occurred as the first event, 27 episodes were reinfections (more than one episode per patient) and three relapses. The rate of reinfection episodes in the group of patients who were primarily cured and those who failed to respond to therapy did not show a significant difference (40.8 vs. 38.9%).

Outcome

Responder Group. Forty-nine of all 67 peritonitis episodes (73.1%) were primarily cured with intraperitoneal cefazolin and gentamicin. In the

Table 2. Causes of peritonitis

Causes of peritonitis	Responder group			Nonresponder group			Total	
	FE	RI	RL	FE	RI	RL	n	%
Unknown	20	12	0	0	1	1	34	50.7
Technique performance	9	5	0	3	1	0	18	26.9
Tunnel infection	0	0	0	5	4	1	10	14.9
Diverticulitis/ diverticulosis	0	3	0	0	1	1	5	7.5
Total	29	20	0	8	7	3	67	100.0

Patients of the responder group were primarily cured with cefazolin and gentamicin and patients of the nonresponder group showed no response to the initial antibiotic combination. In each group it is separately listed, if peritonitis occurred as the first episode (FE), as a reinfection peritonitis (RI) or as relapse (RL).

subgroup of patients without tunnel infections or diverticulitis the primary cure rate was 92.6%. The species-dependent cure rates are listed in table 1.

Nonresponder Group. In 18 episodes (26.9%) the initial treatment failed. Fifteen patients (83.3%) of the nonresponder group were cured after adjusted antibiotic treatment and/or catheter removal, 3 patients died. None of the patients of this group had to be switched to hemodialysis permanently. Three relapses occurred (4.5%), 2 patients had diverticulitis and tunnel infection, respectively, and 1 patient had no predisposing disease.

Ten episodes in the nonresponders were caused by tunnel infections (55.6%), two episodes by diverticulitis (11.1%) and one (5.6%) episode was preceded by a postoperative dislocation of the Tenckhoff catheter (cured after catheter replacement). Five patients (27.8%) had *no predisposing disease* for treatment failure. Two of these 5 patients had *S. aureus* peritonitis and one *S. epidermidis* peritonitis (oxacillin- and gentamicin-resistant strain). They were cured after adjusted antibiotic treatment of 1, 4 and 2 weeks, respectively, with vancomycin (1 g/week i.v.). Two episodes were due to *Pseudomonas* spp. in 1 patient who suffered a relapse. He was finally cured after 4 weeks of intraperitoneal azlocillin (250 mg/l). Seven of the 10 *tunnel infections* were cured after antibiotic treatment of 5–30 days (mean 13.4) and subsequent catheter removal. Two patients with tunnel infection were cured with an extended antibiotic therapy alone. One of these patients had a *S. aureus* tunnel infection and received vancomycin for 3 weeks (1 g/week i.v.). The other patient had a *Pseudomonas aeruginosa* infection and showed a response to mezlocillin (2 × 1 g/day i.v.) and amikacin (125mg/day i.v.) within 9 days. One patient with tunnel infection died of peritonitis-unrelated disorders. Two patients had *diverticulitis* as underlying disease. They were both over 70 years old and polymorbid. Abdominal surgery was indicated in both, but due to their general condition and age they were considered unsuitable for surgery. These 2 patients finally died. Three patients with diverticulosis were primarily cured.

Duration of Treatment

The mean duration of treatment in all 67 episodes with cefazolin and gentamicin was 7.5 days. Patients of the *responder group* received the initial antibiotic combination on average 8.1 days. The mean treatment period for gram-positive peritonitis was 8.2 days (8–16), for gram-negative peritonitis 8.7 days (6–14) and for culture-negative episodes 7.6 days. The *nonresponder group* was treated with cefazolin and gentamicin on average 5.7 days (1–11) and a modified antibiotic regimen was continued thereafter. A modified antibiotic regimen was continued on average 10.4 days (7–56; 56 days in 1 inoperable patient with diverticulitis). The mean duration of the initial therapy in patients with gram-positive peritonitis was 5.4 days with cefazolin/gentamicin and 11.3 days with a modified antibiotic regimen, respectively. Gram-negative peritonitis was treated for an average of 6.4 (cefazolin/gentamicin) plus 8.2 days (adjusted regimen).

Discussion

In the management of CAPD-related peritonitis early antibiotic therapy with subsequent modification on the basis of clinical and microbiological findings is established [2, 5, 10]. For the first-line treatment, an initial antibiotic regimen with a wide antibiotic spectrum, like the combination of an aminoglycoside and a first-generation cephalosporin or an aminoglycoside plus vancomycin was recommended [2, 5, 10]. Cephalosporins in combination with aminoglycosides have a wide antibiotic spectrum and are known for acting synergistically on methicillin-resistant staphylococci, streptococci of the D group, and can prevent the emergence of resistance in pseudomonas [17–19]. This synergistic effect was demonstrated in CAPD fluid as well [16], but it is still controversial if this effect is clinically relevant or only an in vitro phenomenon [17, 18].

Our treatment protocol provides therapeutic serum levels at the end of the first dwell time [11, 12, 14] and mean serum levels at steady state are 50–65 µg/ml for cefazolin [11, 12] and 3.5–5 µg/ml for gentamicin [13–15], as previously reported. These antibiotic levels exceed the minimal inhibitory concentration of cefazolin and gentamicin in CAPD fluid several times for *S. aureus, Escherichia coli* and *Pseudomonas* [16].

The clinical response to cefazolin and gentamicin in our population was variable, depending on the underlying cause and responsible organism of peritonitis. All but two episodes with *S. epidermidis* were successfully treated. The latter two episodes were caused by methicillin (oxacillin)-resistant *S. epidermidis* strains (MRS). The excellent outcome of peritonitis caused by *S. epidermidis* might be partly due to the low number of MRS (20.0%). Two of 4 peritonitis episodes with MRS did not respond to the initial treatment although all MRS were sensitive to cefazolin in vitro. It has been shown that the clinical response of MRS to cephalosporins is poor despite in vitro sensitivity in routine testing due to cross-resistance to cephalosporins [18].

Resistance to either cefazolin or gentamicin occurred in 12 of all 58 bacterial isolates (20.6%) in this evaluation (table 1). Resistance to both drugs did not occur. Cefazolin cover~d all gram-positive organisms but only 37.5% of the gram-negative isolates. All gram-negative organisms were gentamicin-sensitive but resistance of gram-positive organisms to gentamicin occurred in 14.3%. Because neither cefazolin nor gentamicin as single agents could be used with confidence in the initial treatment of peritonitis, only the combination of both drugs appears to provide nearly total cover.

Peritonitis caused by *S. aureus* failed to respond to the initial antibiotic regimen in 10 of 14 patients, in 4 patients the infection could be eradicated. In 8 of the 10 patients peritonitis was caused by tunnel infections.

Cefazolin and gentamicin as the first-line treatment failed in all patients with peritonitis due to tunnel infection but we were able to save two catheters (20%) with an adjusted and extended antibiotic treatment without removing the catheter. Until further clinical experience is available with this approach it must be emphasized to remove the catheter early, as recently recommended [2, 10].

Table 3. Outcome of patients treated with cephalosporins and aminoglycosides/vancomycin

Antibiotic(s)	Route of application	Number of patients	Duration days	Cure rate %	Ref. No.
Antibiotic combinations					
Cephalothin/tobramycin	i.p.	12	n.d.	100	3
Cefamandole/netilmicin	i.p.	29	n.d.	62	6
Vancomycin/tobramycin	i.p.	38	12	84	23
Vancomycin/tobramycin	i.p.	39	10	90	24
Vancomycin/netilmicin	i.p.	35	n.d.	100	25
Vancomycin/ceftazidim	i.p.	64	14	98	26
Vancomycin/ceftazidim	i.p.	102	n.d.	92	27
Cefazolin monotherapy					
Cefazolin	i.p.	43	7–10	84	20
Cefazolin	i.p.	134	14	67	21
Cefazolin	i.p.	29	10	58	22

n.d. = Data not reported.

Gram-negative peritonitis episodes were primarily cured in 64.3%, including two episodes due to *Pseudomonas* spp. Culture-negative peritonitis showed a response in 100% (n = 11) of the patients. The overall cure rate of 73.1% seems to be low; however, we did not preselect our patients and therefore 14.9% of the peritonitis episodes caused by tunnel infection and 3.0% by diverticulitis were included. We also applied a very strict definition of treatment success and considered a cure only in patients who were successfully treated with the initial antibiotic regimen. Taking this into account, the cure rate in the patients without tunnel infection or diverticulitis was 92.6%.

Previous studies with a first-generation cephalosporin plus an aminoglycoside showed cure rates of 62% and 100%, respectively (table 3). Querin and Poisson [6] reported a clinical response to cefamandole and netilmicin in 62% of the patients (n = 29). In the report of Williams et al. [3], 100% of the patients (n = 12) were cured with the combination of cefazolin and tobramycin. Cefazolin plus gentamicin has not been studied prospectively so far. Studies of patients with peritonitis revealed that only 58–84% of the patients showed a response to a monodrug protocol of cefazolin (table 3) [20–22]. These results suggest a beneficial effect from the addition of an aminoglycoside to the cephalosporin. The low response rate of the monodrug protocols might in part be explained by the low cefazolin dose (50 mg/l dialysate and 500 mg/day, respectively) used in two of the studies [20, 21].

In studies with a combination of vancomycin plus a third-generation cephalosporin or plus an aminoglycoside, cure rates of 84–100% were obtained in patients without tunnel infection or bowel disease (table 3). The addition of vancomycin (increased audiovestibular toxicity) or the addition of a third-generation cephalosporin (increased costs) to an aminoglycoside does not result in a significant improvement of the response rate compared to our protocol.

In order to minimize the potential side effects of gentamicin (audiovestibular toxicity, nephrotoxicity), we discontinued gentamicin when the peritonitis-causing organism was susceptible to cefazolin. Gentamicin was only continued when the microorganism was resistant to cefazolin or when the culture was negative. With this approach only 26.9% of the patients received both drugs for the whole treatment period. No patient suffered from manifest audiovestibular impairment.

Since there are no clinical trials determining the optimal duration of antibiotic treatment in peritonitis, we used the daily monitoring of the WBC in the dialysate effluent to evaluate the duration of treatment. Antibiotic therapy was discontinued when the WBC was $\leq 100/\mu l$ for a period of 3 consecutive days. With this individual schedule the mean time of antibiotic therapy was 8.1 days in the patients who were primarily cured. A relapse occurred in 4.5% of the patients and in 1 of these patients the WBC decreased $\leq 100/\mu l$ but cultures remained positive. These results indicate that a sufficient period of antibiotic treatment might be shorter than 10–14 days as recommended by other investigators (table 3). Before this approach for the determination of the optimal duration of therapy can be generally recommended our results have to be confirmed by other investigators.

References

1   Nolph KD, Lindblad AS, Novak JW: Current concepts. Continuous ambulatory peritoneal dialysis. N Engl J Med 1988;318:1595–1600.
2   Keane WF, Everett ED, Fine RN, Golper TA, Vas SI, Peterson PK: CAPD related peritonitis management and antibiotic therapy recommendations. Periton Dial Bull 1987;7:55–68.
3   Williams P, Khanna R, Vas S, Layne S, Pantalony D, Oreopoulos DG: The treatment of peritonitis in patients on CAPD: To lavage or not? Periton Dial Bull 1980;1:14–17.

4 Prowant B, Nolph K, Ryan L, Twardowsky Z, Khanna R: Peritonitis in continuous ambulatory peritoneal dialysis: Analysis of an 8-year experience. Nephron 1986;43:105–109.

5 Peterson PK, Matzke G, Keane WF: Current concepts in the management of peritonitis in patients under continuous ambulatory peritoneal dialysis. Rev Infect Dis 1987;9:604–612.

6 Querin S, Poisson M: Cefamandole and netilmicin as first line treatment of CAPD related peritonitis (abstract). Periton Dial Bull 1987;(suppl)7:61.

7 Oreopoulos DG, Williams P, Khanna R, Vas SI: Treatment of peritonitis. Periton Dial Bull 1981;(suppl)1:17–22.

8 Steurer J, Muench R, Kuhlmann U: Therapie der Peritonitis bei kontinuierlicher ambulanter Peritonealdialyse. Dt Med Wochenschr 1982;107:828–830.

9 Schmid E, Augustin R, Machleidt C, Kuhlmann U: Diagnostik und Therapie der Peritonitis bei CAPD. Mitt Klin Nephrol 1987;16:161–174.

10 Bint AJ, Finch RG, Gokal HJ, Goldsmith HJ, Junor B, Oliver D: Diagnosis and management of peritonitis in continuous ambulatory peritoneal dialysis. Lancet 1987;i:845–849.

11 Paton WT, Manuel A, Cohen LB, Walker SE: The disposition of cefazolin and tobramycin following intraperitoneal administration in patients on continuous ambulatory peritoneal dialysis. Periton Dial Bull 1983;3:73–76.

12 Bunke CM, Aronoff GR, Brier ME, Sloan RS, Luft FC: Cefazolin and cephalexin kinetics in continuous ambulatory peritoneal dialysis. Clin Pharmacol Ther 1983;33:66–72.

13 Somani P, Shapiro RS, Stockard H, Higgins JT: Unidirectional absorption of gentamicin from peritoneum during continuous ambulatory peritoneal dialysis. Clin Pharmacol Ther 1982;32:113–121.

14 Pancorbo S, Comty C: Pharmacokinetics of gentamicin in patients undergoing continuous ambulatory peritoneal dialysis. Antimicrob Agents Chemother 1981;19:605–671.

15 DePaepe M, Belpaire F, Bogaert M, Lameire N, Ringoir S: Gentamicin for treatment of peritonitis in continuous ambulatory peritoneal dialysis. Lancet 1981;ii: 424–425.

16 Loeppky C, Tarka E, Everett ED: Compatibility of cephalosporins and aminoglycosides in peritoneal dialysis fluid. Periton Dial Bull 1983;3:128–129.

17 Klastersky J: Concept of empiric therapy with antibiotic combinations. Indications and limits. Am J Med 1986;80(suppl 5C):2–12.

18 Klastersky J, Van der Auwera P: Cephalosporins, vancomycin, aminoglycosides and other drugs, especially in combination, for the treatment of methicillin-resistant staphylococcal infections. J Antimicrob Chemother 1986;17(suppl A):19.

19 Bourque M, Quintiliani R, Tilton R: Synergism of cefazolin-gentamicin against enterococci. Antimicrob Agents Chemother 1976;10:157–163.

20 Phan HT, Evans JR, Cutler RE: Monodrug therapy for CAPD associated peritonitis (abstract). Periton Dial Bull 1986;(suppl)6:15.

21 Flanigan MJ, Freeman RM, Lawton WJ: Vancomycin is superior to cefazolin for treatment of CAPD peritonitis (abstract). Kidney Int 1988;33:245.

22 Koenig U, Mueller U, Binswanger U: Behandlung der Peritonitis während kontinuierlicher ambulanter Peritonealdialyse (CAPD) mit Co-Trimoxazol, Cefazolin oder Vancomycin (English abstract). Klin Wochenschr 1987;65:562–570.

23 Gruer LD, Turney JH, Curley J, Michael J, Adu D: Vancomycin and tobramycin in
    the treatment of CAPD peritonitis. Nephron 1985;41:279–282.
24 Bennet-Jones D, Wass H, Mawson P, Taube D, Neild G, Ogg C, Cameron JS,
    Williams DG: A comparison of intraperitoneal and intravenous/oral antibiotics in
    CAPD peritonitis. Periton Dial Bull 1987;7:31–33.
25 Brauner L, Kahlmeter G, Lindholm T, Simonsen O: Vancomycin and netilmicin as
    first line treatment of peritonitis in CAPD patients. J Antimicrob Chemother
    1985;15:751–758.
26 Gray HH, Goulding S, Eykyn SJ: Intraperitoneal vancomycin and ceftazidime in the
    treatment of CAPD peritonitis. Clin Nephrol 1985;23:81–84.
27 Beaman M, Salaro L, McGonigle RJS, Michael J, Adu D: Vancomycin and ceftazi-
    dime in the treatment of CAPD peritonitis. Nephron 1989;51:51–55.

Dr. J. Weber, Robert-Bosch-Krankenhaus, ZIM IV,
Auerbachstrasse 110, D–W–7000 Stuttgart (FRG)

Osmotic Agents

La Greca G, Olivares J, Feriani M, Passlick-Deetjen J (eds): CAPD – A Decade of Experience. Contrib Nephrol. Basel, Karger, 1991, vol 89, pp 119–127

Osmotic Agents
An Update

Hannelore Hain, Gerhard Gahl

Division of Nephrology, Department of Internal Medicine,
Universitätsklinikum Rudolf Virchow der Freien Universität Berlin, FRG

An ideal osmotic agent used in peritoneal dialysis should: (1) be nontoxic systemically; (2) be nonimmunogenic; (3) be slowly absorbed; (4) be nontoxic to the peritoneum; (5) be easily metabolized and not cause biochemical or metabolic derangements; (6) not inhibit local defense mechanisms; (7) have physiologic pH and osmolality; (8) exert sustained ultrafiltration; (9) have nutritional value, and (10) be inexpensive and easily manufactured. However, a substance which could meet all these requirements is not available at present. Glucose is the only osmotic agent commercially available for large-scale clinical use but has several disadvantages such as low pH, high osmolality and hyperglycemia. Rapid glucose absorption contributes to hyperlipidemia [1] and ultrafiltration failure in peritoneal dialysis patients [2, 3]. Low pH is related to patient discomfort with inflow of dialysate and inhibits polymorphonuclear phagocytosis as does the high osmolality of the dialysis solution [4]. It is not surprising, therefore, that with derangements of glucose and lipid metabolism in peritoneal dialysis, along with hyperglycemia, hyperosmolality and obesity, alternatives to glucose have been sought for use as osmotic agents in peritoneal dialysis.

Osmotic Agents

Table 1 illustrates a number of osmotic agents which have been tried as substitutes for glucose in peritoneal dialysis solutions.

Albumin has numerous characteristics which might be considered ideal for an osmotic agent [5]. It is nontoxic systemically and does not cause biochemical or metabolic derangements. Because of its high molecular weight (68,000 daltons) albumin is absorbed slowly from the peritoneal

Table 1. Disadvantages of alternative osmotic agents

Albumin	expense
Amino acids	expense; long-term effectiveness?
Glycerol	hypertriglyceridemia
Fructose	hypertriglyceridemia
Peptides	long-term effectiveness?
Plasma substitutes	retention; allergic reactions
(dextran, gelatin, hydroxyethyl starch)	
Polyglucose	retention
Sugar alcohols	hyperosmolal states
(mannitol, sorbitol, xylitol)	
Synthetic polymers	toxicity
(dextran sulfate, polyacrylate, polyethyleneamine)	

cavity and exerts a sustained oncotic effect. However, albumin is currently too expensive to be considered a substitute for glucose in peritoneal dialysis.

Amino acid solutions appear to be viable alternatives to glucose. It has been demonstrated by Williams et al. [6] that a 2% solution of amino acids produces net ultrafiltration equivalent to a 4.25% glucose solution. The same group demonstrated that by the end of 6 h of dwell, 90% of the amino acids had been absorbed, providing an important source of protein to patients undergoing peritoneal dialysis. Prolonged use of 1% amino acid solutions alternated with dialysate containing glucose for 6 months in 6 CAPD patients improved their nutritional status and was well tolerated [7]. Pedersen et al. [8] reported on alternate use of amino acid and glucose solutions in 6 patients for 3 months. The amino acid solution seemed to induce some beneficial alterations in the plasma amino acid concentrations in the uremic patient. However, serum triglycerides continued to increase in spite of the amino acid supplementation and the serum urea increased slightly. Despite the obvious benefits, the high cost of amino acids does not allow widespread use, and more studies are needed to evaluate long-term effectiveness.

Glycerol appeared to be an attractive agent for dextrose substitution in peritoneal dialysis solutions, since it did not require insulin for metabolism and the calculated caloric load for a similar ultrafiltration could potentially be 30% lower than with dextrose. Furthermore, the pH of the glycerol dialysis solution is substantially higher than the pH of the dextrose-containing dialysate [9, 10]. De Paepe et al. [9] reported chronic studies in diabetics and found that use of glycerol was associated with an initial drop in the need for insulin. However, after 3–4 months increased doses of insulin were necessary, but there was better control of glucose homeostasis. Furthermore, there is a risk of cumulation: glycerol levels in plasma showed a peak at 4 h and slowly decreased but did not normalize after an 8-hour dwell. Because of hypertriglyceridemia and the possibility of hyperosmolal states, glycerol is not suitable for replacing glucose as an osmotic agent.

Fructose has also been used for peritoneal dialysis [11, 12] in order to reduce insulin requirements, because it is metabolized predominantly in the liver and independently of insulin. Fructose has the same molecular weight as glucose and has similar osmotic characteristics. It does not appear to provide any advantage over glucose other than the lower insulin doses and may be more potent than glucose in producing hypertriglyceridemia.

Klein et al. [13] reported on the use of *peptides* in rabbits. After enzymatic hydrolysis of milk whey protein they prepared charged peptides. These peptides were compared with 2.5% glucose and shown to provide superior ultrafiltration and reduced uptake (3%) of the osmotic agent from the dialysate after a 60-min dwell. Any peptides that are absorbed should be rapidly metabolized [14]. The resulting amino acids may be of benefit to the patient being treated with CAPD by reducing the impact of protein and amino acid losses on the patient's nutritional status [15, 16]. Further studies will be required to confirm this possibility.

Plasma substitutes such as gelatin, dextran and hydroxyethyl starch (HES) are widely used in Europe. Twardowski et al. [17] reported acute rat studies with 5.5 and 10% *gelatin* isocyanate (Haemaccel) solutions infused intraperitoneally. They recorded sustained ultrafiltration for up to 6 h. The ultrafiltration volume of 5.5% Haemaccel solution was similar to that of 4.25% glucose. Haemaccel 10% yielded even higher ultrafiltration [17]. Gelatin seems to be advantageous for peritoneal dialysis solutions because of its molecular weight of 20,000–35,000 daltons. It is easily metabolized, and the elimination half-life ($t_{1/2}$) of Haemaccel is 985 min in patients with minimal residual renal function undergoing haemodialysis [18]. However, when used as a plasma substitute, Haemaccel has been associated with anaphylactoid reactions in 0.038% of the patients [19]. Thus, the possibility of allergic reactions and cumulation prohibits use of gelatin. We investigated plasma substitutes such as 10% *HES* and 10% *dextran* for use as peritoneal dialysis solutions in nonuremic rats [20, 21]. As compared to 2.3% glucose both substances yielded a significantly sustained ultrafiltration for up to 6 h of dwell (fig. 1, 2). However, lower concentrations

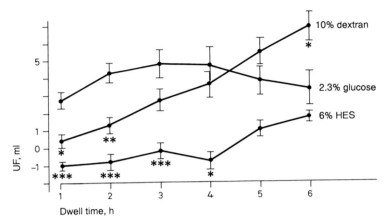

Fig. 1. Mean ultrafiltration (UF) volumes ± SD with different osmotic agents after 6 h dwell in nonuremic rats [20]. Initial volume = 20 ml. n = 6 rats with each osmotic agent. ***p < 0.01; **p < 0.02; *p < 0.05.

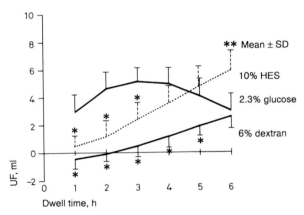

Fig. 2. Mean ultrafiltration (UF) volumes ± SD with different osmotic agents after 6 h dwell in nonuremic rats [21]. *p < 0.01; **p < 0.02.

of 6% dextran and 6% HES did not show any advantage over glucose. Despite their large molecular weight almost 40–60% of dextran and HES were absorbed, probably due to absorption by the lymphatics. Unfortunately, the possibility of allergic reactions prohibits use of both solutions on an ambulatory basis.

Many research groups have used *glucose polymer* solutions in man and animals as substitutes for glucose [22–25]. The substance is a solution of glucose oligosaccharide derived from acid hydrolysis of corn starch. Because of the higher molecular weight the absorption rate from the abdomen is lower than that of glucose. An 8% polymer solution produced ultrafiltration rates similar to those of 4.25% glucose in humans and dogs [22, 23]. Mistry et al. [26] reported on the use of a high-molecular-weight polymer (20,000) as an osmotic agent in CAPD. They compared dialysate containing 5% glucose polymer with 1.36% glucose in 5 nondiabetic patients during a single 6-hour dwell. This study demonstrated that only 14.4% of glucose polymer had been absorbed at the end of the exchange as compared to 61.5% of glucose. Because of the large molecular size, the rate of absorption through the peritoneal membrane is limited, thus allowing more sustained ultrafiltration in a physiological range of dialysate osmolality. There was no difference between the two solutions with regard to caloric load to the patient. However, since human plasma does not contain maltase activity, metabolism might be impaired in uremia [27]. The glucose polymer was broken down to maltose by circulating amylase, resulting in a sevenfold increase in serum levels by the end of dialysis. No short-term side effects of such levels have been reported. However, more studies are needed to evaluate long-term effectiveness.

Mannitol, sorbitol and *xylitol* were considered useful in diabetic patients undergoing peritoneal dialysis, since their metabolism is independent of insulin [28–31]. However, chronic administration of these sugars resulted in hyperosmolal states, and both lactic acidosis and hyperuricemia were demonstrated in patients treated with xylitol for up to 6 months [30].

Three *polyanions* have been tried in animals: polyacrylate, polyethylene-amine and dextran sulfate. Although they have a slow absorption rate and high osmotic driving force, intraperitoneal bleeding and sudden death in animals prohibit their clinical use [32].

Biocompatibility of Osmotic Agents

Several authors (Verbrugh, Keane, Lamperi) have reported that commercial peritoneal dialysis solutions severely endanger peritoneal defenses through defective complement-mediated opsonization and lysis of bacteria [33–35]. Furthermore, interleukin-1, prostaglandins, and leukotrienes have been identified as inflammatory parameters in the setting of peritoneal dialysis. It was recently postulated that chronic overstimulation of peritoneal macrophages (PM) may result in fibrosis and loss of ultrafiltration [36–38]. Since eicosanoids have been identified as mediators of inflammation, they have also been used as parameters of biocompatibility in the setting of hemodialysis [39, 40]. This concept is not commonly applied to peritoneal dialysis at present.

Thus, the purpose of our recent study was to investigate whether alternative osmotic agents (polyglucose, amino acids, glycerol, bicarbonate/glucose, gelatin, hydroxyethyl starch) provoke greater eicosanoid release by PMs than glucose [41]. Fifty milliliters of sterile dialysate containing different osmotic agents were injected intraperitoneally into nonuremic guinea pigs. After 4 h of dwell time, prostaglandin E_2 (PGE_2), thromboxane B_2 (TXB_2) and leukotriene B_4 (LTB_4) production was analyzed in peritoneal effluents using specific radioimmunoassays after liquid extraction. Cyclooxygenase products were generated with all osmotic agents: PGE_2 concentrations ranged from 0.9 to 2.8 ng/4 h, and TXB_2 levels ranged from 39 to 49 ng/4 h. In addition, the lipoxygenase product LTB_4 was found in concentrations between 1.8 and 3.5 ng/4 h. There were no significant differences in eicosanoid release among the osmotic agents. Thus, in this experimental setting, alternative osmotic agents do not offer advantages or disadvantages over glucose with respect to their potential for releasing inflammatory mediators.

Future Development

Although glucose has several disadvantages it will continue to be the mainstay of peritoneal dialysis due to the lack of suitable alternatives. However, for clinical use it might be desirable to prescribe solutions containing large molecules such as polyglucose for sustained ultrafiltration, especially in patients with ultrafiltration failure caused by rapid glucose absorption. Furthermore, it may be possible to prescribe individualized dialysates, with amino acid combinations or peptides which would meet the patient's particular nutritional requirements. Solutions containing mixtures of small and large molecules would induce high initial ultrafiltration and also sustained ultrafiltration. The concentration of each component of the mixture could be decreased to lower the metabolic load and side effects. Amino acids, glucose polymers and possibly peptides seem to be promising agents with potential future use in peritoneal dialysis.

References

1 Cattran D: The significance of lipid abnormalities in patients receiving dialysis therapy. Periton Dial Bull 1983;3:29–32.

2 Verger C: Relationship between peritoneal membrane structure and its permeability: clinical implications; in Khanna R, et al (eds): Advances in Continuous Ambulatory Peritoneal Dialysis. Toronto, Peritoneal Dialysis Bulletin, Inc, 1985, pp 87–95.

3 Wideroe TE, Smeby LC, Mjaland S, Dahl K, Berg KJ, Aas TW: Long-term changes in transperitoneal water transport during continuous ambulatory peritoneal dialysis. Nephron 1984;38:238–247.

4 Duwe AK, Vas SI, Weatherhead JW: Effects of the composition of peritoneal dialysis fluid on chemiluminescence, phagocytosis and bactericidal activity in vitro. Infect Immun 1981;33:130–135.

5 Daniels FH, Nedev ND, Cataldo T, et al: The use of polyelectrolytes as osmotic agents for peritoneal dialysis. Kidney Int 1988;33:925–929.

6 Williams PF, Marlis EB, Anderson GH, et al: Amino acid absorption following intraperitoneal administration in CAPD patients. Periton Dial Bull 1982;2: 124–130.

7 Bruno M, Bagnis C, Marangella M, et al: CAPD with an amino acid dialysis solution: A long-term, cross-over study. Kidney Int 1989;35:1189–1194.

8 Pedersen FB, Dragsholt C, Laier E, et al: Alternate use of amino acid and glucose solutions in CAPD. Periton Dial Bull 1985;5:215–218.

9 De Paepe M, Matthijs E, Peluso F, Dolkart R, Lameire N: Experience with glycerol as the osmotic agent in peritoneal dialysis in diabetic and non-diabetic patients; in Keen H, Legrain M (eds): Prevention and Treatment of Diabetic Nephropathy. MTP Press, Boston, 1983, pp 299–313.

10 Heaton A, Ward MK, Johnston DG, Alberti KGMM, Kerr DNS: Glycerol instead of glucose as an osmotic agent in CAPD; in Maher JF, Winchester JF (eds): Frontiers in Peritoneal Dialysis. Field Rich, New York, 1986, pp 255–260.

11 Robson MD, Levi J, Rosenfeld JB: Hyperglycemia and hyperosmolality in peritoneal dialysis. Its prevention by the use of fructose. Proc Eur Dial Transplant Assoc 1969;6:300–306.

12 Raja RS, Kramer MS, Manchanda R, Lazaro N, Rosenbaum JL: Peritoneal dialysis with fructose dialysate. Prevention of hyperglycemia and hyperosmolality. Ann Intern Med 1973;79:511–517.

13 Klein E, Ward RA, Williams TE, et al: Peptides as substitute osmotic agents for glucose in peritoneal dialysate. Trans Am Soc Artif Intern Organs 1986;32: 550–553.

14 Bennett HPJ, McMartin C: Peptide hormones and their analogues: Distribution, clearance from the circulation, and inactivation in vivo. Pharmacol Rev 1979;30:247–292.

15 Blumenkrantz MJ, Gahl GM, Kopple JD, et al: Protein losses during peritoneal dialysis. Kidney Int 1981;19:593–602.

16 Kopple JD, Blumenkranz MJ, Jones MR, Moran JK, Coburn JW: Plasma amino acid levels and amino acid losses during continuous ambulatory peritoneal dialysis. Am J Clin Nutr 1982;36:395–402.

17 Twardowski ZJ, Hain H, Moore HL, McGary TJ, Keller RS: Sustained ultrafiltration (UF) with gelatin dialysate during long dwell peritoneal dialysis exchanges; in

Maher JF, Winchester JF (eds): Frontiers in Peritoneal Dialysis. Field Rich, New York, 1986, pp 249–254.

18 Köhler H, Kirch W, Fuchs P, Stalder K, Distler A: Elimination of hexamethylene diisocynate cross-linked polypeptides in patients with normal or impaired renal function. Eur J Clin Pharmacol 1978;14:405–412.

19 Ring J, Messmer K: Incidence and severity of anaphylactoid reactions to colloid volume substitutes. Lancet 1977;ii:466–469.

20 Hain H, Kampf D, Schnell P, et al: Ultrafiltration patterns of dextran and hydroxy-ethylstarch during long dwell peritoneal dialysis exchanges in non-uremic rats. Proc IVth Int Symp Peritoneal Dialysis, Venice, 1987, in press.

21 Hain H, Schütte W, Pustelnik A, et al: Ultrafiltration and absorption characteristics of hydroxyethylstarch and dextran during long dwell peritoneal dialysis exchanges in rats; in Khanna R, Nolph KD, Prowant BF, et al (eds): Advances in Peritoneal Dialysis. Toronto, Peritoneal Dialysis Bulletin, Inc, 1989, pp 28–30.

22 Higgins JT Jr, Gross ML, Somani P: Patient tolerance and dialysis effectiveness of a glucose polymer-containing dialysis solution. Periton Dial Bull 1984;4(suppl 3):131–133.

23 Rubin J, Klein E, Jones Q, Planch A, Bower J: Evaluations of a polymer dialysate. Trans Am Soc Artif Organs 1983;29:62–66.

24 Winchester JF, Stegnik LD, Ahmad S, et al: Comparison of glucose polymer and dextrose as osmotic agents in continuous ambulatory peritoneal dialysis; in Maher JF, Winchester JF (eds): Frontiers in Peritoneal Dialysis. Field Rich, New York, 1986, pp 231–240.

25 Mistry CD, Gokal R, Mallick NP: Glucose polymer as an osmotic agent in CAPD; in Maher JF, Winchester JF (eds): Frontiers in Peritoneal Dialysis. Field Rich, New York, 1986, pp 231–240.

26 Mistry CD, Mallick NP, Gokal R: The use of large molecular weight glucose polymer (MW 20,000) as an osmotic agent in continuous ambulatory peritoneal dialysis (CAPD); in Khanna R, et al (eds): Advances in Continuous Ambulatory Peritoneal Dialysis. Periton Dial Bull 1986;7–11.

27 Weser E, Sleisinger MH, Dickstein M, et al: Metabolism of circulating disaccharides in man and in the rat. J Clin Invest 1967;46:499–505.

28 Raja RM, Moros JG, Kramer MS, Rosenbaum JL: Hyperosmolal coma complicating peritoneal dialysis with sorbitol dialysate. Ann Intern Med 1970;73:993–994.

29 Vidt DG: Recommendations on choice of peritoneal dialysis solutions (editorial). Ann Intern Med 1973;78:144–146.

30 Bazzato G, Coli U, Landini S, et al: Xylitol and low dosages of insulin: new perspectives for diabetic uremic patients on CAPD. Periton Dial Bull 1982;2:161–164.

31 Phanichphant S, Govithrapong P: Short-term effect of 4% hypertonic glucose as compared to 4% mixed hypertonic mannitol solution in conventional peritoneal dialysis. Nephron 1985;40:322–328.

32 Twardowsky ZJ, Moore HL, McGary TJ, Poskuta M, Hirszel P, Stathakis C: Polymers as osmotic agents for peritoneal dialysis. Periton Dial Bull 1984;4(suppl 3):125–131.

33 Verbrugh HA, van Bronswijk H, van der Meulen J, Oe PL, Verhoef J: Phagocytic defense against CAPD peritonitis. Contrib Nephrol. Basel, Karger, 1987, vol 57, pp 85–91.

34 Keane WF, Comty CM, Verbrugh HA, Peterson PK: Opsonic deficiency of peritoneal dialysis effluent on continuous ambulatory peritoneal dialysis. Kidney Int 1984;25:539–543.

35 Lamperi S, Carozzi S, Nasini MG: Peritoneal membrane defense mechanism in CAPD. Contrib Nephrol. Basel, Karger, 1987, vol 57, pp 69–78.

36 Shaldon S, Dinarello ACH, Wyler DJ: Inductions of interleukin-1 during CAPD. Contrib Nephrol. Basel, Karger 1987, vol 57, pp 207–212.

37 Foegh ML, Maddox YT, Ramwell PW: Human peritoneal eosinophils and formations of arachidonate cyclooxygenase products. Scand J Immunol 1986;23:599–603.

38 Du JT, Foegh M, Maddox Y, Ramwell PW: Human peritoneal macrophages synthesize leukotrienes B_4 and C_4. Biochim Biophys Acta 1983;753:159–163.

39 Shaldon S: Future trends in biocompatibility aspects of hemodialysis and related therapies. Clin Nephrol 1986;26:13–16.

40 Mahiout A, Jörres A, Hiss R, Meinhold H, Kessel M: Effects of blood-dialyser interaction on prostaglandins in uremic patients and in healthy man. Nephrol Dial Transplant 1987;6:546–550.

41 Hain H, Jörres A, Kögel B, et al: Prostaglandin E_2, thromboxane B_2, and leukotriene B_4 release from peritoneal macrophages by different osmotic agents in nonuremic guinea pigs. Trans Am Soc Artif Organs 1988;34:429–432.

Dr. Hannelore Hain, Freie Universität Berlin,
Universitätsklinikum Rudolf Virchow, Standort Charlottenburg,
Division of Nephrology, Spandauer Damm 130, D–W–1000 Berlin 19 (FRG)

La Greca G, Olivares J, Feriani M, Passlick-Deetjen J (eds): CAPD – A Decade
of Experience. Contrib Nephrol. Basel, Karger, 1991, vol 89, pp 128–133

Galactose-Containing CAPD Solutions: Kinetics and Long-Term Effects in Rats

J.J. Lasserre[a], P. Drescher[a], V. Steudle[b],
M. Strauch[a], N. Gretz[a, 1]

[a]Clinic of Nephrology, University of Heidelberg, Klinikum Mannheim;
[b]Fresenius AG, Oberursel/Taunus, FRG

For many years now glucose has proved to be a safe and effective osmotic agent in CAPD solutions. However, metabolism of diabetic patients on CAPD is often complicated by hyperglycemia. This experience has motivated the search for an alternative to glucose.

A number of alternative agents such as fructose [1], xylitol [2], sorbitol [3], glycerol [4] and amino acids [5] have been used. Data are also available on large molecular weight substances like albumin [6, 7], dextran [8], gelatin [9, 10], polyanionic and polycationic polymers [10], and glucose polymers [11, 12].

However, the majority of these substances are ineffective, or lead to systemic accumulation of final breakdown products, or toxicity, or allergic reaction.

Up to now galactose has not been examined as a candidate for replacing glucose in CAPD solutions. Because of its metabolism it might be, in theory, a reasonable alternative to glucose.

In fact, galactose is a stereoisomer of glucose (fig. 1). Its metabolism leads either to glucose or, mainly, to glycogen formation.

In addition, galactose increases the glycogen production from galactose [13–16].

[1] The authors are indebted to Mrs. I. Sellger and Mrs. U. Helbig for their excellent technical help in performing the laboratory analyses.

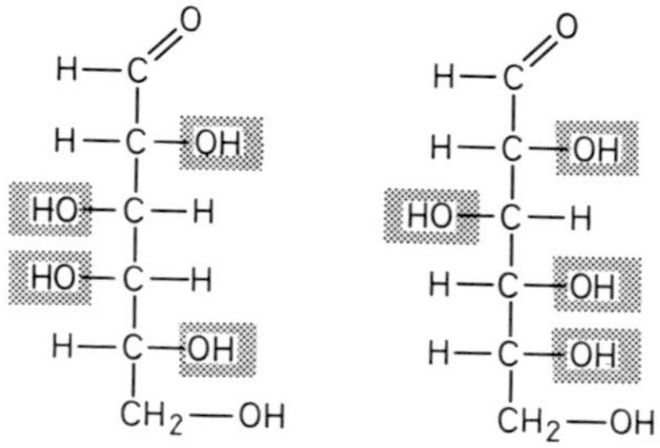

Fig. 1. Galactose and glucose molecule.

Table 1. Composition of the CAPD solution

Sodium, mmol/l	134.0
Calcium, mmol/l	1.75
Magnesium, mmol/l	0.5
Chloride, mmol/l	103.5
Lactate, mmol/l	35.0
Galactose, g/l	15.0
Osmolarity, mosmol/l	354

The aim of this study was to assess the galactose absorption from the peritoneal cavity, the conversion of galactose into glucose and the potential toxicity of galactose.

Animals and Methods

Twelve male Sprague-Dawley rats weighing at least 400 g received a Tenckhoff CAPD catheter (Fresenius) as described elsewhere [17]. The catheter implantation was performed under antiseptic, but not aseptic conditions. The animals were allowed to recover from the operation for 4 weeks.

All 12 animals were subjected to a long-term evaluation. 20 ml of 1.5% galactose-containing CAPD solution was infused daily through the capped catheter for 4 weeks. During infusion the rats were anesthetized with ether.

Table 1 depicts the composition of the galactose solution. Since the fluid was completely absorbed, a rat received about 300 mg/day (750 mg/kg/day) of galactose. After the 4th week the animals were sacrificed and histology of peritoneum, kidney and liver was obtained.

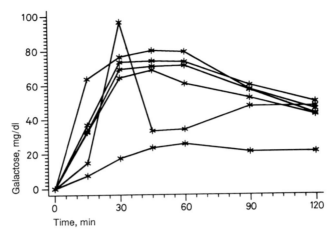

Fig. 2. Individual course of the plasma concentration of galactose (mg/dl), over time following the intraperitoneal instillation of 20 ml of a galactose-containing CAPD solution.

In addition to the long-term study, we performed a kinetic study in 6 of the above rats. For that purpose the animals were anesthetized by using a ketamine/diazepam mixture. Then blood sampling was performed at 0, 10, 20, 30, 45, 60, 90 and 120 min after the peritoneal infusion. Blood was drawn from the retroorbital plexus.

Plasma galactose concentration was determined by using the 'Test-Combination Galactose' (Boehringer Mannheim, FRG). The glucose levels were analyzed by the reflo check system (Boehringer Mannheim).

Statistical analysis was performed by using the SAS system [18, 19].

Results

Kinetic Study

The course of plasma galactose concentration in the individual rats is depicted in figure 2. The plasma galactose levels showed a rapid increase during the first 30–45 min, followed by a continuous slow decrease afterwards. In one animal no significant rise occurred due to the enwrapment of the catheter following a peritonitis episode. Thus, a free distribution in the peritoneal cavity was not possible and absorption was delayed.

In contrast to the rapid increase in plasma galactose concentration, a delayed increase of glucose plasma levels was observed (fig. 3). No changes in

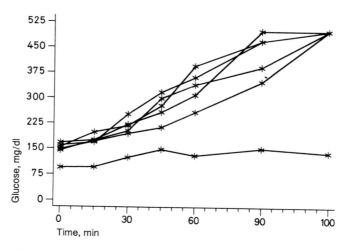

Fig. 3. Individual course of the plasma concentration of glucose (mg/dl) over time following the intraperitoneal instillation of 20 ml of a galactose-containing CAPD solution.

plasma glucose concentration were recorded in the rat with the delayed galactose absorption.

No signs of acute toxicity were observed.

Long-Term Study

During the study 4 of 12 rats died of peritonitis. The remaining 8 were sacrificed after 4 weeks. The histological evaluation of peritoneum, liver and kidney was uneventful in the surviving rats.

No signs of chronic toxicity were observed.

Discussion

Glucose is the common osmotic agent in CAPD solutions. However, the rapid carbohydrate load due to the continuous glucose absorption from dialysate may lead to a further increase of plasma glucose levels in diabetic CAPD patients.

Galactose is an epimer of glucose with the same osmotic capacity. After the intraperitoneal infusion of the galactose-containing CAPD solution, a steady increase of plasma galactose levels occurred during the first 30–

45 min, followed by a continuous decrease afterwards. The increase in plasma galactose concentration confirms that galactose diffuses through the peritoneal membrane. The subsequent decrease indicated that continuous accumulation did not occur and galactose was metabolized.

In contrast to the rapid increase in plasma galactose concentration, glucose levels showed a delayed increase with a steady rise up to the end of the observation period (120 min).

Despite the fact that galactose is supposed to be metabolized to glycogen [13–16, 20], unexpectedly high plasma glucose levels were recorded. Perhaps a stress reaction due to anesthesia could have shifted the galactose metabolism from glycogen to glucose production [21]. This phenomenon could be partially responsible for the excessive plasma glucose levels.

In the kinetic study no signs of acute toxicity occurred. In the long-term study no signs of chronic toxicity (liver failure) were observed either.

Thus, we conclude that galactose at this low a concentration is a nontoxic substance. Our experimental protocol was unsuccessful to confirm the metabolic advantages of this substance over glucose. Further studies are needed to prove that galactose is a suitable alternative to glucose.

References

1   Raja RM, Kramer MS, Manchanda R, Lazaro N, Rosenbaum JL: Peritoneal dialysis with fructose dialysate: Prevention of hyperglycaemia and hyperosmolality. Ann Intern Med 1976;79:511–517.
2   Bazzato G, Coli U, Landinis S, Fracasso A, Morachiello P, Righetto F, Scanferla F: Xylitol and low dosage of insulin: New perspectives for diabetic uraemic patients on CAPD. Periton Dial Bull 1982;2:161–164.
3   Raja RM, Moros JG, Kramer MS, Rosenbaum JL: Hyperosmotic coma complicating peritoneal dialysis with sorbitol dialysate. Ann Intern Med 1970;73:993–994.
4   Daniels FH, Leonhard EF, Cortell S: Glucose and glycerol compared as osmotic agents for peritoneal dialysis. Kidney Int 1984;25:20–25.
5   Oreopoulos DG, Crassweller P, Kaartirzoglou A, Ogilvie R, Zellermann G, Rodella H, Vas SI: Amino acids as an osmotic agent in continuous peritoneal dialysis; in Legrain M (ed): Continuous Ambulatory Peritoneal Dialysis. Amsterdam, Excerpta Medica, 1979, pp 335–340.
6   Khanna R, Twardowski ZJ, Oreopoulos, DG: Osmotic agents for peritoneal dialysis. Int J Artif Organs 1986;9:387–390.
7   Rottembourg J, Brouard R, Issad B, Allouadie M, Ghali B, Boudjemaa A: Role of acetate in loss of ultrafiltration during CAPD; in Augustin R (ed): Peritonitis in CAPD. Contrib Nephrol. Basel, Karger, 1987, vol 57, pp 197–206.
8   Gjessing J: Use of Dextran as a dialysing fluid in peritoneal dialysis. Acta Med Scand 1969;185:237–239.

9   Twardowski ZJ, Khanna R, Nolph KD: Osmotic agents and ultrafiltration in peritoneal dialysis. Nephron 1986;42:93–101.
10 Twardowski ZJ, Moore H, McGary T, Poskuta M, Hirszel P, Stathakis C: Polymer as osmotic agents in peritoneal dialysis. Periton Dial Bull 1984;4:125–131.
11 Mistry CD, Gokal R, Mallik NP: Glucose polymer as an osmotic agent in CAPD; in Maher JF, Winchester JF (eds): Frontiers in Peritoneal Dialysis. New York, Field, Rich, 1986, pp 241–248.
12 Winchester JF, Stegink LD, Ahmad S, Gross M, Hammeke M, Horowitz AM, Maher JF, Pollak V, Rakowski T, Schreiber M, Singh S, Somani P, Vidt D: A comparison of glucose polymer and dextrose as osmotic agents in CAPD; in Maher JF, Winchester JF (eds): Frontiers in Peritoneal Dialysis. New York, Field, Rich, 1986, pp 231–240.
13 Kliegman RM, Miettinen EL, Kalhan SC, Adam PAJ: The effect of enteric galactose on neonatal canine carbohydrate metabolism. Metabolism 1981;30:1109–1114.
14 Kliegman RM, Miettinen EL, Morton S: Potential role of galactokinase in neonatal carbohydrate assimilation. Science 1983;220:302–304.
15 Kliegman RM, Morton, S: Galactose assimilation in pups of diabetic canine mothers. Diabetes 1987;36:1280–1285.
16 Kliegman RM, Sparks JW: Perinatal galactose metabolism. J Pediatr 1985;6: 831–841.
17 Gretz N, Lasserre JJ, Drescher P, Mall K, Strauch M: Experimental CAPD: A rat model; in La Greca G, Olivares J, Feriani M, Passlick-Deetjen J (eds): CAPD – A Decade of Experience. Contrib Nephrol. Basel, Karger, 1991, vol 89, pp 43–46.
18 SAS/GRAPH User's Guide: Version 5 Edition. Cary, SAS Institute Inc., 1985.
19 SAS User's Guide: Basics, Version 5 Edition. Cary, SAS Institute Inc., 1985.
20 Pribylowa J, Kozlova J: Glucose and galactose infusions in newborns of diabetic and healthy mothers. Biol Neonate 1979;36:193–197.
21 Sparks J, Glinsman W: Regulation of rat liver glycogen synthesis and activities of glycogen cycle enzymes by glucose and galactose. Metabolism 1976;25:47–55.

J.J. Lasserre, MD, Clinic of Nephrology, University of Heidelberg,
Klinikum Mannheim, D–W–6800 Mannheim (FRG)

La Greca G, Olivares J, Feriani M, Passlick-Deetjen J (eds): CAPD – A Decade of Experience. Contrib Nephrol. Basel, Karger, 1991, vol 89, pp 134–146

High Osmolar Amino Acid Solution: An Alternative to Glucose?

J. Passlick-Deetjen, R. Koch, B. Grabensee[1]

Department of Nephrology, University of Düsseldorf, FRG

Despite the fact that CAPD has been established for a period of over 10 years now, several metabolic problems have emerged from the use of glucose as the sole osmotic agent.

The continuous absorption of glucose from the dialysate leads to reduced appetite and inadequate nutritional intakes. As a consequence, CAPD patients may show low levels of total serum protein, albumin and transferrin. The daily loss of protein (5–15 g/24 h) [1] and amino acids (AA; 1.2–3.5 g/24 h) [2, 3] into the dialysate may also contribute to the protein malnutrition. A further problem is the aggravation of hyperinsulinemia and hypertriglyceridemia as well as the decreased levels of high-density lipoproteins [4]. As long as these abnormalities may be related to the glucose load it seems reasonable to replace glucose by a different osmotic agent. AA, for example, may possibly combine less adverse effects with nutritional benefits.

This study was planned to investigate whether an AA solution produces adequate ultrafiltration volumes and a sufficient removal of urea and creatinine. Moreover, we wanted to show to which extent the AAs influence the blood levels of urea (BUN), insulin and AAs and the loss of protein into the dialysate.

Patients and Methods

Eight patients (4 male and 4 female) with end-stage renal failure were studied. The cause of renal failure was glomerulonephritis (4 patients) or diabetic nephropathy (2 patients) and in 2 cases unknown.

[1] The authors wish to acknowledge the assistance of Mr. Beutner and Mrs. Maier (Fresenius AG) in the analysis of amino acids.

Table 1. Composition of the AA solution (values are mmol/l)

L-Histidine	11.75
L-Isoleucine	32.39
L-Leucine	54.04
L-Methionine	13.90
L-Valine	30.20
L-Lysin hydrochloride	19.57
L-Phenylalanine	11.04
L-Threonine	15.03
L-Malic acid	3.79
Sodium chloride	99.00
Calcium chloride	1.75
Magnesium chloride	0.50
Sodium lactate	35.00
Glucose monohydrate	27.75

The patients had been on CAPD for an average of 31 months. Their age ranged from 37 to 65 years. None of them had a residual renal function. All were using 1.5 liters glucose (GL) solution (1.36% Dianeal®, Baxter) two, three or four times a day. High osmolar solution (3.86% Dianeal®, Baxter) was used once (5 patients) or twice (2 patients) a day.

Three patients had no history of peritonitis, 3 had one episode and 2 had two episodes (mean rate of peritonitis: 1 per 41 months). None of these episodes had occurred within 4 weeks before the study.

The investigation started in the morning after the patients had fasted for 10 h. During the night they had used a 1.36% glucose-containing solution, which was drained and replaced by 1.5 liters of the AA or GL solution. The dwell time ranged from 1 to 6 h on 12 different days.

Thus, each patient served as his own control. Between two investigations there was always a period of 3 days. The patients fasted during the first 4 h of the study, thereafter they received a standard breakfast containing 3 g of protein. Venous blood and dialysate samples were taken before and immediately after the instillation of the dialysis fluid, again after half an hour and at the end of each dwell time.

After the dialysate had been drained, the total volume was measured. Serum and dialysate were analyzed for creatinine, BUN, electrolytes, glucose, insulin, proteins and AAs (plasma).

Solutions

We studied an AA solution containing 2.59% essential amino acids (EAA) and 0.55% glucose monohydrate (CAPD 3AS, Fresenius, Bad Homburg, FRG). The exact composition is given in table 1. The 3.86% GL solution served as a control. The electrolyte composition of the solutions did not differ except for sodium, which was 2 mmol higher in the AA solution. Osmolality (AA solution: 514 ± 2 mosm/kg; GL solution: 486 ± 1 mosm/kg) and pH (AA solution: 5.7 ± 0.1; GL solution 5.1 ± 0.1) of the AA solution were also slightly higher.

Amino Acid Measurement

Samples of 2 ml EDTA-plasma and 5 ml dialysate were deproteinized with sulfosalicylic acid, kept cool at 4 °C for 10 min and centrifuged for 10 min. 1 ml of deproteinized plasma was mixed with 1 ml Li-citrate-buffer and stored at −20 °C until it was analyzed. The supernatant of the dialysate samples was kept frozen under the same conditions. An amino acid analyzer Beckman 6300 (Beckman Instruments Inc., USA) was used to determine the AA concentrations.

Measurement of Creatinine, Protein and Insulin

Creatinine in serum and dialysate was measured manually by enzymatic methods (Boehringer Mannheim Diagnostics). Total protein analysis was also performed manually by the Biuret method, while albumin and immunoglobulins were analyzed by a laser nephelometer (Behring). Insulin concentrations were determined by radioimmunoassay (Pharmacia Insulin RIA 100).

Statistical Methods

Paired t tests were used to compare either the measurements at a certain dwell time with the baseline values or the data received by the alternate use of AA or GL solution at certain dwell times.

Results

The AA solution was well tolerated by the patients except for two, who complained about slight abdominal discomfort or pain immediately after the instillation of the dialysate.

Ultrafiltration was higher with the AA solution compared to the GL solution (fig. 1), though the difference was significant only after 1, 3 and 6 h. Maximum ultrafiltration was reached after 3 and 4 h with the AA solution and after 4 and 5 h with the GL solution.

The slight difference in osmolality between the solutions disappeared already after a short dwell time. Serum osmolality was found to be significantly higher after a dwell time of 2 h, when the AA solution was used (fig. 2).

The dialysate to plasma ratio of BUN was significantly higher with the AA solution at every hour of dialysis (fig. 3), while the equilibration of creatinine showed a significant difference only after 4 and 6 h (fig. 3). This had no effect on serum creatinine levels.

The equilibration of insulin (5,807 daltons), β_2-microglobulin (11,800 daltons) and albumin (66,290 daltons) during AA and GL dialysis showed no difference. Quantitative elimination of total proteins, β_2-microglobulin, albumin, IgG (150,000 daltons) and IgA (160,000 daltons) was not different either (fig. 4).

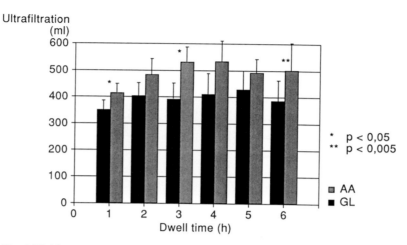

Fig. 1. Fluid removal with a 2.59% AA solution in comparison to 3.86% GL solution in 8 CAPD patients.

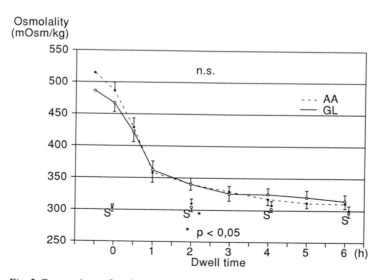

Fig. 2. Comparison of peritoneal and serum osmolality over a 6-hour dwell time with AA and GL dialysates.

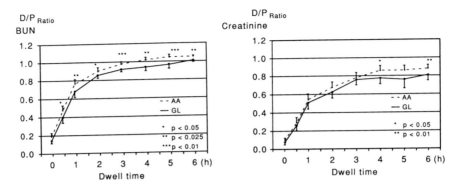

Fig. 3. Comparison of BUN and creatinine equilibration during a 6-hour dwell time with AA and GL solutions.

Table 2. Effect of the AA and GL solutions on plasma levels of the EAA during different dwell times in 8 patients on CAPD

AA (normal values) μmol/l	Dwell time				
	0 h	2 h	4 h	6 h	
Leucine	92 ± 7	82 ± 7	96 ± 14	85 ± 9	GL
(90–170)	86 ± 8	860 ± 114	465 ± 62[c]	337 ± 71	AA
Isoleucine	46 ± 8	57 ± 6	52 ± 10	50 ± 9	GL
(43–89)	54 ± 6	477 ± 72	260 ± 35[c]	173 ± 23	AA
Valine	137 ± 14	122 ± 13	136 ± 18	127 ± 17	GL
(165–298)	136 ± 13	828 ± 81	617 ± 70[d]	465 ± 38	AA
Lysine	145 ± 9	144 ± 12	147 ± 9	147 ± 11	GL
(129–236)	150 ± 10	461 ± 40	302 ± 19[d]	257 ± 15	AA
Methionine	28 ± 6	33 ± 6	31 ± 6	27 ± 7	GL
(17–46)	28 ± 4	291 ± 54	195 ± 23[e]	150 ± 21	AA
Phenylalanine	58 ± 3	50 ± 7	56 ± 5	64 ± 4	GL
(40–77)	53 ± 8	247 ± 25	168 ± 15[d]	188 ± 27	AA
Histidine	73 ± 5	72 ± 7	72 ± 5	77 ± 7	GL
(67–116)	77 ± 5	175 ± 20	112 ± 10[c]	98 ± 5	AA
Threonine	99 ± 11	97 ± 17	92 ± 12	97 ± 15	GL
(76–139)	114 ± 17	313 ± 35	298 ± 54[c]	287 ± 60	AA

Normal values from [29].
4 h vs. 0 h: [c]p < 0.005; [d]p < 0.001; [e]p < 0.0005.

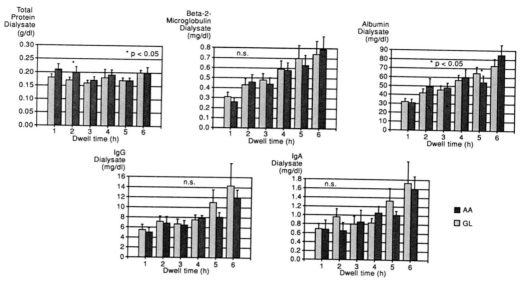

Fig. 4. Comparison of the elimination of total protein, β_2-microglobulin, albumin, IgG and IgA using AA and GL solutions.

Regarding basal plasma levels of AA, in our patient group, only valine levels were lower in plasma compared to normal subjects (table 2). The levels of the remaining EAAs were within the normal range. Regarding the nonessential amino acids (NEAA) only serine and tyrosine were slightly reduced, whereas plasma levels of proline, citrulline and glycine were elevated (table 3). The EAA/NEAA ratio was (normal values [3] in parentheses): 0.43 ± 0.001 (0.53 ± 0.10), the tyrosine/phenylalanine ratio 0.73 ± 0.002 (0.97 ± 0.33) and the glycine/serine ratio 3.75 ± 0.10 (2.28 ± 0.52).

During dialysis most of the EAAs and some of the NEAAs showed a slight decrease in the plasma levels (tables 2, 3) using the 3.86% GL solution.

During the administration of the AA solution the plasma concentration of the EAAs reached their peak concentration 1 or 2 h after instillation had started, e.g. the plasma level of histidine rose twofold, whereas that of methionine rose tenfold (table 2).

Though there were no NEAAs present in the solution, plasma levels of alanine, citrulline, ornithine and arginine rose significantly after 1, 2 and 3 h at the same time. There was a decrease in serine, proline, glycine and taurine (table 3).

Table 3. Effect of the AA and Gl solutions on plasma levels of the NEAA during different dwell times in 8 patients on CAPD

AA (normal values) μmol/l	Dwell time				
	0 h	2 h	4 h	6 h	
Aspartic acid	10 ± 1	10 ± 1	9 ± 1	10 ± 1	GL
(2–9)	12 ± 2^a	12 ± 2	14 ± 3	16 ± 4^a	AA
Serine	69 ± 5	64 ± 7^b	62 ± 11	62 ± 12	GL
(78–130)	65 ± 11	68 ± 12	$53 \pm 5^{f+}$	$62 \pm 6^{b**}$	AA
Glutamic acid	44 ± 11	39 ± 9	44 ± 10	43 ± 11	GL
(33–53)	53 ± 14	48 ± 14	54 ± 10	85 ± 30^a	AA
Proline	275 ± 30	248 ± 38	268 ± 35	230 ± 28	GL
(129–192)	261 ± 25	226 ± 35^a	220 ± 20^c	244 ± 19	AA
Glycine	267 ± 20	247 ± 31^a	239 ± 14^c	255 ± 20	GL
(133–261)	268 ± 20	$189 \pm 26^{e*}$	$189 \pm 23^{e+}$	$185^{f*} \pm 19^{f*}$	AA
Alanine	358 ± 39	364 ± 38	323 ± 34	362 ± 43	GL
(186–376)	357 ± 34	$423 \pm 42^{c+}$	$410 \pm 23^{d*}$	390 ± 31	AA
Tyrosine	40 ± 4	40 ± 5	44 ± 9	43 ± 4	GL
(51–83)	39 ± 3	32 ± 3	31 ± 3	43 ± 6	AA
Ornithine	85 ± 6	77 ± 8	82 ± 6	83 ± 9	GL
(36–86)	90 ± 7	$109 \pm 11^+$	$95 \pm 9^+$	$95 \pm 5^+$	AA
Taurine	53 ± 4	46 ± 4	55 ± 5	47 ± 4	GL
(40–90)	$47 \pm 4^+$	43 ± 5	41 ± 4	43 ± 3	AA
Citrulline	87 ± 13	79 ± 14	80 ± 7	74 ± 14^d	GL
(18–35)	86 ± 13	$121 \pm 20^{b*}$	$113 \pm 19^{b+}$	$124 \pm 20^{d**}$	AA
Arginine	81 ± 8	75 ± 11	82 ± 10	84 ± 11	GL
(55–115)	82 ± 10	$106 \pm 12^{d**}$	82 ± 10	78 ± 7^b	AA

AS vs. GL: $^+p < 0.05$; $^*p < 0.025$; $^{**}p < 0.01$; $^{***}p < 0.005$.
2,4,6 h vs. 0 h: $^ap < 0.05$; $^bp < 0.025$; $^cp < 0.01$; $^dp < 0.005$; $^ep < 0.001$; $^fp < 0.0005$.

The absorption of the EAAs of the solution is shown in the upper part of figure 5. The quantity absorbed was dependent on the concentration of the particular amino acid in the dialysate and varied from 2 to 10 g after a dwell time of 6 h, resulting in an uptake of 35 g of AAs, which is nearly 90% of the quantity administered.

The elimination of the EAAs (fig. 5, lower part) while using a 3.86% GL solution showed a direct relation to the particular plasma levels. After a 6-hour dialysis a loss of 166 mg EAAs was found, which means a daily loss of about 650 mg based on four exchanges a day. With respect to the elimination

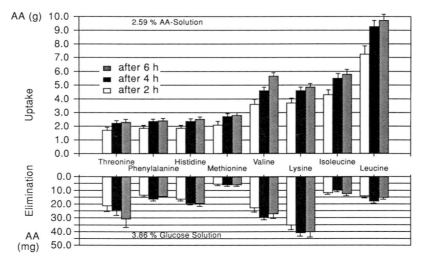

Fig. 5. Uptake of EAA during dialysis with the AA solution in comparison to the elimination of EAA during dialysis with a 3.86% GL solution.

of NEAAs in both solutions it could be noticed that the dialysate concentrations of alanine, ornithine, citrulline and arginine were higher when the AA solution was used.

The effect of the AA solution and the glucose solution on glucose and insulin metabolism was only studied in nondiabetic patients. When using the GL solution, serum glucose rose from 99 mg% to a maximum of 168% during the first 2 h (table 4). With the AA solution the serum glucose levels remained almost unchanged. Using the glucose solution serum insulin concentrations rose from 16.6 to 35.1 µU/ml during the first hour, while the AA dialysate led to an increase in serum insulin to 75 µU/ml. With both solutions serum insulin levels decreased during the following dwell time, however, did not reach the baseline values (table 4).

There was no definite change in BUN levels with GL solution. Using the AA dialysate, BUN showed a slight but not significant increase (table 4).

Discussion

In accordance with other authors [5–9], a more efficient ultrafiltration as well as a higher D/P ratio for urea and creatinine was observed in our

Table 4. Comparison of serum glucose, insulin and BUN concentration using a 2.59% AA solution (+ 55% GL) and a 3.86% GL solution

		Dwell time						
		0 h	1 h	2 h	3 h	4 h	5 h	6 h
Serum glucose, mg/dl	GL	99 ± 4	108 ± 16[++]	168 ± 34[++]	143 ± 32	123 ± 32	120 ± 17	104 ± 7
	AA	98 ± 5	105 ± 21	102 ± 12	94 ± 11	96 ± 13	89 ± 10	96 ± 15
Serum insulin, μU/ml	GL	16.6 ± 1.4	35.1 ± 8.9*	32.8 ± 6.8	31.4 ± 8.2	25.6 ± 7.5[+]	25.3 ± 7.2	31.9 ± 10.6
	AA	17.9 ± 1.2	75.0 ± 17.7	50.7 ± 14.1	40.2 ± 11.3	31.9 ± 9.2	26.3 ± 7.6	19.8 ± 8.8
BUN, mg/dl	GL	60 ± 2	59 ± 5	60 ± 5	58 ± 4	58 ± 4	58 ± 5	59 ± 5
	AA	50 ± 2	63 ± 3	63 ± 5	59 ± 4[a]	60 ± 6[c]	60 ± 5[a]	62 ± 5[b]

GL vs. AA: [+]p < 0.05; [++]p < 0.025; *p < 0.01; **p < 0.005.
BUN, t h vs. 0 h: [a]p < 0.025; [b]0 < 0.005; [c]0 < 0.0005.

patients. This may indicate an alteration of the peritoneal permeability and/ or surface area by the AA solution.

In spite of this fact, the type of solution had no significant influence on the equilibration of insulin, β_2-microglobulin and albumin, which could probably be explained by the higher molecular weight and larger intraindividual variations.

The elimination of proteins was also not different in our patient group, which is in contrast to results that have been formerly reported [5, 10].

Also in contrast to other studies [6, 7,9,11], but in accordance with the recent results of Bergstöm et al. [12] in hemodialysis patients, only valine and serine levels were markedly lower than in normal controls, while proline, glycine, and citrulline were elevated as has already been stated by several authors [5, 12, 13]. Comparable to different other reports, EAA/NEAA tyrosine/phenylalanine, and valine/glycine ratios were low, while the glycine/ serine ratio was high due to impaired transformation of AA and to uncorrected acidosis in uremia [1, 12, 14–19].

During the exchange with the GL solution, a slight decrease in plasma AA levels was observed probably due to the loss of AA into the dialysate, the amount of which was directly correlated to the plasma levels.

After intraperitoneal infusion of the AA solution, plasma EAA levels rose far above concentrations reached after a protein-rich meal [20], but were below the range described to be toxic [21]. Though, in chronic treatment these high levels, e.g. methionine, could aggravate acidosis, which is an undesired effect [22] and may in addition lead to unpredicted amino acid imbalances.

There was no difference concerning the rate of absorption of AA after a dwell time of 6 h compared to other experiences [7]. The quantity of 35 g absorbed amounted to nearly 50% of the daily protein need recommended for a dialysis patient of 70 kg body weight, which could be of nutritional benefit for the patient.

Loss of EAA and NEAA into the dialysate while using the GL solution amounted to 400 mg in 6 h, which results in a loss of 1.6 g/day, similar to the results of former studies [2, 3].

Using the EAA solution, plasma levels of some NEAA increased significantly, probably due to a stimulation of the de novo synthesis by an increased AA supply [23] and due to a disturbance of the hepatic uptake [24]. Simultaneously, elimination of these AA into the dialysate rose.

As could be expected, the small amount of glucose absorbed with the AA solution did not affect serum glucose levels although it led to a significant

26 Hanning RM, Balfe JW, Zlotkin SH: Effectiveness and nutritional consequences of
    amino acid-based vs glucose-based dialysis solutions in infants and children receiv-
    ing CAPD. Am J Clin Nutr 1987;46:22.
27 Yalow RS, Baumann WA: Plasma insulin in health and disease; in Ellenberg M,
    Rifkin H (eds): Diabetes mellitus. New York, Excerpta Medica, 1983, p 119.
28 Blumenkrantz MJ, Kopple JD, Moran SK, Grodstein GP, Coburn JW: Nitrogen and
    urea metabolism during continuous ambulatory peritoneal dialysis. Kidney Int
    1981;20:78.
29 Weidler B: Veränderungen der Plasmaaminosäuren unter invasiven Operationsver-
    fahren und differenten Narkosetechniken; thesis Giessen, 1982, p 69.

Dr. J. Passlick-Deetjen, Science Department, Fresenius AG, Borkenberg 14,
D–W–6370 Oberursel/Taunus (FRG)

La Greca G, Olivares J, Feriani M, Passlick-Deetjen J (eds): CAPD – A Decade
of Experience. Contrib Nephrol. Basel, Karger, 1991, vol 89, pp 147–154

Alternate Use of Amino Acid and Glucose Solutions in CAPD

A Review

Fritz Bangsgaard Pedersen

Department of Nephrology, Odense University Hospital, Denmark

There are several indications and reasons for the use of amino acids (AA) as osmotic agents in peritoneal dialysis fluids. They can be used in order to counteract the loss of AA and protein through the peritoneum and dialysate during intermittent peritoneal dialysis as proposed by Gjessing [1] in 1968. Uremic patients treated by this method may show abnormalities with regard to plasma proteins and AA, which can be partly corrected by adding AA to the dialysis fluid as proposed by Kobayashi et al. [2] in 1979.

In 1979 Oreopoulos et al. [3] suggested that AA could be used as osmotic agents in CAPD instead of glucose.

The nitrogen losses mentioned above, and the metabolic abnormalities disclosed in the uremic population undergoing renal replacement therapy have been considered a challenge in relation to treatment with AA-based solutions [4–6].

In fact, some patients on CAPD do show subtle indices of malnutrition [7] and, when CAPD treatment is extended for more than 1 year, a decrease in total body nitrogen has been reported [8].

During uncomplicated CAPD a weekly loss of 10–30 g of AA and about 70 g of protein across the peritoneal membrane takes place [9, 10]. During the same period 500–2,100 g of glucose are transferred from the dialysate to the bloodstream [9, 10]. By using AA as osmotic agents instead of glucose, this constant glucose overload might be decreased and the hypertriglyceridemia, usually seen in CAPD patients, might be improved [5]. In addition, AA profiles both in plasma and in intracellular AA pools are abnormal and only partially corrected by CAPD [4, 5].

If the above-mentioned abnormalities and side effects during CAPD could be diminished by the use of AA-based solutions a more physiological treatment for children and diabetics could possibly be achieved.

A short review of studies published on AA-based solutions for CAPD will be presented, and suggestions on the future trends will also be given.

Short-Term Studies

The short-term studies published have mainly focused on the osmotic activity of different AA solutions including the transport of the individual AA across the peritoneal membrane, the instant metabolic effect, and the possible side effects and local as well as systemic intolerance.

Though none of the AA solutions used in short-term studies have been identical some general conclusions can be drawn: AA solutions are efficient osmotic agents. Thus, a 2% AA solution induces the same ultrafiltration as a 4.25% glucose-based solution [11], while Lindholm et al. [12] found equivalent volumes of ultrafiltrate when comparing a 2.76% AA solution with a 3.86% glucose-based one. Working with less hypertonic solutions Goodship et al. [13] found smaller but identical ultrafiltrate volumes when comparing a 1% AA solution with a 1.36% glucose solution. The osmolality of various AA concentrations with standard electrolytes is given by Oreopoulos et al. [3], but as mentioned by the authors, the osmotic power produced by different solutions is not only expressed by the osmolality, calculated or measured, but also depends on the degree of absorption and metabolization of the osmotic active substances in the body. Thus, a high content in blood due to high absorption and a slow metabolization will increase the osmotic pressure in blood and thereby counteract the osmotic pressure in the intra-abdominal solution and reduce the ultrafiltration. The osmolality may also change after instillation in the abdomen due to changes in pH and protein binding. The final evaluation of the ultrafiltration capacities of a given CAPD solution have therefore to be based on experimental and clinical observations.

Transperitoneal Transport and Metabolic Consequences

Another general conclusion from short-term studies is: AA solutions remove urea, potassium and creatinine as efficiently as glucose solutions [3, 12, 13].

The AA content may, when absorbed, induce urea production in the liver. A 1% AA solution as used by Goodship et al. [13], resulted in a stable urea level through 6 h while the level increased by 17% during the same period when a 2.7% AA solution was used by Lindholm et al. [12]. In the long-term experiences discussed later 1% AA solutions also resulted in an increased urea level.

The glucose and insulin levels in plasma are influenced differently using AA and glucose solutions. Though some of the carbon chains in AA may be metabolized into glucose only slight increases in blood sugar level were noticed during the use of a 2.7% AA solution [12], while 1% AA solutions seem to have no effect on the glucose level.

Insulin production is increased by both types of solutions [13–15]. Glucose-based solutions do increase blood glucose levels even when used in 1.36% solutions [13].

Serum Amino Acid Imbalance and Amino Acid Transport

Many of the AA, especially the essential ones and among them the branched-chain AA (BCAA) are found in low concentrations in plasma or in the intracellular AA pools in uremics [5, 6]. The BCAA and especially leucine is supposed to be of major importance and able to increase muscle and liver protein synthesis [16, 17]. Therefore, it is of interest to observe whether an improvement in essential AA and BCAA concentrations can be obtained by use of the AA solutions.

In the short-term studies by Oren et al. [15] and Goodship et al. [13] the AA levels increased to a maximum 1–2 h after the instillation. Goodship et al. [13] using a high concentration of BCAA in their AA solution noticed a significant increase in serum levels. In children [14] a not intended, but too high and long-lasting elevation of the serum levels of methionine and phenylalanine was observed using a 2% AA solution (Travasole®).

The postabsorptive levels of AA seems to depend on the relative concentrations of the different AA in the solutions [11], and if present in the solution especially the BCAA do increase their plasma level to a relatively higher extent than the other AA as they are taken up to a smaller degree by the liver [18, 19].

Side Effects and Intolerance

Clinical observations and biochemical results from the short-term studies mentioned above indicate that AA solutions are generally well tolerated, however slight abdominal discomfort or pain were experienced by patients following intraperitoneal administration by both a Dianeal 3.86% glucose solution and a 2.76% AA solution [12]. The use of 25 mmol/1 of acetate as buffer may explain why some of the patients experienced more discomfort or pain when using AA solutions. The low pH in some hypertonic solutions also seems to provoke discomfort, as observed in children [14].

Recently, Steinhauer et al. [20] reported an augmented peritoneal PGE_2 release accompanied by an augmented protein loss through the dialysate using a 2.6% AA dialysis solution when compared to the PGE_2 release using a conventional 4.25% glucose-based solution. The clearance rates of creatinine, urea, potassium and phosphate were identical for the two solutions while the ultrafiltration diminished slightly during instillation of the AA dialysate. It has to be mentioned that the AA solution also contained glucose.

The risk of a continuous PGE_2 stimulation using AA solutions has to be taken into consideration in the future as it might indicate the presence of a slight, chronic irritation produced by the dialysis fluid.

Long-Term Studies

The first long-term study in which AA-based dialysis solutions were used for CAPD appeared in 1983 [15]. Six patients were studied over 4 weeks. A 1% AA solution was used alternately with dialysate containing glucose. The AA solution used contained 9 essential AA and 4 nonessential AA (NEAA) of which glycine and alanine were present in relatively high concentration. The AA solution was well tolerated, and with respect to the AA in plasma the low concentrations of valine, isoleucine and leucine observed before treatment remained so during the study, while glycine increased and alanine decreased, though the infused amount of the latter was high. The tyrosine/alanine ratio decreased after using AA solutions for 4 weeks. Plasma triglycerides tended to fall, while plasma insulin and glucagon remained elevated and unchanged. No change in bicarbonate was noticed, but serum-urea-nitrogen (BUN) increased from 64 to 103 mg%. Serum transferrin rose, while serum albumin remained constant. A slight increase in total body nitrogen content as measured in vivo by neutron activation was demonstrated, but no change in total body potassium content occurred.

The next long-term study appeared in 1985 [21]. Six patients were treated for 3 months using a 1% AA solution alternately with a 1.36% Dianeal glucose solution. If necessary hypertonic 4.25% glucose solutions were used during the night. 7.5 mmol/1 of sodium bicarbonate was added to each AA bag to increase pH to about 6.6. The AA solution contained 10 essential and 6 nonessential AA. This AA solution was also well tolerated, but, in variance with the results from the study of Oren et al. [15], a rise in the blood concentration of the BCAA during the 3-month study period was noticed. In contrast also to the study by Oren et al. [15], the serum triglyceride level continued to increase, while serum transferrin remained unchanged as did serum albumin. Glycosylated hemoglobin, Hb_{A1c}, also remained stable and normal. As in the study by Oren et al. [15], a significant increase in BUN was observed, a finding also noticed during AA solutions used in the short-term studies mentioned above.

In 1985, Schilling et al. [22] published the results from a prospective, controlled study in which 1% AA solutions were evaluated for their ability to counteract the catabolic effect of peritonitis in CAPD patients. During 4 weeks 12 patients used AA solutions alternately with glucose solutions, while 10 patients continued regular dialysis with glucose-based solutions only. Four of the patients receiving AA solutions withdrew from the study due to poor appetite, which also were noticed by 5 other patients in this group. Only 3 of 10 patients using glucose solutions complained of loss of appetite. The nitrogen balance was similar in the two groups despite AA supplementation in one of them. Blood urea increased markedly in the AA group, while serum albumin remained low. The opposite changes were noticed in the cases of peritonitis treated as usual with glucose-based solutions. Fasting plasma AA levels remained unaltered by the AA instillations. With reference to the study by Steinhauer et al. [20], mentioned above, and in which an increased concentration of PGE_2 and protein was seen in patients treated with AA solutions, it has to be noticed that the protein excretion was identical in the two groups with peritonitis whether they were treated by AA or glucose solutions.

From the present study by Schilling et al. [22], it might be feared that AA solutions are not to be recommended for use in patients with peritonitis, irrespective of their great and negative nitrogen metabolism.

The long-term studies, though few, indicate that 1% AA solutions can be used for periods as long as 3 months without essential problems or patient discomfort. However, no persistent and beneficial effect on the glucose and lipid-fat metabolism has been demonstrated with certainty until now. The blood-urea level increases in short-term as well as long-term studies using AA solutions, indicating that part of the AA administered is used directly for urea production when absorbed. Though sufficient uptake of nitrogen by the peritoneal route takes place during treatment with AA solutions, it has not been shown with certainty whether the AA absorbed may turn into an increased protein mass laid down in organs or muscles. AA solutions seem rather unsuitable as CAPD fluids in the treatment of patients with peritonitis as the nitrogen balance remains unaffected as the patients develop anorexia.

Some of the more concentrated AA solutions (2%) seem to be unsuitable for use in children, and in some patients contribute to the development of abdominal pains and discomfort.

Future Trends

The papers published until now on the use of AA solutions in CAPD have mainly been pilot studies evaluating the tolerance and major side effects of the AA solutions under study. The AA solutions have never been complete as some AA as glutamine are unstable in solution and during heating. Valuable knowledge concerning the change in serum levels of the different AA after peritoneal instillation has nevertheless been obtained, though the ideal mixture has still not been found. It is difficult to find clinically usable and noninvasive methods for repeated application to demonstrate the incorporation of the infused AA into proteins, peptides and AA pools in the different organs.

Still more work has to be done to prove that the AA solutions are inert to the peritoneal membranes, leukocytes and monocytes in the abdominal cavity.

The AA imbalance found in plasma or intracellular AA pools in uremia and during dialysis is still not proven to be a result of AA imbalance per se, malnutrition, increased catabolism or insufficient supply. Other mechanisms which can result in changes in the AA turnover as proposed by Garber et al. [23] in 1984 have to be taken into consideration. The increased muscle proteolysis found in uremia by these authors might be explained by hyperparathyroidism and would presumably remain uninfluenced by AA infusions.

Recently, infusions containing alanyl-glutamine dipeptides have been shown to be effective by reducing the negative nitrogen balance in man after major surgery [24]. The daily protein loss, postoperatively and during treatment with conventional AA solutions, was reduced further and significantly by glutamine supplementation. As glutamine secretion by the muscles seems to be increased in uremia [23], it will be interesting to follow this trend. As certain AA, such as the BCAA, appear to stimulate the synthesis of both glutamine and alanine, the earlier demonstration of a low BCAA content in plasma and in intracellular AA pools may possibly be related to the increased metabolism of glutamine in uremia.

References

1   Gjessing J: Addition of amino acids to peritoneal-dialysis fluid. Lancet 1968;ii: 812–813.
2   Kobayashi K, Manji T, Hiramatsu S, et al: Nitrogen metabolism in patients on peritoneal dialysis. Contr Nephrol. Basel, Karger, 1979, vol 17, pp 93–100.
3   Oreopoulos DG, Crassweller P, Katirtzoglou A, et al: Amino acids as an osmotic agent (instead of glucose) in continuous ambulatory peritoneal dialysis, in: Legrain M (ed): Continuous Ambulatory Peritoneal Dialysis. Amsterdam, Excerpta Medica, 1980, pp 335–340.
4   Bergström J: Protein catabolic factors in patients on renal replacement therapy. Blood Purif 1985;3:215–236.
5   Lindholm B, Bergström J: Metabolic effects of peritoneal dialysis; in La Greca G, Chiaramonte S, Fabris A, et al (eds): Peritoneal Dialysis. Milano, Wichtig Editore, 1986, pp 111–128.
6   Randerson DH, Chapman GV, Farrell PC: Amino acid and dietary status in CAPD patients; in Atkins RC, Thomson NM, Farrell PC (eds): Peritoneal Dialysis. Edinburgh, Churchill-Livingstone, 1981, pp 179–191.
7   Sombolos K, Berkelhammer C, Baker J, et al: Nutritional assessment and skeletal muscle function in patients on continuous ambulatory peritoneal dialysis. Periton Dial Bull 1986;6:53–58.
8   Heide B, Pierratos A, Khanna R, et al: Nutritional status of patients undergoing continuous ambulatory peritoneal dialysis (CAPD). Periton Dial Bull 1983;3:138–141.
9   Gahl GM, Baeyer HV, Riedinger RF, et al: Caloric intake and nitrogen balance in patients undergoing CAPD; in Moncrief JW, et al (eds): CAPD Update. New York, Masson 1981, pp 87–93.
10 Blumenkrantz MJ, Schmidt RW: Managing the nutritional concern of the patient undergoing peritoneal dialysis; in Nolph KD (ed): Peritoneal Dialysis. The Hague, Martinus Nijhoff, 1981, pp 275–308.
11 Williams, PF, Marliss EB, Anderson GH, et al: Amino acid absorption following intraperitoneal administration in CAPD patients. Periton Dial Bull 1982;2:124–130.
12 Lindholm B, Werynski A, Bergström J: Peritoneal dialysis with amino acid solutions: Fluid and solute transport kinetics. Artif Org 1988;12:2–10.
13 Goodship THJ, Lloyd S, McKenzie PW, et al: Short-term studies on the use of amino acids as an osmotic agent in continuous ambulatory peritoneal dialysis. Clin Sci 1987;73:471–478.
14 Hanning RM, Balfe JW, Zlotkin SH: Effectiveness and nutritional consequences of amino acid-based vs. glucose-based dialysis solutions in infants and children receiving CAPD. Am J Clin Nutr 1987;46:22–30.
15 Oren A, Wu G, Anderson GH, et al: Effective use of amino acid dialysate over four weeks in CAPD patients. Periton Dial Bull 1983;3:66–73.

16 Buse MH, Reid SS: Leucine. A possible regulator of protein turnover in muscle. J Clin Invest 1975;56:1250–1261.

17 Mortimor GE, Pösö AK: Mechanism and control of deprivation-induced protein degradation in liver: Role of glucogenic amino acids; in Häussinger D, Sies H (eds): Glutamine metabolism in mammalian tissues. Berlin, Springer, 1984, pp 138–157.

18 Wahren J, Felig P, Hagenfeldt L: Effect of protein ingestion on splanchnic and leg metabolism in normal man and in patients with diabetes mellitus. J Clin Invest 1976;57:987–999.

19 Souba WW, Smith RJ, Wilmore DW: Review. Glutamine metabolism by the intestinal tract. J Parent Ent Nutr 1985;5:608–617.

20 Steinhauer HB, Lubrich-Birkner I, Kluthe R, et al: Amino acid dialysate stimulates peritoneal prostaglandin E$_2$ generation in humans; in: Khanna R, Nolph KD, Prowant BF, et al (eds): Advances in Continuous Ambulatory Peritoneal Dialysis 1988. Toronto, Peritoneal Dialysis Bulletin Inc., 1988, pp 21–26.

21 Pedersen FB, Dragsholt C, Laier E, et al: Alternate use of amino acid and glucose solutions in CAPD. Periton Dial Bull 1985;215–218.

22 Schilling H, Wu G, Pettit J, et al: Use of amino acid containing solutions in continuous ambulatory peritoneal dialysis patients after peritonitis: Results of a prospective controlled trial. Proc EDTA-ERA 1985;22:421–425.

23 Garber AJ, Allen SJ, Moretti-Rojas J, et al: Cyclic nucleotide regulation of glutamine metabolism in sceletal muscle; in Häussinger J, Sies H (eds): Glutamine Metabolism in Mammalian Tissues. Berlin, Springer, 1984, pp 205–222.

24 Stehle P, Mertes N, Puchstein CH, et al: Effect of parenteral glutamine peptide supplements on muscle glutamine loss and nitrogen balance after major surgery. Lancet 1989;i:231–233.

Fritz Bangsgaard Pedersen, MD, Department of Nephrology,
Odense University Hospital, DK–5000 Odense C (Denmark)

La Greca G, Olivares J, Feriani M, Passlick-Deetjen J (eds): CAPD – A Decade of Experience. Contrib Nephrol. Basel, Karger, 1991, vol 89, pp 155–160

Sodium Modelling in CAPD

A. Colombi

Renal Unit of the Department of Medicine,
Kantonsspital, Lucerne, Switzerland

It has long been recognized that some patients on CAPD treatment do have problems with sodium balance. This does not only concern diabetics, although the tendency for sodium and water retention is more often observed in this patient group. Many patients with increased extracellular volume suffer from hypertension. Moreover, an abnormal distribution of water has been noted in CAPD patients with a higher intracellular fraction [1]. Even in the absence of overt edema, a decreasing hematocrit points to an extracellular volume overload. Water and salt retention is obvious when, after successful renal transplantation, these patients lose 5–10 kg of body weight during the first 2 weeks.

Sodium and water excretion along the peritoneal capillary is best described by the Nolph hypothesis [2] with the well-known hydrostatic and oncotic pressure gradients from the arterial to the venous side and with an increasing diameter of the endothelial junctions in the same direction. The physiologic consequences are a predominant ultrafiltration in the arterial and diffusion in the venous limb of the capillary. Since sodium is primarily eliminated by convective transport, this would be an explanation for the famous sieving effect resulting in an ultrafiltrate containing 100 mmol/l sodium or less.

In order to describe fluid movements in the peritoneum properly, lymphatic drainage must be included. In the rat, peritoneal lymphatic flow was found to be about 25 µl/kg/min [3]. For an adult man of 70 kg body weight this would correspond to approximately 1.75 ml/min or 2,520 ml/day. Since the cranial part of the peritoneum is especially rich in lymphatics, more fluid is reabsorbed by this system in the supine position.

In CAPD, total sodium transport can be determined by total sodium in the effluent minus total sodium in the inflow dialysate. The diffusive fraction

Table 1. Ultrafiltration volume (UF) per bag and per day obtained with dialysis solutions of different glucose concentration in CAPD patients

Volume ml	Glucose %	Osmolality mosm/l	Patients n	UF/4 h ml/bag	UF/day ml/24 h
1 × 2,000	2.3	401	20	305 ± 134	–
1 × 2,000	4.25	503[1]	22	324 ± 62	–
1 × 2,000	4.25	512	22	679 ± 137	–
5 × 2,000[2]	1.5	358	50	248 ± 124	1,026 ± 187
4 × 2,000[2]	1.5	358	45	248 ± 124	717 ± 432

[1] 130 mmol/l sodium.
[2] In 24 h.

is calculated from serum sodium minus dialysate inflow sodium multiplied by the inflow volume. With a dialysate containing 132 mmol/l sodium the diffusive fraction is about one third of total sodium eliminated. However, in order to get more precise information on sodium transport and balance in an individual patient, we measured sodium in serum, dialysate and urine.

Methods

In 19 patients on CAPD during 2–48 months, 24 h urine volume was measured and sodium concentration assessed. Dialysate effluent volumes were also measured and total peritoneal sodium transport was calculated from the difference between inflow and outflow concentrations. This was done with dialysate solutions of different osmolality (358–512 mosm/l) and sodium concentration (134 and 130 mmol/l). Total sodium elimination (urinary and peritoneal) was evaluated with the patients being on a standard diet containing 100 mmol/day (2.3 g) of sodium.

Results

With a dialysate containing 134 mmol/l sodium, ultrafiltration volume after a dwell time of 4 h was 248 ± 124 ml/2-liter bag in the 1.5% solution, 305 ± 134 ml/2-liter bag in the 2.3% solution and 679 ± 137 ml/2-liter bag in the 4.25% solution (table 1). In patients using 4 × 2 liters of 1.5% dialysate with an osmolality of 358 mosm/l, ultrafiltration was 717 ± 432 ml/day.

Table 2. Mean calculated sodium excretion (mmol/l) by ultrafiltration (UF) and urine output in patients on CAPD treated with 4 × 2 liters/day 1.5% glucose solution: dialysate sodium at inflow 134 mmol/l (mean urine sodium concentration 70 mmol/l)

UF ml/24 h	Urine volume, ml/24 h										
	0	100	200	300	400	500	600	700	800	900	1,000
1,200	124	131	138	145	152	159	166	173	180	187	194
1,100	111	118	125	132	139	146	153	160	167	174	181
1,000	98	105	112	119	126	133	140	147	154	161	168
900	85	92	99	106	113	120	127	134	141	148	155
800	72	79	86	93	100	107	114	121	128	135	142
700	59	66	73	80	87	94	101	108	115	122	129
600	46	53	60	67	74	81	88	95	102	106	116
500	33	40	47	54	61	68	75	82	89	99	103
400	20	27	34	41	48	55	62	69	76	83	90
300	7	14	21	28	35	42	49	56	63	70	77
200	+6	1	8	15	22	29	36	43	50	57	64
100	+19	+12	+5	2	9	16	23	30	37	44	51
0	+32	+25	+18	+11	+4	3	10	17	24	31	38

Mean urine volume in these 19 patients was 418 ± 264 ml/day. Thus total fluid removal using low osmolality solutions exclusively was 1,135 ml/day not including perspiratio insensibilis. These fluid losses permit a fluid intake of at least 1,500 ml/day.

With serum sodium values around 138 mmol/l and a dialysate concentration of 134 mmol/l, peritoneal sodium elimination was 98 mmol/1,000 ml of ultrafiltrate (table 2). Only when the ultrafiltrate exceeded 300 ml/day did the sodium balance become negative. Urinary sodium concentration was rather constant in this population with 70 mmol/l and contributed a considerable amount to total sodium excretion. With a mean ultrafiltration volume of 700 ml/day and a mean urinary volume of 600 ml/day, total sodium elimination was also 100 mmol/day. With the introduction of a low sodium dialysate containing 130 mmol/l, the proportion of diffusive sodium transport increased by 32 mmol/day using 4 × 2 liters (table 3). If during the years of CAPD residual urinary volume decreases to 100 ml/day, the low sodium dialysate can compensate for this loss of residual function. However, ultrafiltration is somewhat lower with this dialysis solution due partially to the lower osmolality; a higher glucose concentration could be desirable therefore.

The two broken lines in figure 1 describe the conditions concerning ultrafiltrate and urine volume at which a sodium elimination of 100 mmol/

Table 3. Mean calculated sodium excretion by ultrafiltration (UF) and urine output in patients on CAPD treated with 4 × 2 liters/day 1.5% glucose solution: dialysate sodium at inflow 130 mmol/l (mean urine sodium concentration 70 mmol/l)

UF ml/24 h	Urine volume, ml/24 h										
	0	100	200	300	400	500	600	700	800	900	1,000
1,000	130	137	144	151	158	165	172	179	186	193	200
900	117	124	131	138	145	152	159	166	173	180	187
800	104	111	118	125	132	139	146	153	160	167	174
700	91	98	105	112	119	126	133	140	147	154	161
600	78	85	92	99	106	113	120	127	134	141	148
500	65	72	79	86	93	100	107	114	121	128	135
400	52	59	66	73	80	87	94	101	108	115	122
300	39	46	53	60	67	74	81	88	95	102	109
200	26	33	40	47	54	61	68	75	82	89	96
100	13	20	27	34	41	48	55	62	69	76	83
0	0	7	14	21	28	35	42	49	56	63	70

day might be expected. The upper line refers to a dialysate containing 134 mmol/l sodium and the lower line to a concentration of 130 mmol/l dialysate (inflow concentration). For any given urine volume up to 1,000 ml the ultrafiltration volume required for a sodium loss of 100 mmol/day can be derived.

Discussion

In contrast to hemodialyzed patients, those on CAPD are often promised a liberal diet. As to protein and potassium these hopes can easily be held, but regarding sodium and water the promises are often limited. As long as residual urine volume exceeds 1,000 ml/day and ultrafiltration is in the range of 700 ml/day, sodium elimination is more than 130 mmol/day, corresponding to a normal salted diet. However, as urine volume decreases with time, although this happens slower than in hemodialyzed patients [4], down to 500 ml/day, total sodium elimination decreases to 100 mmol/day. This now corresponds to the sodium content of a moderately salt-restricted diet.

Serious sodium balance problems arise in the anuric patient undergoing CAPD treatment. In these cases dietary salt restriction alone is usually inefficient to compensate for the low sodium excretion by the average

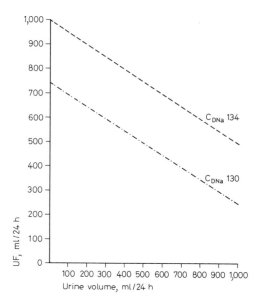

Fig. 1. Conditions for 100 mmol/day sodium excretion by CAPD using a dialysis solution of 134 mmol/l sodium (upper line) and 130 mmol/l sodium (lower line). For any residual urine volume the required ultrafiltrate volume can be derived.

ultrafiltration rate. This rate must be increased by using high osmolar solutions or by choosing a dialysate containing 130 mmol/l sodium. With this dialysate, 800 ml/day of ultrafiltrate will also guarantee a daily sodium excretion of 100 mmol.

Conclusion

For CAPD patients with a residual urine production over 500 ml/day and a peritoneal ultrafiltration rate of 1,000 ml/day, no salt restriction is required when using a dialysate with 134 mmol/l of sodium. However, when patients become anuric in this condition and the ultrafiltration rate is around 800 ml/day, the diffusive sodium transport fraction must be increased by using solutions with a lower sodium concentration. The concentration should preferably be 130 mmol/l in order to allow a sodium intake of 100 mmol/day.

References

1   Panzetta G, Guerra U, D'Angelo A, et al: Body composition and nutritional status in patients on CAPD. Clin Nephrol 1985;23:18–29.

2   Nolph K, Miller FN, Pyle WK, et al: A hypothesis to explain the ultrafiltration characteristics of peritoneal dialysis. Kidney Int 1981;20:543.

3   Barrowman JA, Granger DN: Lymphatic drainage of the peritoneal cavity; in Bengmark S (ed): The Peritoneum and Peritoneal Access. London, Wright, 1989, pp 85–93.

4   Rottembourg J, et al: CAPD – 3 years of experience treating 100 patients. Z Urol Nephrol 1983;76:191.

A. Colombi, MD, Renal Unit of the Department of Medicine,
Kantonsspital, CH–6000 Lucerne (Switzerland)

La Greca G, Olivares J, Feriani M, Passlick-Deetjen J (eds): CAPD – A Decade of Experience. Contrib Nephrol. Basel, Karger, 1991, vol 89, pp 161–174

Peritoneal Transport of Macromolecules in Patients on CAPD

R.T. Krediet, D.G. Struijk, G.C.M. Koomen, D. Zemel,
E.W. Boeschoten, F.J. Hoek, L. Arisz

Renal Unit, Academic Medical Centre, Amsterdam, The Netherlands

Small quantities of serum proteins are always present in the effluent of patients treated with continuous ambulatory peritoneal dialysis (CAPD). The amount of total protein that is lost by the dialysis procedure ranges from 5 to 15 g per 24 h [1–4]. Although local synthesis of some of the proteins can possibly occur in some conditions [2, 5], it is generally assumed that the dialysate proteins mainly originate from the blood by passage through the peritoneal membrane. It is still controversial whether convection or diffusion is the main transport mechanism of macromolecules [6–8].

The magnitude of the peritoneal transport of a solute is dependent on the effective peritoneal surface area and the intrinsic permeability of the peritoneal membrane to that particular solute. The former is the part of the anatomical peritoneal surface area that actually participates in solute transport. It is probably considerably smaller than the anatomical peritoneal surface area [9] that is assumed to equal more or less body surface area [10, 11]. It is also likely that the effective surface area is not constant, but can vary depending on the peritoneal blood flow and the number of peritoneal capillaries perfused. This can be illustrated by the opposite effects of nitroprusside and indomethacin on the protein concentration in peritoneal dialysate [12, 13].

Lymphatic absorption by the subdiaphragmatic lymph vessels is probably the most important mechanism for the transport of intraperitoneally administered macromolecules out of the peritoneal cavity to the circulation [14, 15].

In this paper a review will be given on various aspects of our studies on the peritoneal transport kinetics of macromolecules in CAPD patients. Data will be presented on the variability of clearances, the role of systemic disease,

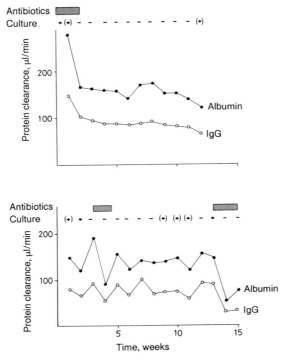

Fig. 1. The time course of the peritoneal clearances of albumin and IgG in the 2 patients studied weekly for 3 months. Culture results of the dialysate and antibiotic treatment are also indicated: (+) indicates an initially negative culture that only became positive after more than 48 h of incubation.

the changes observed in various other conditions, the role of electric charge, the relationship between clearances and molecular size and the effect of the transport route to and from the peritoneal cavity.

Variability of Protein Clearances

The time course of the peritoneal clearances of albumin and IgG, measured once a week during a follow-up period of 3 months, in two patients, is shown in figure 1. The excretion of the proteins in the effluent was determined in a 24-hour collection of dialysate. Every nightbag was cultured to be sure whether – subclinical – peritonitis was present or not. It is obvious that clearance variations occur in the absence of peritonitis. No marked differences are present between the shapes of the albumin and IgG lines. When coefficients of variation were calculated the following values were found: albumin clearance 25%, IgG clearance 26%, IgG/albumin clearance ratio 10%. Omitting the data during collections with positive culture reduced these figures to 19% for albumin clearance and 22% for IgG clearance. This led us to investigate the variability of protein clearances in 14 stable CAPD patients who were studied at least 3 times (mean 4.1) with an interval of 4 months between the studies. Mean follow-up was 13.4 months (range 8–21). None of the patients had peritonitis 2 weeks prior to or 1 week after the study. All studies were done under strictly standardized conditions with dialysate glucose 1.36%, dwell time exactly 4 h and prerinsing of the peritoneal cavity. Mean coefficient of variation for albumin clearance was 26% (range 11–41), for IgG clearance 34% (range 21–48), for the IgG/albumin clearance ratio 14% (8–23) and for the serum concentrations of both proteins 9%. Such high coefficients of variation have also been found by others for dialysate concentrations [16, 17]. Not surprisingly, we were unable to find any relationship between dialysate IgG concentration and peritonitis incidence in our patients [18]. This is in accordance with the findings of some other groups [17, 19]. The validity of studies showing a relationship between dialysate IgG concentration and peritonitis incidence [20–22] can be questioned, as no data on variability are given.

Our finding that the variability of the IgG/albumin clearance ratio was always lower than the clearances themselves suggests that marked day-to-day alterations do occur in the effective peritoneal surface area, but that the intrinsic permeability of the peritoneal membrane to macromolecules (as judged from the IgG/albumin clearance ratio) is less variable during the follow-up time of the study.

Role of Systemic Disease

CAPD is an adequate form of renal replacement therapy in patients with systemic diseases [23]. Vascular abnormalities are present in many of these diseases. When the peritoneal microvessels are involved, peritoneal transport rates of solutes could be influenced. In the past, reduced clearances of low-molecular-weight solutes have been described in a limited number of patients treated with intermittent peritoneal dialysis for renal failure caused

Table 1. Mean peritoneal protein clearances (μl/min/1.73 m^2) in patients with a primary renal disease and in patients with systemic disease

	PRD (n = 13)	SLE (n = 4)	SS (n = 1)	DM (n = 15)	AMY (n = 4)
Albumin	67	73	76	88*	128**
Transferrin	53	56	n.d.	71*	99**
IgG	34	34	42	47*	68**
C$_3$	29	35	n.d.	44*	85*
Alpha$_2$-macroglobulin	12	9	n.d.	14	25*

*p < 0.05, **p < 0.01, when compared to PRD.
PRD = Primary renal disease; SLE = systemic lupus erythematosus; SS = systemic sclerosis; DM = diabetes mellitus; AMY = amyloidosis; n.d. = not done.

by malignant hypertension, diabetic nephropathy, systemic lupus erythematosus (SLE) and systemic sclerosis [24, 25]. We have studied peritoneal protein clearances in 13 CAPD patients with a primary renal disease, 15 with diabetic nephropathy caused by type 1 diabetes melitus [26], 4 with SLE, 4 with amyloidosis [27, 28] and 1 with systemic sclerosis [unpubl.]. The results are summarized in table 1. Peritoneal protein clearances are somewhat higher in diabetic patients than in those with a primary renal disease and markedly elevated in the patients with amyloidosis. In the latter patient group amyloid could be detected in the peritoneal microvessels.

When only losses of total protein are analyzed in diabetic patients [4], no statistically significant differences from nondiabetic patients have been found. This was confirmed for albumin loss in our study. However, conclusions based on total protein loss or even total protein clearances may be misleading, as the diabetic patients in our study had lower serum albumin and higher serum alpha$_2$-macroglobulin concentrations than those with a primary renal disease [26].

Effect of Various Conditions

The effective peritoneal surface area is dependent on the number of perfused capillaries. Furthermore, the peritoneal blood flow is part of the splanchnic blood flow. These facts suggest that alterations in splanchnic blood flow can influence the effective peritoneal surface area and thus

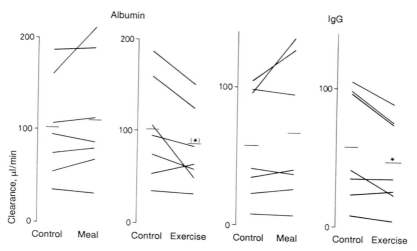

Fig. 2. The effects of a meal and exercise on peritoneal clearances of albumin and IgG in 7 CAPD patients. (*) 0.05 < p < 0.1, *p < 0.05.

peritoneal protein clearances. As splanchnic blood flow is increased after a meal [29] and decreased during exercise [30], we have investigated both conditions in a group of 7 CAPD patients [31]. They were studied on 3 consecutive days. On all 3 days the patients avoided heavy exercise and in the morning two 2-hour exchanges were made: from 8 to 10 a.m. and from 10 to 12 noon. During the first day no food was given until noon. On the second day their first meal (700–1,200 kcal) was taken at 10 a.m. On the third day a light breakfast was allowed. Between 10 and 12 noon of day 3 the patients exercised on a bicycle ergometer: they exerted themselves as much as they could during 3 periods of 10 min each.

The results are given in figure 2: the increase after a meal was only marginal, but a significant decrease in the clearance of IgG was found after exercise. The lack of increase after a meal may be explained by the results of Granger et al. [32]. Using radioactive microspheres in cats, they have shown that commercial peritoneal dialysis solutions dramatically increase blood flow to the mesentery, omentum, intestinal serosa and the parietal peritoneum. No significant alterations were found in the blood perfusion of the major abdominal organs or the blood flow through the coeliac and superior mesenteric arteries. Thus, it may be that peritoneal blood flow during CAPD

Table 2. Effect of peritonitis and of a 3-litre dialysate exchange on peritoneal protein transport, mean ± SEM [33, 34]

	Mass transfer area coefficient, ml/min	
	peritonitis	recovery
Beta$_2$-microglobulin	2.92 ± 1.09	1.24 ± 0.35**
Albumin	0.26 ± 0.13	0.11 ± 0.05**
IgG	0.16 ± 0.06	0.06 ± 0.03**
	2 litres	3 litres
Beta$_2$-microglobulin	1.29 ± 0.54	1.29 ± 0.48
Albumin	0.12 ± 0.04	0.11 ± 0.03
IgG	0.07 ± 0.02	0.07 ± 0.02

** $p < 0.01$.

is so high that the increment of splanchnic blood flow caused by a meal is too small to lead to an increase in effective peritoneal surface area.

The effects of peritonitis and of a 3-litre dialysate exchange on the peritoneal transport of proteins have been described elsewhere [26, 33, 34]. The protein clearances are summarized in table 2. During peritonitis the clearances of all measured serum proteins were increased more than twofold when compared with the situation after recovery. No evidence was found for local synthesis of proteins like IgG and complement C_3. Increasing the dialysate volume from 2 to 3 litres had no effect on peritoneal protein clearances. Clearances of albumin and IgG were also measured in 4 patients who developed sclerosing peritonitis [35]. It appeared that the time course of these clearances paralleled that of the low-molecular-weight solutes.

Role of Electric Charge

The transport of macromolecules across a membrane is dependent on their size, shape and charge. Especially the fixed negative charge in the glomerular basement membrane inhibits the passage of negatively charged serum proteins [36]. Using ruthenium red, fixed negative charges have been demonstrated on the luminal surface of the peritoneal vascular endothelium

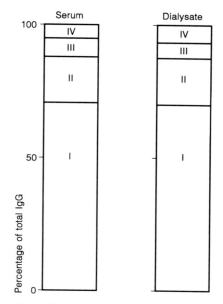

Fig. 3. The distribution of the various subclasses in serum and dialysate of 5 CAPD patients.

of rats [37]. To analyze the importance of negative charge on the peritoneal transport of macromolecules we have studied the transport of IgG subclasses and of a polydisperse neutral dextran solution. IgG can be divided into 4 subclasses with different mean iso-electric points: they range from 7 for class IV to 9.5 for class I. Using an ELISA technique we studied serum and dialysate concentrations (2-litre exchanges, glucose 1.36%, dwell time 4 h) in 5 CAPD patients. The results are shown in figures 3 and 4. No differences were found in the distribution of the various subclasses in serum and dialysate, while a linear relationship was present between the relative concentrations in these two fluids.

The effect of electric charge on the transport of various macromolecules cannot be analyzed on the basis of their molecular weight alone as this does not take the role of the shape of a macromolecule into account. Therefore, the Einstein-Stokes or effective diffusion radius must be used. It is the radius of an imaginary sphere with the same free diffusion coefficient as the protein it is compared to. The relationship between the Stokes radius (r) and the free diffusion coefficient in water (D_w) is given by the equation: $D_w = RT/6\pi\eta rN$,

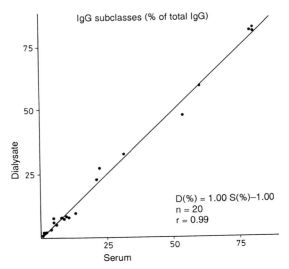

Fig. 4. The linear relationship between the serum and dialysate concentrations of the 4 IgG subclasses in 5 CAPD patients, relative to the total IgG concentration.

in which R is Boltzmann's gas constant, T the absolute temperature, η the viscosity of the solution, and N is Avogadro's number.

We compared the peritoneal transport of serum proteins and a poly-disperse neutral dextran solution in 13 CAPD patients. In 6 of them the study was continued until the exchange that was instilled at 38 h after the intravenous administration of dextran 70. This exchange was drained at 46 h [38]. Using gel permeation chromatography dextran fractions of various Einstein-Stokes radii could be compared with proteins of almost identical radii. As shown in table 3, no evidence was found that the peritoneal membrane is a charge-selective barrier to the transport of macromolecules. Protein clearances were even higher than dextran clearances in the 3- to 7-hour study. These differences had disappeared in the 38- to 46-hour study. This can be explained by assuming that the peritoneal interstitium is a third compartment between blood and dialysate. In this compartment equilibrium between blood and dialysate is present for serum proteins, but initially not for dextran.

From our studies with neutral dextran and IgG subclasses it can be concluded that the peritoneal membrane is a size-selective, not a charge-selective, barrier to the transport of macromolecules.

Table 3. Peritoneal clearance ratios of protein and corresponding dextran fractions in the 6 patients who were studied up to 46 h after the administration of dextran [38]

	Protein/dextran clearance ratio	
	3- to 7-hour study	38- to 46-hour study
Albumin/dextran 37 Å	1.25	1.01
Transferrin/dextran 43 Å	1.70	1.10
IgG/dextran 54 Å	1.44	0.95
Alpha$_2$-macroglobulin/ dextran 90 Å	1.17	0.70

Relationship between Clearances and Molecular Size

Power curve fitting has been used to describe the relationship between solute clearances (C) and their molecular weights (MW): $C = aMW^b$, or ln C = b ln MW +ln a, in which a and b are constants [39, 40]. We could also fit our data on protein transport using a power curve [26, 33, 34]. An exponential type of curve, instead of a linear one, when protein clearances and molecular weight were plotted on a double logarithmic scale has been found by Steinhauer et al. [13]. When free diffusion coefficients of serum proteins were plotted against molecular weight, the power fit could also be applied [26]. However, the slope of the regression lines of protein clearances was much steeper than that of the free diffusion coefficients [26]. This suggested a mechanism of size-selective restricted diffusion for the peritoneal transport of serum proteins.

In the study using intravenously administered polydisperse neutral dextran it was possible to analyze peritoneal clearances of 18 dextran fractions with Einstein-Stokes radii ranging from 30 to 90 Å [38]. It appeared that the relationship between dextran clearances and radii was not linear when plotted on a double logarithmic scale. It can be deduced from Stokes equation that by definition a linear relationship is present between the reciprocal of the free diffusion coefficients in water of macromolecules and their Einstein-Stokes radii. When diffusion is the transport mechanism of macromolecules across the peritoneal membrane, a linear relationship should be obtained when the reciprocal of the clearance is plotted against the Einstein-Stokes radius. Using this plot we found correlation coefficients ranging between 0.95 and 1.00 for both the dextran fractions and the serum proteins. The slopes of the lines were far above the slope of the line for the free diffusion coefficients. The finding again points to a size selective restricted diffusion as the main mechanism for the peritoneal transport of macromolecules from blood to dialysate. Above radii of 70 Å the dependency of clearance on molecular size is less marked [38]. It may be that these large solutes pass through a small number of very large pores that cannot discriminate with respect to size.

Transport to and from the Peritoneal Cavity

The passage of macromolecules from the blood in the peritoneal capillaries to the dialysate in the peritoneal cavity is transcapillary across the endothelial cells and capillary basement membrane, through the interstitial tissue and across the mesothelial cells. Transport in the opposite direction, i.e. out of the peritoneal cavity, is only partly transcapillary but probably mainly takes place by uptake in the subdiaphragmatic lymphatic vessels. Their terminal parts or lacunae are situated between bundles of collagenous fibres and are covered by mesothelial cells. Gaps or stomata are present in the junctions of these cells. Most of the lymph passes via the substernal ducts associated with the internal mammary vessels to the anterior mediastinal lymph nodes and from these into the circulation via the right lymphatic duct [41].

It is well known from studies using intraperitoneally administered macromolecules for the measurement of peritoneal fluid kinetics that the recovery of these solutes averages between 80 and 90% irrespective of the kind of solute used: either radiolabeled serum albumin or autologous haemoglobin [42–44]. We compared the outward clearance of intraperitoneally administered autologous haemoglobin (MW 68,000) to the inward clearance of albumin (MW 69,000). Mean haemoglobin clearance was 1.49 ml/min and mean albumin clearance 0.12 ml/min [45]. Higher outward clearances than inward clearances have also been reported in rabbits for neutral dextran [46]. Both studies suggest that lymphatic uptake is the most important way for the disappearance of macromolecules from the peritoneal cavity, as has been pointed out by Nolph and co-workers [14, 15].

Lymphatic absorption is essentially a convective process. If so, no relationship between the Einstein-Stokes radii of neutral dextran fractions and their clearance should be present. We investigated this hypothesis by the administration of a polydisperse solution of dextran 70 into the dialysate of 9 CAPD patients and performing gel permeation chromatography of the effluent [47]. In all patients the maximum of the dextran distribution curve before inflow was found at the same Stokes radius as after drainage. No relationship was found between clearances and Stokes radii. This supports the hypothesis that the disappearance of macromolecules from the peritoneal cavity is essentially size-independent.

Conclusions

From the above-mentioned studies it can be concluded that the trans-peritoneal passage of macromolecules from the blood to the dialysate is a process of size- not charge-dependent restricted diffusion. Its magnitude is probably determined by the effective peritoneal surface area. Marked variations occur in this surface area, not only between patients but also at various points of time in 1 patient. The disappearance of intraperitoneally administered macromolecules is about ten times higher than the transcapillary diffusion and is not dependent on molecular size. Lymphatic absorption is the most likely transport mechanism.

Acknowledgments

The studies on the peritoneal transport of macromolecules that were performed in the renal unit of the Academic Medical Centre, Amsterdam, were partly supported by the Dutch Kidney Foundation (Nierstichting Nederland: grant C86.597) and by Baxter Nederland B.V. Mrs. K. Berkinshaw is acknowledged for her contribution to the exercise and meal studies. All studies were done with the excellent technical assistance of Mrs. M.J. Langedijk, Mrs. M.B. Kerssens and A.C.J. Leegwater. The determination of the IgG subclasses was performed in the laboratory for clinical immunology of the Academic Medical Centre, head Dr. T.A. Out. Mrs. Y. Robberse is acknowledged for the preparation of the manuscript.

References

1   Blumenkrantz MJ, Gahl GM, Kopple JD, et al: Protein losses during peritoneal dialysis. Kidney Int 1981;19:593–602.
2   Dulaney JT, Hatch FE: Peritoneal dialysis and loss of proteins: A review. Kidney Int 1984;26:253–262.
3   Young GA, Brownjohn AM, Parsons FM: Protein losses in patients receiving continuous ambulatory peritoneal dialysis. Nephron 1987;45:196–201.

4   Rubin J, Walsh D, Bower JD: Diabetes, dialysate losses and serum lipids during continuous ambulatory peritoneal dialysis. Am J Kidney Dis 1987;10:104–108.

5   Boesken WH, Schuppe HC, Seidler A, et al: Peritoneal membrane permeability for high and low molecular weight proteins (H/LMWP) in CAPD; in Maher JF, Winchester JF (eds): Frontiers in Peritoneal Dialysis. New York, Field Rich, 1986, pp 47–52.

6   Krediet RT, Arisz L: Fluid and solute transport across the peritoneum during continuous ambulatory peritoneal dialysis (CAPD). Periton Dial Int 1989;9:15–25.

7   Leypoldt JK, Parker HR, Frigon RP, et al: Molecular size dependence of peritoneal transport. J Lab Clin Med 1987;110:207–216.

8   Rippe B, Stelin G: Simulations of peritoneal solute transport during CAPD. Application of two-pore formalism. Kidney Int 1989;35:1234–1244.

9   Henderson LW: The problem of peritoneal membrane area and permeability. Kidney Int 1973;3:409–410.

10 Wegner G: Chirurgische Bemerkungen über die Peritonealhöhle mit besonderer Berücksichtigung der Ovariotomie. Archs Klin Chir 1877;20:51–155.

11 Esperanca MJ, Collins DL: Peritoneal dialysis efficiency in relation to body weight. J Paediatr Surg 1966;1:162–169.

12 Nolph K, Ghods A, Brown P, et al: Effects of nitroprusside on peritoneal mass transfer coefficients and microvascular physiology. Trans Am Soc Artif Intern Organs 1977;23:210–217.

13 Steinhauer HB, Schollmeyer P: Prostaglandin-mediated loss of proteins during peritonitis in continuous ambulatory peritoneal dialysis. Kidney Int 1986;29: 584–590.

14 Nolph KD, Mactier R, Khanna R, et al: The kinetics of ultrafiltration during peritoneal dialysis: The role of lymphatics. Kidney Int 1987;32:219–226.

15 Mactier RA, Khanna R, Twardowski Z, et al: Contribution of lymphatic absorption to loss of ultrafiltration and solute clearances in continuous ambulatory peritoneal dialysis. J Clin Invest 1987;10:461–466.

16 van Bronswijk H: Microbial invasion and peritoneal defence in CAPD patients; clinical, microbiological and cytological studies; thesis, Free University, Amsterdam, 1988, pp 33–48.

17 Holmes CJ, Chapman J, Aono F: Longitudinal study of humoral immune factors in CAPD effluent (abstract). Periton Dial Int 1989;9(suppl 1):81.

18 Zemel D, Struijk DG, Krediet RT, et al: No relationship between dialysate IgG and peritonitis incidence (abstract). Nephrol Dial Transplant 1989;4:755–756.

19 McGregor SJ, Brock JH, Briggs JD, et al: Relationship of IgG, C_3 and transferrin with opsonising and bacteriostatic activity of peritoneal fluid from CAPD patients and the incidence of peritonitis. Nephrol Dial Transplant 1987;2:551–556.

20 Keane WF, Peterson PK: Host defence mechanisms of the peritoneal cavity and continuous ambulatory peritoneal dialysis. Periton Dial Bull 1984;4:122–127.

21 Lamperi S, Carozzi S: Defective opsonic activity of peritoneal effluent during continuous ambulatory peritoneal dialysis (CAPD): importance and prevention. Periton Dial Bull 1986;6:87–92.

22 Coles GA, Alobaidi HMM, Topley N, et al: Opsonic activity of dialysis effluent predicts those at risk of *Staphylococcus epidermidis* peritonitis. Nephrol Dial Transplant 1987;2:359–365.

23 Cantaluppi A: CAPD and systemic diseases. Clin Nephrol 1988;30(suppl 1):S8–S12.

24 Nolph KD, Stolz ML, Maher JF: Altered peritoneal permeability in patients with systemic vasculitis. Ann Intern Med 1971;75:753–755.

25 Brouw ST, Ahearn DJ, Nolph KD: Reduced peritoneal clearances in scleroderma increased by intraperitoneal isoproterenol. Ann Intern Med 1973;78:891–894.

26 Krediet RT, Zuyderhoudt FMJ, Boeschoten EW, et al: Peritoneal permeability to proteins in diabetic and non-diabetic continuous ambulatory peritoneal dialysis patients. Nephron 1986;42:133–140.

27 Krediet RT, Berkinshaw K, Boeschoten EW, et al: Clinical aspects of peritoneal permeability. Neth J Med 1985;28:424–434.

28 Krediet RT, Boeschoten EW, Zuyderhoudt FMJ, et al: Permeability of the peritoneum to proteins in CAPD patients with systemic disease; in Davison AM, Guillon PJ (eds): Proceedings of the European Dialysis and Transplant Association-European Renal Association. London, Baillière Tindall, 1985, vol 22, pp 405–409.

29 Brandt JL, Castleman L, Ruskin HD, et al: The effect of oral protein and glucose feeding on splanchnic blood flow and oxygen utilization in normal and cirrhotic subjects. J Clin Invest 1955;34:1017–1025.

30 Wade OL, Combes B, Childs AW, et al: The effect of exercise on the splanchnic blood flow and splanchnic blood volume in normal man. Clin Sci 1956;15:457–463.

31 Krediet RT: Peritoneal permeability in continuous ambulatory peritoneal dialysis patients; thesis, University of Amsterdam, 1986, pp 89–102.

32 Granger DN, Ulricht M, Perry MA, et al: Peritoneal dialysis solutions and feline splanchnic blood flow. Clin Exp Pharmacol Physiol 1984;11:473–482.

33 Krediet RT, Zuyderhoudt FMJ, Boeschoten EW, et al: Alterations in the peritoneal transport of water and solutes during peritonitis in continuous ambulatory peritoneal dialysis patients. Eur J Clin Invest 1987;17:43–52.

34 Krediet RT, Boeschoten EW, Struijk DG, et al: Differences in the peritoneal transport of water, solutes and proteins between dialysis with two and with three litre exchanges. Nephrol Dial Transplant 1988;2:198–204.

35 Krediet RT, Struijk DG, Boeschoten EW, et al: The time course of peritoneal transport kinetics in continuous ambulatory peritoneal dialysis patients who develop sclerosing peritonitis. Am J Kidney Dis 1989;13:299–307.

36 Brenner BM, Hostetter TH, Humes HD: Molecular basis of proteinuria of glomerular origin. N Engl J Med 1978;298:826–833.

37 Gotloib L, BarSella P, Jaichenko J, et al: Ruthenium red-stained polyanionic fixed charges in peritoneal microvessels. Nephron 1987;47:22–28.

38 Krediet RT, Koomen GCM, Koopman MG, et al: The peritoneal transport of serum proteins and neutral dextran in CAPD patients. Kidney Int 1989;35:1064–1072.

39 Lasrich M, Maher JM, Hirszel P, et al: Correlation of peritoneal transport rates with molecular weight: a method for predicting clearances. ASAIO J 1979;2:107–113.

40 Popovich RP, Moncrief JW, Pyle WK: Transport kinetics; in Nolph KD (ed): Peritoneal Dialysis, ed 3. Dordrecht, Kluwer, 1989, pp 96–116.

41 Khanna R, Mactier R, Twardowski ZJ, et al: Peritoneal cavity lymphatics. Periton Dial Bull 1986;6:113–121.

42 Daugirdas JT, Ing TS, Gandhi VC, et al: Kinetics of peritoneal fluid absorption in patients with chronic renal failure. J Lab Clin Med 1980;95:351–361.

43 Krediet RT, Boeschoten EW, Zuyderhoudt FMJ, et al: Simple assessment of the efficacy of peritoneal transport in continuous ambulatory peritoneal dialysis patients. Blood Purif 1986;4:194–203.

44 De Paepe M, Belpaire F, Schelstraete K, et al: Comparison of different volume markers in peritoneal dialysis. J Lab Clin Med 1988;111:421–429.

45 Krediet RT, Struijk DG, Boeschoten EW, et al: Measurement of intraperitoneal fluid kinetics in CAPD patients by means of autologous haemoglobin. Neth J Med 1988;33:281–290.

46 Hirzel P, Shea-Donohue T, Chakrabarti E, et al: The role of the capillary wall in restricting diffusion of macromolecules. Nephron 1988;49:58–61.

47 Krediet RT, Struijk DG, Koomen GCM, et al: The disappearance of macromolecules from the peritoneal cavity during continuous ambulatory peritoneal dialysis (CAPD) is not dependent on molecular size. Periton Dial Int 1990;10:147–152.

R.T. Krediet, MD, Dialysis Unit, Academic Medical Centre,
Meibergdreef 9, NL–1105 AZ Amsterdam (The Netherlands)

La Greca G, Olivares J, Feriani M, Passlick-Deetjen J (eds): CAPD – A Decade of Experience. Contrib Nephrol. Basel, Karger, 1991, vol 89, pp 175–185

Calcium Metabolism in Patients on CAPD and Hemodialysis

P. Kurz[a], *T. Tsobanelis*[a], *U. Ewald*[b], *P. Roth*[b], *E. Werner*[b], *J. Vlachojannis*[a]

[a]St. Markus Hospital, and [b]Gesellschaft für Strahlen- und Umweltforschung, Frankfurt/M., FRG

With progression of renal insufficiency, disorders of calcium homeostasis increase. Normalization cannot be reached in the majority of patients even under dialysis treatment. The reasons for this are the vitamin D deficiency, the parathyroid hormone (PTH) and vitamin D resistance of the uremic bone [1], as well as the loss of the excretory function of the kidney as the organ controlling the calcium balance. Thus, irrespective of the dialysis method, progress of secondary hyperparathyroidism is observed. However, there are contradictory findings concerning the progression of renal bone disease under the different forms of dialysis. A majority of authors observed an improvement of osteomalacia under CAPD treatment [2, 3], whereas no differences could be detected with regard to the development or progression of osteitis fibrosa. These comparative studies were based on histological and/or radiological findings.

The histological picture of renal osteopathy is the morphological manifestation of the underlying disorder in calcium homeostasis. Calcium metabolism can only be studied by means of tracer kinetic investigations [4]. Investigations of calcium kinetics with ^{45}Ca and ^{47}Ca allow the calculation of intestinal calcium absorption, the rate of clearance of calcium from the plasma, calcium retention in the bone and the calculation of the compartments involved in calcium homeostasis.

For comparison of calcium kinetics under CAPD and HD treatment, a total of 38 patients who had been under dialysis for at least 6 months was investigated. The calcium kinetic parameters were correlated with laboratory and clinical data.

Patients and Methods

Thirty-eight patients on chronic dialysis were investigated (23 hemodialysis and 15 CAPD patients). The mean age was 60.9 ± 11.1 years for the hemodialysis group, and 62.7 ± 11.7 years for the CAPD group. 70% of the HD patients were women as compared to 40% of the CAPD group. The percentage of diabetics was 26.6% (4/15) in the CAPD group, as compared to 4.3% in the HD group (1/23). All patients were dialyzed for at least 6 months. None of the patients received vitamin D preparations or calcium supplementation at the time of investigation. Vitamin D and calcium were discontinued at least 4 weeks prior to the calcium kinetic studies. HD patients were dialyzed three times a week for a total of 15 h. Calcium concentration of the dialysate was 1.75 mmol/l. CAPD patients made four exchanges per day using two low (1.36%) and two high (3.86%) glucose solutions. The dialysate calcium concentration was 1.75 mmol/l, the volume instilled was 2,000 ml for each exchange.

The determination of alkaline phosphatase, phosphate and calcium in the serum was carried out according to standard clinical test methods. Intact parathyroid hormone (iPTH) was determined with a two-site assay as described by Blind et al. [5]. $1,25(OH)_2$ vitamin D_3 ($1,25(OH)_2D_3$) and 25(OH) vitamin D_3 ($25(OH)D_3$) were determined according to the method of Scharla et al. [6].

Calcium Kinetics

For investigation of calcium kinetics the patients received approximately 0.45 MBq ^{47}Ca intravenously and approximately 0.2 MBq^{45}Ca per os as tracer. After administration of the tracer, the activities in the first 4 h after application were measured in plasma samples, and a gamma spectrometric measurement of the ^{47}Ca emission was made in a whole-body counter; further measurements were made on the 1st, 7th, 14th, 21st and 28th days after application.

The following parameters of calcium kinetics were calculated from the measurements: (1) The fractional intestinal absorption from the isotope concentration ratio of the tracers in the plasma [7]. (2) The rate of disappearance of ^{47}Ca within the first 24 h after injection, interpreted as calcium plasma clearance. (3) The long-term whole-body retention of ^{47}Ca over 28 days for characterization of mineralization in the bone calcium pool. (4) The size of the different compartments involved in calcium homeostasis according to a modified four-compartment model (fig. 1).

Results

Clinical and Laboratory Data

The mean duration of dialysis treatment was 23.5 ± 17.4 months in the CAPD group (range: 6–60 months). The duration of treatment for the HD patients averaged 52.3 ± 29.2 months (range: 6–100 months) ($p < 0.05$).

Table 1 summarizes the laboratory data of the HD and CAPD group. Serum calcium and $1,25(OH)_2D_3$ did not differ in the two groups. iPTH was higher in the HD group, but this difference was not significant. Significant

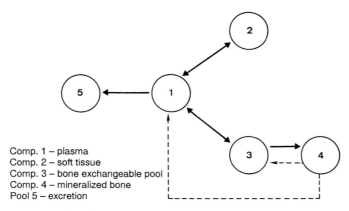

Comp. 1 – plasma
Comp. 2 – soft tissue
Comp. 3 – bone exchangeable pool
Comp. 4 – mineralized bone
Pool 5 – excretion

Fig. 1. Modified four-compartment model of blood-bone calcium kinetics. The total exchangeable calcium pool is formed by compartments 1–3.

Table 1. Biochemical data in CAPD and HD patients

	HD patients	CAPD patients
iPTH (1.2–6.0 pmol/l)	53.8 ± 52.9	32.8 ± 34.7
1,25(OH)$_2$D$_3$ (35–90 ng/l)	24.2 ± 9.9	25.2 ± 12.4
25(OH)D$_3$ (50–300 nmol/l)	133.8 ± 150.6*	45.8 ± 63.2
Calcium (2.1–2.6 mmol/l)	2.4 ± 0.2	2.3 ± 0.2
Phosphate (0.8–1.6 mmol/l)	2.0 ± 0.4**	1.7 ± 0.3
Alkaline phosphatase (<190 U/l)	237.2 ± 210.6*	96.8 ± 76.4

Values are reported as mean ± SD.
The numbers in parentheses denote the normal range.
*p < 0.05; **p < 0.01.

Table 2. Calcium kinetic data in both groups of dialysis patients

	HD patients	CAPD patients
Intestinal Ca absorption (72 ± 9%)	46.2 ± 12.5	44.4 ± 15.6
Ca retention (43.2 ± 5.8%)	40.0 ± 22.3	30.5 ± 11.6
Ca clearance (2.57 ± 0.15 ml/min)	3.1 ± 1.1	2.7 ± 0.5
Exchangeable Ca pool (2.8 – 7.7 g)	15.2 ± 17.3*	7.0 ± 1.5

Values are reported as mean ± SD.
The numbers in parentheses denote the normal range.
*$p < 0.05$.

differences were only found in the $25(OH)D_3$ levels, the serum concentration of the alkaline phosphatase, and in the serum phosphate levels ($p < 0.05$, $p < 0.05$ and $p < 0.01$, respectively).

Calcium Kinetic Data

The results of the calcium kinetic studies and the values of the total exchangeable calcium pool are shown in table 2. The correlations of the different parameters with iPTH are shown in figures 2–4.

Intestinal calcium absorption was lowered in both groups owing to the subnormal $1,25(OH)_2D_3$ concentration. Calcium absorption in the CAPD group was only slightly less than in the HD group (44.4 vs. 46.2%). None of the CAPD patients displayed calcium absorption in the normal range, although 4 had $1,25(OH)_2D_3$ levels in the lower range of normal. Two of the 23 HD patients showed a normal intestinal calcium absorption. One of these patients had a normal $1,25(OH)_2D_3$ level.

The calcium retention after 28 days was lower in the CAPD group than in the HD group (30.5 vs. 40.0%), but this difference was not statistically significant. Eleven of 23 HD patients had lowered retention values despite the presence of secondary hyperparathyroidism (mean iPTH: 20.8 pmol/l). Four patients had normal values for calcium retention. The mean iPTH value for this subgroup was 36.7 pmol/l. Eight patients showed retention values above the normal range. None of these patients had iPTH values less than 55 pmol/l. Three of 15 CAPD patients had a raised calcium retention. In 2 patients, it was in the normal range and the remaining 10 patients had subnormal retention values.

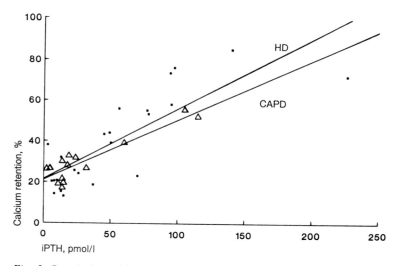

Fig. 2. Correlation of iPTH concentrations with the calcium retention for both groups of dialysis patients (r = 0.80 for HD and r = 0.65 for CAPD patients).

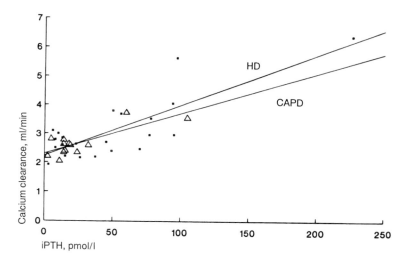

Fig. 3. Correlation of iPTH concentrations with the calcium clearance (r = 0.87 for HD and r = 0.77 for CAPD patients).

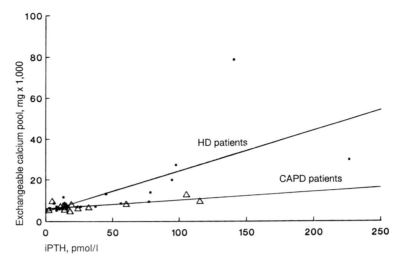

Fig. 4. Correlation of iPTH levels with the size of the exchangeable calcium pool (r = 0.86 for HD and r = 0.52 for CAPD patients).

A good correlation between the iPTH concentration and the retention values (r = 0.80 for HD and r = 0.65 for CAPD) was found in both groups (fig. 2). The lower values of overall retention in the CAPD group were hence a result of the lower iPTH levels. Good correlations between the serum alkaline phosphatase and the iPTH concentration and between the phosphatase and the calcium retention were only found in the HD group.

The clearance rate of calcium from the serum reflects the rapid mixing of serum calcium within the exchangeable calcium pool. The value of 3.1 in the HD group did not differ significantly from that in the CAPD group (mean: 2.7). The difference results from the different severity of secondary hyperparathyroidism in the two groups (table 1).

A good correlation between the iPTH and the clearance values (r = 0.87 for HD and r = 0.77 for CAPD patients) was also found here in the two groups (fig. 3). Five of the HD patients had a normal calcium clearance. The mean iPTH value for this subgroup was 31.6 pmol/l. On the other hand, almost half of the CAPD patients had a normal calcium clearance (7 of 15). The mean iPTH concentration in these patients was 19.4 pmol/l.

Besides the plasma, the actual soft tissue and the bone exchangeable pool are contained in the total exchangeable calcium pool (fig. 1). In the HD

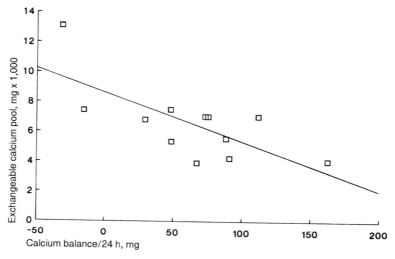

Fig. 5. Correlation of the total exchangeable calcium pool with the daily calcium balance achieved with a standard CAPD regime in 12 CAPD patients (r = –0.75).

group, the mean size of this pool was more than twice as large as the upper range of normal (mean: 15.2 g). On average, CAPD patients showed an exchangeable calcium pool which was in the upper range of normal (mean: 7.0 g). This difference was statistically significant (p < 0.05). The serum iPTH concentration correlated positively with the size of the exchangeable calcium pool in both groups (fig. 4). However, this correlation was very much closer in the HD group (r = 0.86) than in the CAPD group (r = 0.52). A positive correlation between the exchangeable calcium pool and the duration of dialysis treatment was found only in the HD group (r = 0.45).

Transperitoneal Calcium Balance in CAPD Patients
The daily calcium balance which was attained with a standard CAPD regime correlated negatively with the size of the exchangeable calcium pool (r = –0.75). Calcium balance was negative in 2 patients who had an exchangeable calcium pool well above the normal range (fig. 5). The calcium of the exchangeable pool is in contact with the dialysate side via the plasma. There is a calcium transport via the peritoneal membrane based on different passive processes.

Discussion

On the one hand, our findings show that the calcium kinetic parameters in HD and CAPD patients show marked but equidirectional alterations as compared to patients with normal or only slightly reduced renal function [8]. On the other hand, the differences observed between the various dialysis groups are small with regard to most parameters of calcium kinetics and are attributable to differences in the iPTH status and/or the duration of treatment. However, the significant difference in the size of the exchangeable calcium pool has to be emphasized.

The calcium retention after 28 days is a parameter for calcium turnover in the bone [9]. Since the osteoclastic release of the tracer plays a negligible role over this period, calcium retention correlates very well with the mineralization rate which depends on the one hand on the number of osteoblasts and on the other hand on their activity. The number of osteoblasts is controlled via PTH, and the activity of the individual cell is controlled via vitamin D [10]. As there was no difference in the $1,25(OH)_2D_3$ status of the two groups, the differences in calcium retention are therefore most probably the result of the different iPTH status between the two groups. In a study by Vincenti et al. [11], in uremic diabetics lower PTH levels have been found than in nondiabetics. In our study the number of diabetics was higher in the CAPD group (4/15) than in the HD group (1/23) but the difference in iPTH status remained even after consideration of the nondiabetics on their own.

Losses of PTH via the peritoneum have been repeatedly described with CAPD. These are reported to amount to 10–15% of the serum levels [12]. Delmez et al. [12] reported a peritoneal PTH clearance of 1.5 ml/min. There is still no unanimous view on the clinical significance of this finding. A further cause of the different severity of secondary hyperparathyroidism might be attributable to the greatly differing duration of treatment (52.3 vs. 23.5 months in HD and CAPD patients, respectively). However, a correlation of the serum iPTH levels with the duration of dialysis treatment was not found either in the HD or in the CAPD group.

From the ratio of the serum activity after tracer application to the 24-hour value, calcium clearance constitutes a parameter of the rapid mixing of the tracer within the exchangeable calcium pool. This parameter is PTH dependent. Both groups showed a good positive correlation of this value with the iPTH levels and the observed differences between CAPD and HD in this context are also to be regarded as a consequence of the different iPTH concentration. Similar to the correlation curve for calcium retention, a displacement of the correlation curve to the right to higher iPTH values was found for the calcium clearance. Irrespective of the dialysis procedure, higher PTH levels are necessary in the situation of end-stage renal failure in order to bring the two calcium kinetic parameters into the normal range compared to controls with normal kidney function. For iPTH levels between 25 and 40 pmol/l the calcium kinetic parameters were within the normal range. The correlation curves were almost identical for both groups and parameters, which underlines the independence of these parameters of the form of dialysis.

The significant difference in the size of the exchangeable calcium pool is especially striking in this investigation. This difference is even more remarkable since iPTH and $1,25(OH)_2D_3$ levels, as well as the kinetic parameters, do not differ significantly. In controls with normal kidney function the external regulation of the exchangeable calcium pool is possible via intestinal and renal mechanisms. An internal regulation of the exchangeable calcium pool is possible via the process of mineralization (calcium displacement from compartment 3 to 4) or via osteoclastic calcium release (calcium displacement from compartment 4 to 3) (fig. 1).

In contrast to healthy controls, hemodialysis patients succeed in regulating the exchangeable calcium pool only via the intestinal tract and internally via calcium shifts between the exchangeable bone compartment and mineralized bone. Owing to the PTH and vitamin D resistance [1] of the uremic bone, however, there are limits to the enhancement of mineralization, i.e. reducing the size of the exchangeable calcium pool via calcium shifts into mineralized bone. This assumption is further supported by the observation of Reeve [9] in osteoporotic patients treated with PTH where he found that the decrease of the transit time of calcium in the exchangeable pool is not to be explained solely on the basis of an increase of calcium accretion in bone.

Owing to the inadequate possibility of regulating the exchangeable calcium pool and owing also to the continuous calcium stress by each hemodialysis treatment with a dialysate calcium concentration of 1.75 mmol/l, an increase of the exchangeable pool is to be expected in HD patients. The significance of the form of dialysis for the increase of this calcium pool is supported by the dependence of the pool size on duration of treatment. The increase of the exchangeable calcium pool with time on dialysis treatment was only observed in HD patients.

CAPD patients had a significantly smaller exchangeable calcium pool. In contrast to HD patients, a weak but negative correlation with the duration of treatment was found. Via the transperitoneal calcium flux, CAPD patients have the possibility of adapting the calcium balance to the current status of the exchangeable calcium pool. With the increase of this pool, the daily calcium balance became negative under a standard CAPD regime. This might explain why, for a given iPTH level, CAPD patients displayed a lower size of the exchangeable calcium pool than HD patients (fig. 4). This observation is of clinical interest to the extent that the soft tissue compartment is a component of the exchangeable calcium pool and extraosseous calcifications are a frequent complication of chronic dialysis treatment. The peritoneal calcium flux might prevent a rapid increase of the exchangeable calcium pool under CAPD treatment.

In order to be able to define the effect of the dialysis procedure on calcium kinetics, a prospective investigation is required to establish whether this difference from HD patients is manifested in a reduced rate of soft tissue calcifications under CAPD treatment.

References

1   Massry SG, Stein R, Garty J, et al: Skeletal resistance to the calcemic action of parathyroid hormone in uremia: Role of 1,25(OH)2D3. Kidney Int 1976;9:467–474.
2   Gokal R, Ramos JM, Ellis HA, et al: Histological renal osteodystrophy, and 25-hydroxycholecalciferol and aluminum levels in patients on continuous ambulatory peritoneal dialysis. Kidney Int 1983;23:15–21.
3   Cassidy MJD, Owen JP, Ellis HA, et al: Renal osteodystrophy and metastatic calcification in long-term continuous ambulatory peritoneal dialysis. Q J Med 1985; 213:29–48.
4   Neer R, Berman M, Fisher L, et al: Multicompartmental analysis of calcium kinetics in normal adult males. J Clin Invest 1967;46:1364–1379.
5   Blind E, Schmidt-Gayk H, Scharla S, et al: Two-site assay of intact parathyroid hormone in the investigation of primary hyperparathyroidism and other disorders of calcium metabolism compared with a midregion assay. J Clin Endocrinol Metab 1988;67:353–360.
6   Scharla S, Schmidt-Gayk H, Reichel H, et al: A sensitive and simplified radioimmunoassay for 1,25-dihydroxyvitamin D3. Clin Chim Acta 1984;142:325–338.
7   Roth P, Werner E: Interrelations of radiocalcium absorption tests and their clinical relevance. Mineral Electrolyte Metab 1985;11:351–357.
8   Malluche HH, Werner E, Ritz E: Intestinal absorption of calcium and whole-body calcium retention in incipient and advanced renal failure. Mineral Electrolyte Metab 1978;1:263–270.
9   Reeve J: The turnover time of calcium in the exchangeable pools of bone in man and the long-term effect of a parathyroid hormone fragment. Clin Endocrinol 1978;8:445–455.

10   Malluche HH, Matthews C, Faugere MC, et al: 1,25-dihydroxy-vitamin D maintains bone cell activity, and parathyroid hormone modulates bone cell number in dogs. Endocrinology 1986;119:1298–1304.
11   Vincenti F, Arnaud SA, Recker R, et al: Parathyroid and bone response of the diabetic patient to uremia. Kidney Int 1984;25:677–682.
12   Delmez JA, Slatopolsky E, Martin KJ, et al: Minerals, vitamin D, and parathyroid hormone in continuous ambulatory peritoneal dialysis. Kidney Int 1982;21:862–867.

Dr. P. Kurz, St. Markus-Krankenhaus, II. Medizinische Klinik,
Wilhelm-Epstein-Strasse 2, D–W–6000 Frankfurt/Main 50 (FRG)

Clinical Experiences in Peritoneal Dialysis

La Greca G, Olivares J, Feriani M, Passlick-Deetjen J (eds): CAPD – A Decade of Experience. Contrib Nephrol. Basel, Karger, 1991, vol 89, pp 186–189

Subcutaneous Recombinant Human Erythropoietin Treatment of Children Undergoing Peritoneal Dialysis

Richard N. Fine[1]

UCLA Center for the Health Sciences, Los Angeles, Calif., USA

Anemia is a frequent clinical manifestation in children with chronic renal insufficiency. It is usually noted when the glomerular filtration rate (GFR) falls below 20 ml/min/1.73 m^2 [1]. In the past, the etiology of the anemia of uremia was thought to be multifactorial [2]; however, the recent studies demonstrating the beneficial effect of recombinant human erythropoietin (r-HuEpo) on the hemoglobin level in adult patients undergoing hemodialysis has emphasized the primacy of erythropoietin deficiency as the cause of the anemia associated with renal failure [3].

Since limited data were available both detailing the use of r-HuEpo in pediatric patients as well as the use of subcutaneous (s.c.) r-HuEpo in patients undergoing peritoneal dialysis, we initiated a study in September 1987 to treat children over the age of 12 years who were undergoing continuous cycling peritoneal dialysis (CCPD), with s.c. r-HuEpo [4].

Patient Data

Five patients aged 12–18 years with end-stage renal disease (ESRD) who were undergoing some form of dialysis for periods of 16–65 months prior to initiation of the study and were undergoing CCPD at the time of the study were included. With one exception each patient had had one or more renal transplants prior to initiation of the study and 2 of the 5 patients were anephric. All 5 patients were transfusion-dependent as indicated by the fact that they required 5–18 units of blood in the 6 months prior to initiation of the study.

[1] This manuscript was completed during the time that Dr. Fine was recipient of the United States Senior Research Scientist Award of The Alexander von Humboldt Foundation.

Treatment Protocol

Each patient initially received 150 U/kg of s.c. r-HuEpo (Amgen, Thousand Oaks, Calif.) thrice weekly, which was self-administered at home. When the hematocrit (Hct) level reached 35%, the dosage of r-HuEpo was decreased by 25 U/kg/dose each week. When the Hct reached 40%, the r-HuEpo was discontinued until the Hct level decreased to <40% and then the r-HuEpo was reinstituted at a dose of 150 U/kg/dose once a week to maintain the Hct level at approximately 35%.

Results

All 5 patients responded to r-HuEpo treatment with a sustained increase in their Hct level and were thus able to avoid any subsequent transfusion during the 6-month follow-up period.

The reticulocyte count increased from a mean of 1.6 to 13.0% within a mean of 15 days from the initiation of treatment. The Hct level increased from a mean of 22% to a mean of 33% within 3 weeks of r-HuEpo treatment. All 5 patients exceeded an Hct level of 40% and r-HuEpo had to be discontinued for a period of 14–36 days until the Hct level dropped to <40%. Four of the 5 patients were able to maintain a Hct level in the range of 33–38% for a period of at least 6 months with a once-a-week dosage of 150 U/kg/dose. The remaining patient was found to be iron deficient as indicated by a reduction in the % iron saturation to 16% and required supplemental oral iron therapy. During the period that the patient required supplemental iron therapy thrice weekly r-HuEpo was administered to maintain the Hct level at >30%.

A typical clinical course following r-HuEpo treatment is shown in figure 1.

The only side effect of r-HuEpo noted was the exacerbation of hypertension in 3 previously hypertensive patients. A modest increase in the dosage of antihypertensive medications was therapeutic in each instance.

Pharmacokinetic studies performed prior to the initial dose of r-HuEpo and after 3 weeks of treatment revealed a mean serum half-life of 14.5 h [unpubl. data].

Discussion

The results of this study confirm that r-HuEpo is effective in reversing the anemia of transfusion-dependent patients undergoing dialysis. Utilizing

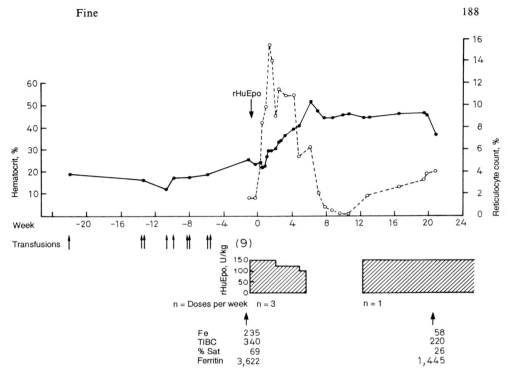

Fig. 1. Typical clinical course following s.c. r-HuEpo treatment. ○ = Reticulocyte count; ● = hematocrit.

the subcutaneous route of administration in patients undergoing CCPD it was noted that the rapidity of the response was greater than that achieved with the same dosage administered intravenously to adult patients undergoing hemodialysis [3].

The fact that the target Hct level could be maintained in 4 of the 5 patients with a once-a-week dosage schedule will certainly be cost effective and was appreciated by the pediatric population studied. This phenomenon in addition to the fact that subcutaneously administered r-HuEpo has a bioavailability seven times greater than that of intraperitoneally administered r-HuEpo [5] indicates that the latter route of administration will be utilized rarely to treat patients, even pediatric patients, undergoing peritoneal dialysis.

The pharmacokinetic studies did not elucidate the mechanism for the prolonged biological effectiveness of subcutaneously administered r-HuEpo in patients undergoing CCPD. A r-HuEpo half-life at the initiation of treatment and after 3 weeks of therapy of 14.5 h does not explain the prolonged biological effect that would permit a once-a-week dosage schedule.

Despite the fact that the rise in the Hct level following initiation of r-HuEpo treatment was rather rapid and the fact that pediatric patients with ESRD have a high incidence of seizure disorders, no patient had a seizure following initiation of r-HuEpo treatment. The only complication was the mild exacerbation of hypertension in 3 of the 5 patients which was easily controlled by a modest adjustment of the dosage of their antihypertensive medications.

The quality of life improved dramatically in each patient following correction of the anemia. Nonspecific clinical manifestations attributable to uremia abated following stabilization of the Hct level to within normal values for patient age. In at least 1 patient the desire for a subsequent renal transplant was minimized because of her general feeling of well-being.

It can be concluded from the results of this study that s.c. r-HuEpo treatment of pediatric patients with ESRD who are undergoing peritoneal dialysis is effective in correcting the anemia, thereby avoiding further transfusions. The effectiveness of a once a week maintenance dosage schedule in maintaining the target Hct level indicates that the subcutaneous route of administration is probably optimal for such patients.

References

1   Chandra, M.; Clemons, G.K.; McVivar, M.I.: Relation of serum erythropoietin levels to renal excretory function: Evidence for lowered set point for erythropoietin production in chronic renal failure. J. Pediat. *113:* 1015–1021 (1988).
2   Eschbach, J.W.; Adamson, J.W.: Anemia in end-stage renal disease. Kidney int. *28:* 1–5 (1985).
3   Eschbach, J.W.; Egrie, J.C.; Downing, M.R.; et al.: Correction of the anemia of end-stage renal disease with recombinant human erythropoietin. New Engl. J. Med. *310:* 73–78 (1987).
4   Sinai-Trieman, L.; Salusky, I.B.; Fine, R.N.: Use of subcutaneous human erythropoietin in children undergoing continuous cycling peritoneal dialysis. J. Pediat. *114:* 550–554 (1989).
5   Macdougall, I.C.; Roberts, D.E.; Nuebert, P.; et al.: Pharmacokinetics of recombinant human erythropoietin in patients on continuous ambulatory peritoneal dialysis. Lancet *i:* 425–427 (1989).

Richard N. Fine, MD, Department of Pediatrics,
State University of New York (Suny) at Stony Brook,
Stony Brook, NY 11794-8111 (USA)

La Greca G, Olivares J, Feriani M, Passlick-Deetjen J (eds): CAPD – A Decade of Experience. Contrib Nephrol. Basel, Karger, 1991, vol 89, pp 190–198

Low Calcium Dialysate Increases the Tolerance to Vitamin D in Peritoneal Dialysis[1]

N.A.T. Hamdy[a, b], *J. Boletis*[a], *D. Charlesworth*[b], *J.A. Kanis*[b], *C.B. Brown*[a]

Departments of [a]Nephrology and Transplantation and [b]Human Metabolism and Clinical Biochemistry, University of Sheffield Medical School, Sheffield, UK

Renal osteodystrophy describes the constellation of disorders of mineral and skeletal metabolism associated with chronic renal failure. It is widely prevalent in patients with renal failure by the time they require dialysis [1, 2], and is an increasing cause of significant morbidity with increasing years on dialysis replacement therapy. Whereas the natural history of renal osteodystrophy is well documented in patients on maintenance haemodialysis, opinions are still divided as to the outcome of bone disease in patients on continuous ambulatory peritoneal dialysis (CAPD). Thus, authors variously report improvement, no change or worsening of osteitis fibrosa and/or osteomalacia [3–7].

Several factors may play a role in any difference in the natural history of bone disease between the two types of dialysis treatments. The continuous nature of CAPD compared to the intermittent one of haemodialysis results in less fluctuations in calcium and phosphate balance in CAPD, and significant amounts of parathyroid hormone (PTH) are removed by CAPD [8]. In CAPD, there is also an obligatory daily loss of protein into the dialysate of 5–12 g [9] which increases the losses of $25(OH)D_3$ and other metabolites of vitamin D by the removal of vitamin D binding protein [9–13]. The lower serum concentrations of $1,25(OH)_2D_3$, $24,25(OH)_2D_3$ and $25(OH)D_3$ result in a greater reduction in intestinal absorption of calcium than seen in haemodialysis patients [7, 10]. This may be compensated in part by an increase in peritoneal mass transfer of calcium when dialysate calcium concentrations of 1.75 mmol/l are used [14–17]. Calcium gain from the

[1] We wish to thank Fresenius Ltd. and the Medical Research Council for their support with this work.

dialysate fluid may thus represent a major source of calcium in patients on CAPD.

Manipulation of extracellular calcium and phosphate concentrations represents the mainstay of treatment in renal osteodystrophy and for this reason, vitamin D and its metabolites have an established role in the medical management of hyperparathyroid bone disease. Thus, a conspicuous effect of the administration of alfacalcidol, calcitriol or dihydrotachysterol is to raise serum calcium concentrations and thereby lower PTH secretion [18–21]. Recently, it has become apparent that $1,25(OH)_2D_3$ may also suppress the secretion of parathyroid hormone by direct genomic actions independently of changes in extracellular calcium concentrations [22–25]. In addition, vitamin D may have direct actions on bone cell function although the evidence for this is still largely indirect and circumstantial [26].

The question arises, whether for any given concentration of serum calcium, patients would benefit by also having high concentrations of vitamin D. However, in patients on CAPD, the use of high concentrations of vitamin D is often precluded by the development of hypercalcaemia when standard dialysate solutions containing 1.75 mmol/l of calcium are used, due to the underlying positive mass transfer of calcium from the dialysate [27]. It is possible, therefore, that the use of low dialysate calcium concentrations with vitamin D might not only permit a higher tolerance to vitamin D, but also be of benefit for the control of PTH secretion and hyperparathyroid bone disease.

In this study, we have compared the effects of two different dialysate calcium concentrations in patients established on CAPD in whom serum calcium was maintained at similar values with the use of maximum tolerable doses of alfacalcidol, the synthetic analogue of $1,25(OH)_2D_3$. In this way, we hoped to assess the differential effects, direct or otherwise, of $1,25(OH)_2D_3$ on the natural history of bone disease in patients on CAPD, independent of the maintenance of calcium homeostasis.

Patients and Methods

We studied 32 randomly selected patients aged 22–68 years, established on CAPD for 3–70 months, using $4 \times 1.5\%$ dextrose exchanges/day with an occasional additional hypertonic exchange (4.25%), and standard dialysate solutions containing 1.75 mmol/l of calcium. No episodes of peritonitis were recorded for at least 1 month before the study to eliminate the effect of abnormal peritoneal permeability, and no patients had taken vitamin D metabolites or calcium supplements for at least 3 months before the study.

Patients were randomly allocated to standard (1.75 mmol/l; n = 16) or low (1.00 mmol/l; n = 16) dialysate calcium.

In both groups, maximum tolerable doses of alfacalcidol were used to maintain serum calcium at the upper limit of the normal laboratory reference range (2.12–2.63 mmol/l).

Aluminium-containing phosphate binders (up to a maximum of 1.5 g/day) were used to control serum phosphate and serum aluminium was closely monitored to detect any risk of toxicity.

Biochemistry

Serum measurements were made at the start of the study and at regular intervals thereafter. Serum calcium (adjusted for an albumin of 42 g/l), phosphate, alkaline phosphatase activity and liver transaminases were estimated using a standard Technicon SMAC, and serum aluminium was measured by electrothermal atomic absorption spectrophotometry [28].

Parathyroid hormone was measured using an antiserum recognising the mid-region (44–68) of the human parathyroid molecule [29]. The inter-assay variation (coefficient of variation) was 10% and the intra-assay variation 7.5%. The upper limit of the normal reference range is 135 pmol/l and the upper limit of detection of the assay is 1,000 pmol/l. Dilutions of serum were made before analysis where appropriate.

Mass Transfer Studies

Net calcium fluxes to and from the dialysate were examined by using simple mass transfer studies whereby dialysate samples were taken before and after the completion of an exchange and measured for calcium content (Ca_1 and Ca_2). Dialysate volumes were assessed by accurately weighing the dialysis bags before and after an exchange (V_1 and V_2). Calcium mass transfer (MT) was calculated using the following formula:

$$MT = (Ca_1 \times V_1) - (Ca_2 \times V_2).$$

To standardise the procedure, mass transfer studies were performed in all patients on the first (1.5% dextrose) exchange of the day and following the use of an overnight empty bag.

Mass transfer studies were conducted at the start of the study and after 6 months of treatment.

Assessment of Bone Mass

Bone mineral density was assessed by dual photon absorptiometry of the lumbar spine (L2-L4) using a Gadolinium-153 source (Nuclear Data 2100 scanner). The technique provides accurate and reproducible measurements of bone mineral density, with a coefficient of variation of 1.2% at this site in our laboratory.

Measurements were made at the start of the study and at 6 months.

Histological Assessment

Trans-iliac bone biopsies were obtained from all patients under local anaesthesia using a Meunier manual trephine (8 mm) at the start of the study, and will be repeated at its completion after a year of treatment. Secondary hyperparathyroidism (osteitis fibrosa: OF) was diagnosed by an increase in the erosion surfaces, number of osteoclasts and active osteoid surfaces associated with variable fibrosis in marrow cavities. Histological data are not included in this inital report.

Table 1. Demographic details, serum biochemistry, peritoneal mass transfer of calcium and bone mineral density measurements at the start of the study, showing no significant difference between patients allocated to standard (1.75 mmol/l) or low (1.00 mmol/l) dialysate calcium

	1.75 mmol/l (n = 16)	1.00 mmol/l (n = 16)
Demographic details		
Age, years	55 ± 2	55 ± 3
Male/female ratio	11 : 5	13 : 3
Months on CAPD	25 ± 7	23 ± 5
Biochemistry		
Serum calcium, mmol/l	2.46 ± 0.03	2.46 ± 0.03
Serum phosphate, mmol/l	2.21 ± 0.15	2.09 ± 0.15
Serum alkaline phosphatase, IU/l	89 ± 5	107 ± 9
Serum iPTH, pmol/l	1,214 ± 249	1,802 ± 506
Mass transfer		
Calcium, mmol/exchange	0.58 ± 0.05	0.42 ± 0.06
Bone mass		
BMD, g/cm^2	1.16 ± 0.07	1.07 ± 0.06

Results

The study duration is 1 year, and is still in progress. We report here the results of the initial 6 months of treatment including early effects on serum biochemistry, mass transfer of calcium and bone mass measurements.

There was no significant difference in age, sex or time on dialysis between the two groups. The two groups were also well matched for starting serum values, calcium mass transfer and bone mineral density measurements (table 1). All patients had normal liver transaminases and changes in alkaline phosphatase activity were considered to be bone derived.

At 6 months, patients on low dialysate calcium tolerated significantly higher doses of alfacalcidol than patients on standard dialysate calcium (0.88 vs. 0.36 µg/day; $p < 0.02$), with no significant difference in serum calcium between the two groups at this time (2.64 ± 0.03 vs. 2.62 ± 0.03 mmol/l) (fig. 1).

The increased tolerance to alfacalcidol in patients on the low dialysate regime was due to the significant peritoneal efflux of calcium observed in this group compared to patients on standard dialysate (−0.67 ± 0.09 vs. +0.3 ± 0.05 mmol; $p < 0.0001$).

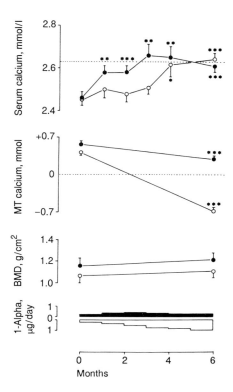

Fig. 1. Sequential changes in serum calcium and mean doses of alfacalcidol (μg/day) showing that patients on low dialysate calcium (○) tolerated significantly higher doses of the metabolite than patients on standard dialysate calcium (●) whilst maintaining comparable serum calcium concentrations. The negative mass transfer of calcium resulting from the use of low dialysate calcium was not associated with any loss in bone mass. *** p < 0.001, ** p < 0.01, * p < 0.01.

There were no changes in bone mineral density of the lumbar spine in either group after 6 months of treatment, suggesting that despite their significant losses of calcium to the dialysate fluid, patients on the low calcium dialysate maintained calcium balance by increasing their intestinal absorption of calcium.

As expected, there was an increase in serum phosphate in both groups, albeit not significant, due to the enhanced intestinal absorption of phosphate with the use of vitamin D metabolites. However, a similar rise in serum phosphate was demonstrated in both groups despite the significantly larger

Table 2. Mean changes (± SEM) in serum (mmol/l) and mass transfer values (mmol/exchange) for calcium and phosphate in 32 patients before and after 6 months of using either standard (1.75 mmol/l: n = 16) or low (1.00 mmol/l: n = 16) dialysate concentrations of calcium and maximum tolerable doses of alfacalcidol

	1.75 mmol/l		1.00 mmol/l	
	before	6 months	before	6 months
Serum calcium	2.46 ± 0.03	2.62 ± 0.03***	2.46 ± 0.03	2.64 ± 0.03***
MT calcium	+0.58 ± 0.05	+0.32 ± 0.05**	+0.42 ± 0.06	−0.67 ± 0.09***
Serum phosphate	2.21 ± 0.15	2.34 ± 0.13	2.03 ± 0.14	2.32 ± 0.12
MT phosphate	−3.18 ± 0.21	−3.27 ± 0.24	−2.64 ± 0.24	−3.07 ± 0.24
Dose alfacalcidol	0	0.39 ± 0.07	0	0.90 ± 0.18
Dose Alu-cap	0.82 ± 0.19	0.89 ± 0.19	0.37 ± 0.15	0.82 ± 0.18
Serum aluminium	28 ± 10	35 ± 13	13 ± 3	22 ± 5

Mean doses of alfacalcidol (µg/day) and the aluminium-containing phosphate binder, Alu-Cap (g/day), are also shown for the two time points as well as the mean changes in serum aluminium (µg/l). *** $p < 0.0005$, ** $p < 0.005$, * $p < 0.01$.

doses of alfacalcidol tolerated by patients on the low dialysate calcium. This was due to the more marked loss of phosphate to the dialysate fluid in patients on the low dialysate calcium (table 2). Thus, neither group required a significant increase in the dose of aluminium-containing phosphate binders and there was also no significant rise in serum aluminium (table 2).

The effect of the two different dialysate regimes on parameters of bone disease were not as clear-cut. Whereas patients on the standard calcium dialysate regimen showed a decrease in alkaline phosphatase activity and parathyroid hormone concentrations at the 6-month time point, this was less marked in patients on the low dialysate calcium despite the greater doses of alfacalcidol tolerated by this group.

Discussion

Our findings so far suggest that the use of low dialysate calcium provides a mechanism for tolerating high doses of vitamin D metabolites in patients on CAPD, without the risk of inducing sustained hypercalcaemia. Hypercalcaemic episodes occurred commonly but with equal frequency in both groups since the aim of the study was to give the maximum dose of alfacalcidol that could be tolerated. Due to the short half-life of the metabolite, these episodes readily responded to a decrease in dosage.

Our results also suggest that in the low dialysate group, the net calcium loss in the dialysate was not associated with any bone loss over the period of observation. Thus, calcium balance was probably maintained by the increase in intestinal absorption of calcium resulting from the higher doses of alfacalcidol used.

One potential concern with the use of larger doses of alfacalcidol is the associated increase in phosphate absorption and the resulting hyperphosphataemia. Whereas hyperphosphataemia could aggravate hyperparathyroid bone disease, the use of aluminium-containing binders to control it may also have adverse effects on bone. Neither of these concerns seemed to be substantiated in the patients studied, at least for the duration of observation, suggesting that any tendency to increase serum levels of phosphate or aluminium was counteracted by increased peritoneal losses of either to the dialysate fluid.

The lack of effect of the higher doses of alfacalcidol on bone turnover as measured by alkaline phosphatase activity or parathyroid hormone concentrations over the period of the study may be time-related. Thus, significant changes in serum calcium and indeed in doses of alfacalcidol only occurred after 4 months from the start of the study and a favourable effect of the combined regime is likely to be delayed.

Whereas there is little doubt that low calcium dialysate solutions provide a mechanism to increase the doses of vitamin D metabolites tolerated, it is too early at this stage to assess the long-term effects of this combined regime on the progression of hyperparathyroid bone disease. Notwithstanding, vitamin D deficiency has been shown to play a major role in the development of hyperparathyroidism in renal failure, indirectly by its effects on extracellular calcium and phosphate concentrations, as well as directly by its effects on parathyroid cell function. It seems logical, therefore, to suppose that correction of this deficiency might alter favourably the progression of bone disease in CAPD patients. Our initial results indicate that vitamin D deficiency may be more adequately corrected with the use of low dialysate calcium solutions, but whether this would beneficially affect hyperparathyroid bone disease must await histological assessment and a longer-term experience.

References

1   Malluche, H.H.; Ritz, E.; Kutschera, J.; Hodgson, M.; Seiffert, U.; Shoeppe, W.: Bone histology in incipient and advanced renal failure. Kidney int. *9:* 355–362 (1976).

2 Cundy, T.; Hand, D.J.; Oliver, D.O.; Woods, C.G.; Wright, F.W.; Kanis, J.A.: Who gets renal bone disease before beginning dialysis? Br. med. J. *290:* 271–275 (1985).

3 Buccianti, G.; Bianchi, M.L.; Valenti, G.: Progress of renal osteodystrophy during continuous ambulatory peritoneal dialysis. Clin. Nephrol. *22:* 279–283 (1984).

4 Zuchelli, P.; Catizone, L.; Casanova, S.; Fusaroli, M.; Fabbri, L.; Ferrari, G.: Renal osteodystrophy in CAPD patients. Mineral Electrolyte Metab. *10:* 326–332 (1984).

5 Cassidy, M.J.D.; Owen, J.P.; Ellis, H.A.; Dewar, J.; Robinson, C.J.; Wilkinson, R.; Ward, M.K.; Kerr, D.N.S.: Renal osteodystrophy and metastatic calcification in long-term continuous ambulatory peritoneal dialysis. Q. Jl. Med. *54:* 29–48 (1985).

6 Delmez, J.A.; Fallon, M.D.; Bergfeld, M.A.; Gearing, B.K.; Dougan, C.S.; Teitelbaum, S.L.: Continuous ambulatory peritoneal dialysis and bone. Kidney int. *30:* 379–384 (1986).

7 Shusterman, N.H.; Wasserstein, A.G.; Morrison, G.; Audet, P.; Fallon, M.D.; Kaplan, F.: Controlled study of renal osteodystrophy in patients undergoing dialysis: Improved response to continuous ambulatory peritoneal dialysis compared with haemodialysis. Am. J. Med. *82:* 1148–1156 (1987).

8 Delmez, J.; Martin, K.; Harter, H.; et al.: The effects of continuous peritoneal dialysis (CAPD) on parathyroid hormone (PTH) and mineral metabolism. Kidney int. *19:* 114 (1985).

9 Katirtzoglou, A.; Oreopoulos, D.G.; Husdan, H.; et al.: Reappraisal of protein losses in patients undergoing CAPD. Nephron *26:* 230–233 (1980).

10 Gokal, R.; Ramos, J.M.; Ellis, H.A.; Parkinson, I.; Sweetman, V.; Dewar, J.; Ward, M.K.; Kerr, D.N.S.: Histological renal osteodystrophy and 25-hydroxy-cholecalciferol and aluminium levels in patients on continuous ambulatory peritoneal dialysis. Kidney int. *23:* 15–21 (1983).

11 Aloni, Y.; Shany, S.; Chaimovitz, C.: Losses of 25-hydroxyvitamin D in peritoneal fluid: possible mechanism for bone disease in uraemic patients treated with chronic ambulatory peritoneal dialysis. Mineral Electrolyte Metab. *9:* 82–86 (1983).

12 Digenis, G.; Khanna, R.; Pierratos, A.; Meema, H.E.; Robinovitch, S.; Petit, J.; Oreopoulos, D.: Renal osteodystrophy in patients maintained on CAPD for more than three years. Periton. Dial. Bull. *3:* 81–86 (1983).

13 Tielemans, C.; Aubry, C.; Dratwa, M.: The effects of continuous ambulatory peritoneal dialysis (CAPD) on renal osteodystrophy; in Gahl, Kessel, Nolph, Advances in peritoneal dialysis, pp. 455–460 (Excerpta Medica, Amsterdam 1981).

14 Shany, S.; Rapoport, J.; Goligorsky, M.; Yankowitz, N.; Zuili, I.; Chaimovitz, C.: Losses of 1,25- and 24-25-dihydroxycholecalciferol in the peritoneal fluid of patients treated with continuous ambulatory peritoneal dialysis. Nephron *36:* 111–113 (1984).

15 Moncrief, J.W.; Popovitch, R.P.; Nolph, K.D.: Additional experience with continuous ambulatory peritoneal dialysis (CAPD). Trans. Am. Soc. artif. internal Organs *24:* 476–483 (1978).

16 Parker, A.; Nolph, K.D.: Magnesium and calcium mass transfer during continuous ambulatory peritoneal dialysis. Trans. Am. Soc. artif. internal Organs *26:* 194–196 (1980).

17 Delmez, J.A.; Slatopolsky, E.; Martin, K.J.; Gearing, B.N.; Harter, H.R.: Minerals, vitamin D and parathyroid hormone in continuous ambulatory peritoneal dialysis. Kidney int. *21:* 862–867 (1982).

18 Kurtz, H.B.; McCarthy, J.T.; Kumar, R.: Hypercalcaemia in continuous peritoneal dialysis (CAPD) patients: Observations on parameters of calcium metabolism; in

Gahl, Kessel, Nolph, Advances in peritoneal dialysis, pp. 467–472 (Excerpta Medica, Amsterdam 1981).

19   Kaye, M.; Chatterji, G.; Cohen, E.F.; Sagar, S.: Arrest of hyperparathyroid bone disease with dihydrotachysterol in patients undergoing chronic haemodialysis. Ann. intern. Med. *73:* 225–233 (1970).

20   Peacock, M. (ed): The clinical uses of 1α-hydroxyvitamin D_3. Clin. Endocrinol. *7:* 1–246 (1977).

21   Coburn, J.W.; Massry, S.G. (eds): Uses and actions of 1,25-dihydroxyvitamin D_3 in uremia. Contr. Nephrol. vol. 18; pp. 1–217 (Karger, Basel 1980).

22   Chertow, B.S.; Baylink, D.J.; Wergedal, J.E.; Su, M.H.H.; Norman, A.W.: Decrease in serum immunoreactive parathyroid hormone in rats and in parathyroid hormone secretion in vitro by 1,25-dihydroxycholecalciferol. J. clin. Invest. *56:* 668–678 (1975).

23   Madsen, S.; Olgaard, K.; Ladefoged, J.: Suppressive effect of 1,25-dihydroxyvitamin D_3 on circulating parathyroid hormone in acute renal failure. J. clin. Endocr. Metab. *53:* 823–827 (1981).

24   Cantley, L.K.; Russell, J.; Lettieri, D.; et al.: 1,25-dihydroxyvitamin D_3 suppresses parathyroid hormone secretion from parathyroid cells in tissue culture. Endocrinology *117:* 2114–2119 (1985).

25   Rusell, J.; Lettieri, D.; Sherwood, L.M.: Suppression by 1,25$(OH)_2D_3$ of transcription of the pre-pro parathyroid hormone gene. Endocrinology *119:* 2864–2866 (1986).

26   Teitelbaum, S.L.; Bergfeld, M.A.; Freitag, J.; Hruska, K.; Slatopolsky, E.: Do parathyroid hormone and 1,25-dihydroxyvitamin D modulate bone formation in uraemia. J. clin. Endocr. Metab. *51:* 247–251 (1980).

27   Hamdy, N.A.T.; Brown, C.B.; Boletis, J.; Boyle, G.; Tindale, W.; Beneton, M.N.C.; Charlesworth, D.; Kanis, J.A.: Mineral metabolism in chronic ambulatory peritoneal dialysis (CAPD); in Coles GA, Davies M, Williams JD (eds.): CAPD: Host Defence, Nutrition and Ultrafiltration. Contr. Nephrol. vol. 85, pp. 100–110 (Karger, Basel, 1990).

28   Gardner, P.; Ottoway, J.; Fell, G.S.; Halls, D.: Determination of aluminium in blood, plasma or serum by electrothermal atomic absorption spectrophotometry. Analyt. chim. Acta *128:* 57–66 (1981).

29   Mallette, L.E.; Tuma, S.N.; Berger, R.E.; Kirkland, J.L.: Radioimmunoassay for the middle region of human parathyroid hormone using an homologous antiserum with a carboxy-terminal fragment of bovine parathyroid hormone as radioligand. J. clin. Endocr. Metab. *54:* 1017–1024 (1982).

Dr. N.A.T. Hamdy, Department of Endocrinology and
Metabolic Diseases, University Hospital Leiden, Rijnsburgerweg 10,
NL-2333 AA Leiden (The Netherlands)

La Greca G, Olivares J, Feriani M, Passlick-Deetjen J (eds): CAPD – A Decade of Experience. Contrib Nephrol. Basel, Karger, 1991, vol 89, pp 199–204

Peritoneal Resting and Heparinization as an Effective Treatment for Ultrafiltration Failure in Patients on CAPD

B. Miranda, R. Selgas, O. Celadilla, J. Muñoz, L. Sánchez Sicilia

Hospital La Paz, Madrid, Spain

CAPD is an effective technique for the management of patients in ESRD. The earlier problems of peritonitis and catheter function have decreased but other long-term problems such as loss of ultrafiltration (UF) and viability of peritoneal membrane are becoming more important [1].

The peritoneal ultrafiltration capacity is the consequence of maintaining an appropriate osmotic gradient for glucose which depends on the preservation of the peritoneal membrane structure [2]. In some cases diaphragmatic lymphatic absorption modulates the final result of measuring net UF [3].

When peritoneal permeability is increased there is a rapid transfer of glucose to the bloodstream resulting in a low UF rate [2]. The anatomical basis of this UF defect is a demesothelization of which the origin could be a deficitary regeneration of mesothelial cells after chronic or acute injuries [4, 5]. Peritoneal regeneration lasts 2–4 weeks, probably according to the degree of injury and its origin [6].

The possibility that this demesothelization favors fibroblasts activation and thereby sclerosing peritonitis, the major influence of this problem on peritoneal dialysis viability and the absence of effective treatment methods, prompted us to evaluate the effect of peritoneal resting to allow cell regeneration together with the antifibrin formation effect of locally instilled heparin.

Material and Methods

Patients

Seven patients out of our 67 current CAPD patients showed progressive loss of UF capacity from October 1987 to November 1988. Their clinical characteristics are dis-

Table 1. Clinical characteristics of patients

Patient	Sex	Age	Months on CAPD at UF failure	Peritoneal antecedents	Renal disease
1	M	55	93	5 peritonitis episodes	unknown
2	F	30	90	4 peritonitis episodes, massive hemoperitoneum, laparotomy	cortical necrosis
3	F	35	63	3 peritonitis episodes	renal tuberculosis
4	M	34	29	3 peritonitis episodes	diabetes type I
5	M	35	45	1 peritonitis episode	diabetes type I
6	F	63	76	4 peritonitis episodes	nephrosclerosis
7	M	73	72	3 peritonitis episodes	renal tuberculosis

played in table 1. They were included in the trial after excluding other causes of poor peritoneal UF such as catheter malfunction, hyperglycemia and peritonitis. According to the data on solute peritoneal equilibration and peritoneal mass transfer coefficient (MTC) determination for small molecules, every patient could be diagnosed as having peritoneal hyperpermeability or membrane failure type I [4].

CAPD Method
For bag exchanges patients used CAPD manual or ultraviolet chamber systems without any disinfectants.

Procedure
CAPD was discontinued and hemodialysis started via central catheter cannulation. Substitute therapy was maintained for 4 weeks and during that period peritoneal care consisted of the infusion of 100 ml of 1.5% dextrose dialysate containing 35 mg (3,500 IU) of heparin, every 3–4 days by the patient himself. After that month, CAPD was resumed as usual.

Peritoneal Functional Parameters
Before and after the peritoneal resting period, urea and creatinine MTCs were determined through a well-known mathematical model described previously [7].

Ultrafiltration capacity was also evaluated before and after the procedure and quantified as net ultrafiltration using a similar CAPD schedule: one 4.25% dextrose exchange with a peritoneal dwell time of 6 h and three 1.5% exchanges with peritoneal dwell times between 4 and 8 h.

Biochemical determinations were carried out by standard methods.

Statistical Analysis
Results are expressed as means ± SDs. Statistical analysis was performed in an IBM PC Computer by the ANOVA method. $p < 0.05$ was considered to have statistical significance.

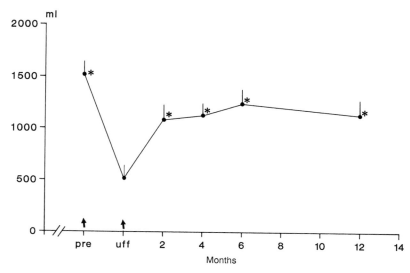

Fig. 1. Net ultrafiltration capacity in 7 patients on CAPD. uff = Ultrafiltration failure. * $p < 0.05$.

Results

The evolution of UF capacity is expressed in figure 1. A progressive decrease in this capacity was observed in every patient during the pre-treatment period (a mean of 60% with respect to previous capacity). After the resting and heparinization procedure, a recovery in the UF capacity was also observed in every patient (a mean of 105%) but to different degrees. In 4 patients the UF recovery was ad integrum. The posttreatment observation period, during which UF capacity remained stable, ranged from 6 to 17 months.

Peritoneal diffusion capacities (MTC) for small molecules, urea and creatinine, showed the following changes: (1) Urea-MTC (fig. 2) values did not show any statistically significant change before and after the procedure. (2) At the time of ultrafiltration failure (UFF) creatinine-MTC values (fig. 2) showed a clear increase with respect to previous ones. After the procedure, a slight decrease was observed.

Discussion

Two different patterns of loss of UF capacity in CAPD patients have been described by Verger [8]. Type I corresponds to the hyperpermeable peri-

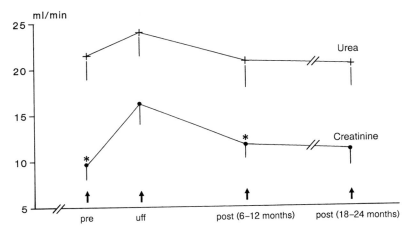

Fig. 2. Peritoneal mass transfer coefficient (MTC) of urea and creatinine in 7 patients on CAPD before and after ultrafiltration failure (uff). * p < 0.05.

toneum and histologically shows a loss of mesothelial microvilli and increased intercell separation. Type II occurs when peritoneal permeability is reduced and is associated with peritoneal sclerosis and multiple adhesions.

Our patients are included in type I UFF with high peritoneal permeability demonstrated by high creatinine-MTC values [9]. The etiology of this failure remains unknown, but may be related to an inability in mesothelium-regenerating capacity after acute or chronic aggressions [6, 10]. There is evidence that in some CAPD patients peritoneal macrophages are in an overstimulated state. They are able to release interleukin I which stimulates fibroblasts toward collagen production and fibrosis initiation [4, 11]. The progressive inflammatory changes induced by these cells would lead to an increased peritoneal permeability (type I UFF) and thereafter to a peritoneum thickening (type II UFF) [5].

Several factors have been implied in the pathogenesis of UFF: acetate in dialysate solutions [12], glucose metabolites in very old or very hot dialysate [4], chlorhexidine [13] and the overuse of hypertonic solutions [5]. A high incidence of peritonitis can also be considered as an aggressor for the peritoneum [14]. Only in 2 patients included in this study was the incidence of peritonitis higher than that of the rest of our CAPD population (1 episode/ 24 patient-months). Furthermore, 6 episodes of peritonitis occurred in the late stages of CAPD, that is, over the 4th year. We have demonstrated that late peritonitis could have a special negative effect on the peritoneum, probably because of the loss of some properties with its long-term use for dialysis [15]. Nevertheless, the relationship between peritonitis and permanent peritoneal functional changes remains controversial [2, 14]. It is remarkable that UFF occurred after the 4th year on CAPD in 6 of the 7 patients; a factor such as time on CAPD could be implied [5].

The management of UFF is not well established. As palliative measures, we employed transfer to IPD, CCPD or diurnal PD with empty peritoneum overnight [4]. Forced diuresis and hemofiltration in order to reduce interstitial edema of the peritoneum resulted in transitory improvements [16]. The administration of calcium channel blockers blunting the fibroblast-increased activation has also been effective for type II UFF [17]. However, the best results reported are those obtained by oral or intraperitoneal phosphatidylcholine administration [18, 19]. Unfortunately, this measure has not been at all effective in our patients [20], probably reflecting the absence of mesothelial cells. The integrity of this layer seems to be necessary for drug action on the peritoneal surface.

According to the observation by Verger and Celicon [21] on peritoneal anatomical restoration in a CAPD patient, most of our patients should have regained a normal structure of the membrane. The medium and long-term observations suggested that this recovery is persistent. Our data on creatinine diffusion capacity changes before and after the procedure may reflect a trend to normalize peritoneal permeability [9]. The concomitant administration of heparin has probably played an important role to avoid the adhesion formation that could preclude the appropriate regeneration of mesothelial cells.

In summary, CAPD patients with type I UFF independent of its suspected origin could be treated by peritoneal resting and heparinization for 4 weeks with the hope of recovering their peritoneal structure, and, consequently, the possibility of maintaining an adequate glucose gradient in order to obtain the desired ultrafiltration capacity.

References

1 Gokal R: Continuous ambulatory peritoneal dialysis (CAPD). Ten years old. Q J Med 1987;242:465–472.
2 Slingeneyer A, Canaud B, Mion C: Permanent loss of ultrafiltration capacity of the peritoneum in long-term peritoneal dialysis. An epidemiological study. Nephron 1983;33:133–138.
3 Nolph KD, Mactier R, Khanna R: The role of lymphatics in the kinetics of net ultrafiltration during peritoneal dialysis; in La Greca G, Chiaramonte S, Fabris A, et al (eds): Peritoneal Dialysis. Milano, Wichtig, 1988, pp 19–22.

4   Henderson I, Gokal R: Loss of ultrafiltration on CAPD; in Gokal R (ed): Continuous Ambulatory Peritoneal Dialysis. London, Churchill-Livingstone, 1986, pp 218–227.

5   Gokal R: Continuous ambulatory peritoneal dialysis; in Maher JF (ed): Replacement of Renal Function by Dialysis. Dordrecht, Kluwer, 1989, pp 590–615.

6   Dobbie JW, Henderson I, Wilson LS: New evidence of the pathogenesis of sclerosing encapsulating peritonitis obtained from serial biopsies; in Khanna R, Nolph KD, Prowant BF, et al (eds): Advances in Continuous Ambulatory Peritoneal Dialysis 1987. Toronto, Peritoneal Dialysis Bulletin Inc, 1987, pp 138–149.

7   Rodriguez-Carmona A, Selgas R, Martinez ME: Characteristics of the peritoneal mass transfer of parathormone in patients under CAPD. Nephron 1984;37:21–24.

8   Verger C: Clinical significance of ultrafiltration alterations on CAPD; in La Greca G, Chiaramonte S, Fabris A, et al (eds): Peritoneal Dialysis. Milano, Wichtig, 1986, pp 91–94.

9   Selgas R, Rodriguez-Carmona A, Martinez ME: Follow-up of peritoneal mass transfer properties in long-term CAPD patients; in Maher JF, Winchester JF (eds): Frontiers in Peritoneal Dialysis. New York, Field Rich, 1986, pp 53–55.

10 Gotloib L, Shostack A, Bar-Sella P, Cohen R: Continuous mesothelial injury and regeneration during long-term peritoneal dialysis. Periton Dial Bull 1987;7:148–155.

11 Lamperi S, Carozzi S: Lymphomonokine disorders and UF loss in CAPD patients; in Khanna R, Nolph KD, Prowant BF, et al (eds): Advances in Continuous Ambulatory Peritoneal Dialysis 1987. Toronto, Peritoneal Dialysis Bulletin Inc, 1987, pp 7–12.

12 Faller B, Marichal JF: Loss of UF in CAPD. A role for acetate. Periton Dial Bull 1984;4:137–142.

13 Oules R, Challah S, Brunner FP: Case control study to determine the cause of sclerosing peritoneal disease. Nephrol Dial Transplant 1988;3:66–69.

14 Verger C, Luzar A, Moore J, Nolph KD: Acute changes in peritoneal morphology and transport properties with infectious peritonitis and mechanical injuries. Kidney Int 1983;23:823–828.

15 Cigarran S, Selgas R, Muñoz J: Peritoneal function parameters after five years on CAPD. Nephrol Dial Transplant 1987;2:452.

16 Bazzato G, Coli U, Landini S: Restoration of UF capacity of peritoneal membrane in CAPD patients. Int J Artif Organs 1984;7:93–96.

17 Lamperi S, Carozzi S: Intraperitoneal verapamil therapy in CAPD patients with ultrafiltration loss; in La Greca G, Chiaramonte S, Fabris A, et al (eds): Peritoneal Dialysis. Milano, Wichtig, 1988, pp 53–56.

18 Di Paolo N, Sacchi G, Capotondo L: Physiolagial role of phosphatidylcholine in peritoneal function; in La Greca G, Chiaramonte S, Fabris A, et al (eds): Peritoneal Dialysis. Milano, Wichtig, 1988, pp 49–52.

19 Breborowicz A, Sombolos K, Rodela H, et al: Mechanisms of phosphatidylcholine action during peritoneal dialysis. Periton Dial Bull 1987;7:6–9.

20 De Alvaro F, Selgas R, Moñoz J: Oral phosphatidylcholine effect on peritoneal MTCs in CAPD patients. EDTA Abstr 1988:93.

21 Verger C, Celicon TB: Peritoneal permeability and encapsulating peritonitis. Lancet 1985:1:986–987.

Rafael Selgas, MD, Servicio de Nefrologia, Hospital La Paz,
Castellana 261, E–28046 Madrid (Spain)

La Greca G, Olivares J, Feriani M, Passlick-Deetjen J (eds): CAPD – A Decade
of Experience. Contrib Nephrol. Basel, Karger, 1991, vol 89, pp 205–213

Arterial Calcification in Diabetic Patients Undergoing CAPD

J.C. Rodríguez-Pérez[a], *N. Vega*[a], *A. Torres*[b], *C. Plaza*[a],
V. Lorenzo[b], *A. Fernández*[a], *L. Hortal*[a], *L. Palop*[a, 1]

[a]Department of Nephrology, Hospital Nuestra Señora del Pino, Las Palmas de
Gran Canaria, Spain; [b]Hospital Universitario, Tenerife, Spain

It has been suggested that arterial calcification in end-stage renal disease
(ESRD) is related to a high calcium × phosphorous (Ca × P) serum product
[1–3], secondary hyperparathyroidism [4], treatment with 1,25 (OH)$_2$ D3
[1, 5], and/or low magnesium serum levels [6].

Some reports [7, 8] have pointed out that these vascular calcifications in
uremic patients are age related, occurring more frequently in the 'over
forties' age group.

Although numerous publications have indicated a greater incidence of
arterial calcification in the diabetic population with ESRD, only a few have
analyzed its incidence, progression or regression in patients treated with
dialysis [6, 9, 10–16].

The etiology of arterial calcification in uremic diabetic patients is still a
controversial subject. Various influences such as age, atheromatosis, diabetic
neuropathy, renal osteodystrophy, vitamin D treatment and hypomagnese-
mia have been reported [5, 6, 8, 13, 17, 18].

In order to clarify these discordant data, the incidence, progression and
regression of arterial calcification (AC) in our group of diabetic patients on
CAPD with a long-term follow-up were analyzed.

The relationship with the neuropathic evolution, bone histomorphom-
etry as well as the possible role of vitamin D treatment both before and after
the patients' admittance to CAPD were studied.

[1] The authors wish to acknowledge Dr. Cereceda for his electrophysiological assistance and Miss Aranzazu Anabitarte for data collection.

Patients and Methods

From January 1981 to December 1988 twenty-six patients (9 females) with diabetic ESRD (mean duration of diabetes 17.3 ± 5.4 years; mean age 51.5 ± 12.7 years) having been on CAPD for various lengths of time took part in the study.

The first evaluation was made the month prior to the admittance to the program, while final studies were made in December 1988 (mean observation period 34.1 ± 17.2 months, range 12–84 months). The number of exchanges for most patients was 4 per day. For patients with lower creatinine the number of exchanges was 3 per day (Baxter, Fresenius Lab.).

All patients were included in an additional study and were randomized for vitamin D treatment (alfacalcidol). Each patient served as his own control.

Patients who had undergone parathyroidectomy or renal transplant were not included.

Radiology

All patients had a radiological metabolic bone survey annually, X-rays were taken of both hands, including the wrist, pelvis including lateral views of the feet and ankles and lumbar region. Post-anterior radiographies of both hands were taken on fine grain film (Kodak M) and industrial film (Kodak type AA) was used for the remainder. These X-rays were scrutinized with a fixed focus magnifier (×6) in order to detect the slightest arterial calcification and its progression or regression.

Arterial calcification was classified in 3 groups, according to the size of the vessels following Cassidy's criteria [19] with some modifications: AC-I: digital and/or arcade vessels in hands and/or feet; AC-II: radial and/or ulnar and/or tibial and/or peroneal; AC-III: aorta and/or iliacs. Initial and final examinations were compared.

Neuropathy

According to Dawson and Scott [20], motor and sensory nerve conduction velocities were recorded by a trained electrophysiologist in the same room and at the same temperature, using surface electrodes or needle electrodes if warranted.

All electrophysiologic studies were evaluated in the dominant half of the body. Motor and sensory nerve conduction were measured in the external sciatic popliteal nerve, the sural nerve and the third finger-hand-wrist segment.

A Medelec MS-92 system with a band width from 2 Hz to 10 kHz and an amplifier and sweep of 5 mV and 5 ms were used for motor nerve conduction and 20 Hz to 2 kHz with amplifier and sweep of 20 µV and 1 ms for sensory nerve conduction.

Bone Histomorphometry

In 7 patients bone biopsies were taken using the transiliac technique. Quantitative analysis and aluminum (aurine-tricarboxylic acid) stain were performed following previously described methods [21, 22]. Histological studies were made of all but 1 patient, due to the deterioration of the sample during the process. All histological forms were classified, with slight modifications, in 4 groups following Sherrard's criteria [23].

Statistical Analyses

A Sigma (Horus Hardware) statistical package was used in an IBM PC-XT computer. Analyses employed were: Student's t test for paired and impaired data, chi-square test and

Table 1. Distribution of arterial calcifications pre- and post-CAPD treatment

	I	II	III	I+II	I+III	II+III	I+II+III
Pre-CAPD							
n	8	9	16	8	7	8	7
%	30.7	34.6	61.5	30.7	26.9	30.7	26.9
Post-CAPD							
n	11	14	21	10	10	12	9
%	42.3	53.8	80.7	38.4	38.4	46.1	34.6

multivariate analysis of variance (Anova 1). Correlations were evaluated by linear regression.

Results

At predialysis examination, the prevalence of major vessel calcification (AC-III) was found to be higher in older patients, with no correlation between age and AC-I and AC-II. There was no apparent relationship between sex of the patient and length of time of diabetes (7–30 years). Sites and distribution of the arterial calcification are depicted in table 1. The differences between pre- and post-CAPD, were not statistically significant; however, a clear association was found between AC-I predialysis and post-CAPD treatment (chi-square = 12.52, p < 0.001). The same relationship was seen in AC-II.

At the initial examination, motor and sensory nerve conduction velocities did not have any clear-cut relationship with any type of arterial calcification (I, II, III). However, although not statistically significant, a decrease in the sensory nerve conduction velocity (3rd finger-hand-wrist segment) in patients with AC-III, could be observed after CAPD treatment. Electrophysiological studies of the peripheral nerves of these patients showed no evidence of progression during CAPD treatment (fig. 1–3). Yet, in 3 patients the sural nerve conduction velocity and in 2 patients the third finger-hand-wrist segment conduction velocity even showed an improvement.

When starting CAPD treatment the bone biopsies of 7 of 26 patients showed evidence of mild forms of renal osteodystrophy. No correlation between the arterial calcifications and any of the morphometric parameters could be observed. After CAPD treatment bone biopsies did not show any

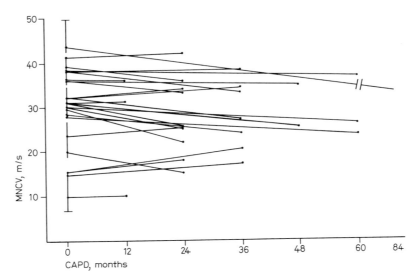

Fig. 1. Motor nerve conduction velocity (MNCV) pre- and post-CAPD (external sciatic popliteal nerve).

modification in 4 patients, one developed osteomalacia and another a mixed form of renal osteodystrophy, both with positive aluminum staining.

The relationship between arterial calcifications (I, II, III) and treatment with alfacalcidol, did not differ significantly in any group after CAPD treatment.

Regression of arterial calcifications was also assessed by sequential comparison of the radiography. Regression of AC-I or AC-II was not found in any patient and regression of iliac calcification was only seen in one.

Discussion

Pathological changes in the arteries of uremic patients undergoing dialysis are extremely common. The results of different studies [7, 8] suggest that these changes represent an acceleration in the normal arterial aging process and that calcification plays an integral role in this arterial disease.

Various studies show that these arterial calcifications are more frequent in diabetic than in nondiabetic patients with ESRD [9, 18, 24–26] with an

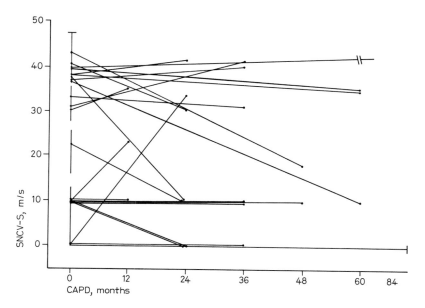

Fig. 2. Sensory nerve conduction velocity (sural nerve, SNCV-S) pre- and post-CAPD.

incidence of 35–60% at the beginning of renal replacement therapy increasing to 60–90% depending on the time of treatment [9–11, 18]. Most studies, however, do not provide an analysis of the large vessels.

In this study, following Cassidy's criteria [19] with some modifications for the classification of arterial calcification, an incidence of calcification of 30.7% for small vessels and 61.5% for large vessels was detected. This increased to 42.3 and 80.7%, respectively, after 12–84 months on CAPD.

According to previous studies [9–11], our results confirm an elevated incidence of arterial calcification in uremic diabetic patients especially after prolonged dialysis treatment. In some of these studies nearly 100% arterial calcification was reported after a mean peritoneal dialysis treatment of 24 months, while in our group of CAPD patients the incidence of all types of calcification was much lower in spite of nearly twice the time on dialysis (table 1).

Although spontaneous regression of arterial calcification in ESRD is considered to be nonexistent [27] or rare [15], Meema and Oreopoulos [18] have recently found regression in 13% of their patients. In this study the only

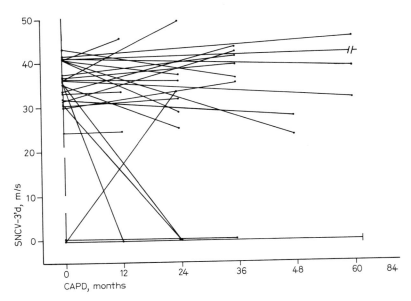

Fig. 3. Sensory nerve conduction velocity (3rd finger-hand-wrist segment, SNCV-3'd) pre- and post-CAPD.

regression of iliac calcification observed was in a 62-year-old patient after 36 months on CAPD.

In contrast to other reports [17, 28, 29], no relationship between arterial calcification and neuropathy was observed either before or after CAPD treatment. But in agreement with other studies [30, 31] our diabetic CAPD population, having been on CAPD for at least 1 year, did not show any evidence of neuropathic progression.

Although it has previously been suggested that a high serum $Ca \times P$ product or secondary hyperparathyroidism are principal factors in the development of arterial calcification in ESRD [1–3], some recent studies [19, 32, 33] have failed to show any relationship. In our study, although neither the $Ca \times P$ product nor the serum magnesium levels were analyzed, a histological bone study in a small group of patients was performed.

In agreement with other studies [34], a predominance of lower bone turnover rate forms with 2 patients having positive aluminum stain (>10% of total trabecular surface) were observed.

Our findings indicate that PTH does not play a role either in the appearance or in the progression of arterial calcification, which is contrary to previous reports [1–4].

There is no evidence [19] either to suggest that vitamin D has any direct effect on the progression or regression of arterial calcification. It appears therefore that arterial calcification is a complication of diabetic patients, especially in those with ESRD after start of treatment, including CAPD. Large vessel calcifications are age related and, although a relationship with neuropathy, bone morphometry and vitamin D treatment could not be observed, it seems that AC-I (small vessels) and AC-II (medium vessels) are a consequence of a summation of various 'risk' factors.

But to identify all risk factors of arterial calcification in diabetics and nondiabetics, both before and after dialysis, it would be desirable to carry out a prospective study.

References

1 Mallick NP, Berline GM: Arterial calcification after vitamin-D therapy in hyper-phosphatemic renal failure. Lancet 1968;ii:13–16.
2 Parfitt AM: Soft tissue calcifications in uremia. Arch Intern Med 1969;124:544–556.
3 Rubini ME, Coburn JW, Massry SG, Shinaberger JH: Renal osteodystrophy. Arch Intern Med 1969;124:663–669.
4 Eastwood JB, Bordier PJ, De Wardener HE: Some biochemical, radiological and clinical features of renal osteodystrophy. Kidney Int 1973;4:128–140.
5 Krogg M, Ejerblad S, Erikson I, Johanson H: Arterial calcification in uremic rats treated with 1α-hydroxycholecalciferol and parathyroidectomy. Scand J Urol Nephrol 1984;18:227–239.
6 Meema HE, Oreopoulos DG, Rapoport A: Serum magnesium level and arterial calcification in end stage renal disease. Kidney Int 1987;32:388–394.
7 Ritz E, Mehls O, Bommer J, Schmidt-Gayk H, Fiegel P, Reitinger H: Vascular calcifications under maintenance hemodialysis. Klin Wochenschr 1977;55:375–378.
8 Ibels LS, Alfrey AC, Huffer WE, Craswell PW, Anderson JT, Weil R III: Arterial calcification and pathology in uremic patients undergoing dialysis. Am J Med 1979; 66:790–796.
9 Meema HE, Oreopoulos DG: Arterial calcifications in patients undergoing chronic peritoneal dialysis, incidence, progression and regression. Periton Dial Bull 1985; 5:241–247.
10 Parsons V, Watkins PJ: Diabetics and the kidney; in Black D, et al (eds): Renal Disease, ed. 4. Oxford, Blackwell, 1979, p 701.
11 Katirtzoglou A, Izatt S, Oreopoulos DG, et al: Chronic peritoneal dialysis in diabetics with end stage renal failure; in Friedman E, et al (eds): Diabetic Renal-Retinal Syndrome. New York, Grune & Stratton, 1980, pp 317–331.

12 Tatler GLV, Baillod RA, Varghese Z, et al: Evolution of bone disease over 10 years in 135 patients with terminal renal failure. Br J Med 1973;iv:315–319.

13 Meema HE, Oreopoulos DG, deVeber GA: Arterial calcifications in severe chronic renal disease and their relationship to dialysis treatment, renal transplant, and parathyroidectomy. Radiology 1976;121:315–321.

14 Eisenberg E, Bartholow PV Jr: Reversible calcinosis cutis: Calciphylaxis in man. N Engl J Med 1963;268:1216–1220.

15 Verberckmoes R, Bouillon R, Krempien BV: Disappearance of vascular calcifications during treatment of renal osteodystrophy. Ann Intern Med 1975;82:529–533.

16 Legrain M, Rottembourg J, Bentchikou A, et al: Dialysis treatment of insulin dependent diabetic patients: Ten years experience. Clin Nephrol 1984;21:72–81.

17 Edmonds ME, Morrison N, Laws JW, Watkins P: Medial arterial calcification and diabetic neuropathy. Br Med J 1982;284:928–931.

18 Meema HE, Oreopoulos DG: Morphology, progression, and regression of arterial and periarterial calcifications in patients with end-stage renal disease. Radiology 1986;158:671–677.

19 Cassidy M, Owen J, Ellis H, Dewar J, Robinson C, Wilkinson R, Ward M, Kerr DN: Renal osteodystrophy and metastatic calcification in long term CAPD. Q J Med 1985;54:29–48.

20 Dawson GD, Scott JW: Recording of nerve action potentials through skin in man. J Neurol Neurosurg Psychiatry 1949;12:259–267.

21 Lorenzo V, Torres A, Gonzalez-Posada J, Pestana M, Rodriguez A, Diaz-Flores L: Prevalencia de las distintas formas histológicas de osteodistrofia renal con especial referencia a la osteomalacia. Nefrologia 1986;6:25–33.

22 Rodriguez-Perez JC, Lorenzo V, Torres A: Efecto de 1 año de tratamiento con diálisis peritoneal continua ambulatoria (DPCA) sobre la histologia ósea del enfermo urémico. Nefrologia 1988;8(suppl):138–143.

23 Sherrard D, Ott S, Maloney N, Andress D, Coburn J: Uremic osteodystrophy: classification, cause and treatment; in Frame B, Potts J (eds): Clinical Disorders of Bone and Mineral Metabolism. Amsterdam, Excerpta Medica, 1983, pp 254–259.

24 Ferrier TM: Radiologically demonstrable arterial calcification in diabetes mellitus. Aust Ann Med 1964;13:222–228.

25 Christensen NJ: Muscle blood flow measured by xenon-133 and vascular calcifications in diabetics. Acta Med Scand 1968;183:449–454.

26 Campbell WL, Feldman F: Bone and soft tissue abnormalities in diabetes mellitus. Am J Roentgenol Radium Ther Med 1975;124:7–16.

27 Schoenfeld P, Humphreys M: A general description of the uremic state; in Brenner B, Rector F Jr (eds): The Kidney. Philadelphia, Saunders, 1976, pp 1438.

28 Sinha S, Munichoodapa CS, Kozak GP: Neuroarthropathy (Charcot joints) in diabetes mellitus. Medicine 1972;51:191–210.

29 Clouse ME, Gramm HF, Legg M, Flood T: Diabetic osteoartropathy. Am J Roentgenol Radium Ther Med 1974;121:22–34.

30 Blair G: Electrophysiologic studies in peripheral nerves of diabetics undergoing CAPD. Periton Dial Bull 1982;2(suppl):53–55.

31 Sunderrajan S, Nolph KD: Longitudinal study of nerve conduction velocities during CAPD. Periton Dial Bull 1985;5:48–50.

32 Coburn JW, Henry DA: Renal osteodystrophy; in Stollerman G (ed): Advances in Internal Medicine. Chicago, Medical Publisher, 1984, vol 30, pp 387–424.

33   De Francisco AM, Ellis HA, Owen JP, Cassidy MJ, et al: Parathyroidectomy in chronic renal failure. Q J Med 1985;55:289–311.
34   Andress D, Kopp J, Maloney N, Coburn J, Sherrard D: Early deposition of aluminum in bone in diabetic patients on hemodialysis. N Engl J Med 1987;316: 292–296.

Dr. J. C. Rodriguez-Perez, Department of Nephrology,
Hospital Nuestra Señora del Pino, E–35004 Las Palmas de Gran Canaria (Spain)

La Greca G, Olivares J, Feriani M, Passlick-Deetjen J (eds): CAPD – A Decade
of Experience. Contrib Nephrol. Basel, Karger, 1991, vol 89, pp 214–223

Effect of Human Recombinant Erythropoietin on Dialysis Efficiency in CAPD

Hjalmar B. Steinhauer, Iris Lubrich-Birkner, Peter Schollmeyer

University of Freiburg, Department of Internal Medicine, Division of Nephrology,
Freiburg i. Br., FRG

Inappropriate low serum levels of erythropoietin are the major cause of anemia in patients with chronic renal failure [1–4]. Further factors affecting the physiological equilibrium between formation and breakdown of erythrocytes are iron deficiency due to chronic blood loss on hemodialysis [5], osteomyelofibrosis associated with hyperparathyroidism [6, 7], diminished iron transfer to the erythroid progenitor cells induced by chronic aluminum toxicity [8], and a shortened red blood cell life [9, 10]. Renal anemia in patients undergoing CAPD is less severe in comparison with patients on hemodialysis [11]. Nevertheless, about 30% of our patients on chronic CAPD develop anemia with hematocrit below 28%.

In a recent short-time study the recombinant human erythropoietin (rHuEPO)-induced correction of anemia in CAPD patients was associated with an increased peritoneal ultrafiltration [12]. Long-term CAPD is supposed to induce peritoneal fibrosis in a minority of patients, resulting in decreased ultrafiltration and diminished solute clearances [13, 14]. If the observed rise in ultrafiltration after rHuEPO-induced correction of anemia is long lasting, rHuEPO therapy may improve fluid balance and dialysis efficiency in patients on maintenance CAPD. In the present study, we investigated the long-term effect of rHuEPO treatment on dialysis efficiency in patients undergoing CAPD.

Patients and Methods

We studied 14 patients (10 females, 4 males; mean age 41.8 ± 4.0 years, range 21–65 years) with end-stage renal failure who had been on CAPD for 25.4 ± 2.9 months (range 10–41 months). The underlying renal disease was chronic glomerulonephritis in 10, chronic interstitial nephritis in 2, polycystic kidney disease in 1, and diabetic nephropathy in 1 patient.

All patients were suffering from renal anemia (hematocrit below 28%). Serum ferritin levels of all participants were above 20 µg/1, vitamin B_{12} and folic acid in serum were in the normal range. Before the onset of rHuEPO treatment they were free from peritonitis for at least 4 weeks. None of the patients were on androgen treatment, immunosuppressive therapy, or steroid medication. One patient was bilaterally nephrectomized. Informed consent was obtained from all patients prior to the trial.

CAPD was performed with dialysis solutions containing 1.5–4.25% glucose monohydrate (Fresenius AG, Bad Homburg, FRG; Baxter Deerfield, Ill., USA) according to the clinical requirements. Twice weekly the patients underwent a study dialysate exchange in the morning with 1.5 liters 1.5% glucose monohydrate and a dwell time of 4 h. These dialysates were used for the analysis of peritoneal ultrafiltration und solute clearances.

After a 2-week run-in period for baseline measurements rHuEPO (Cilag AG, Wiesbaden, FRG) was administered subcutaneously twice weekly in the dose of 50 U/kg body weight (BW). If the hematocrit did not rise for a minimum of 5% per month this dose was increased for 25 U/kg BW every 4 weeks until the target hematocrit of 35% had been achieved. In the event that this hematocrit was exceeded, rHuEPO treatment was discontinued for 4 weeks and restarted on hematocrit below 35% at a maintenance dose of 25 U/kg BW below the last dose.

Blood pressure, heart rate, body temperature, and adverse effects of rHuEPO treatment were monitored twice weekly. Serum and dialysate chemistry, dialysate prostanoids, and hematological profile were measured once weekly. Serum ferritin and transferrin were determined monthly. Net ultrafiltration was calculated from the difference of dialysate bag weight before infusion and after dialysate efflux.

Serum and dialysate chemistry were determined by a multichannel autoanalyzer technique, blood counts were performed on a Coulter counter. Ferritin was measured by enzyme-linked immunoassay (Boehringer Mannheim, Mannheim, FRG), transferrin by radial immunodiffusion (Partigen, Boehringer Mannheim).

The dialysate prostanoids PGE_2, TXB_2 and 6-keto-$PGF_{1\alpha}$ were adsorbed to C18-octadecyl columns (Amprep, Amersham Buchler, Braunschweig, FRG) and sequentially eluted according to the method of Luderer et al. [15] prior to radioimmunological determination. Sensitivity and specificity of the radioimmunoassays used were described recently by our group [16, 17].

Results are expressed as means ± SEM. Data were evaluated by distribution-free Wilcoxon's rank-sum test and linear regression analysis. The null hypothesis was rejected at $p < 0.05$.

Results

Fourteen anemic patients undergoing CAPD were treated with rHuEPO subcutaneously for a total of 168 months (12 months per patient). The initial rHuEPO dose of 50 U/kg BW twice weekly was increased to 67.8 ± 4.9 U/kg BW during the first 3 months of treatment. During the following study time (months 4–12), the mean rHuEPO dose was 48 ± 2 (range 0–125) U/kg BW (fig. 1).

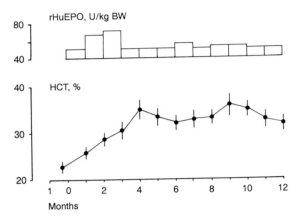

Fig. 1. Hematocrit (HCT) response to subcutaneous rHuEPO and mean dose of rHuEPO twice weekly in 14 CAPD patients.

Subcutaneous administration of rHuEPO was tolerated without severe adverse effects. Seven patients reported slight local pain after the subcutaneous injection which discontinued after a few minutes. Four patients required increased antihypertensive medication. One patient suffered from a flu-like syndrome without a rise in body temperature after 2 weeks of rHuEPO treatment. The symptoms disappeared as the treatment progressed.

A continuous rise in hematocrit was noted within the first 3 months of rHuEPO application. During the following study period hematocrit remained widely unchanged (range 31.3–34.1%) (fig. 1).

The improvement of hematocrit was paralleled by an increase of hemoglobin and red blood cells ($p < 0.03$). Leukocytes and platelet count were not affected by rHuEPO (table 1).

Mean serum ferritin decreased continuously during the first 3 months ($p < 0.05$). Throughout the following study period it returned to the initial range (table 1). In 3 patients ferritin concentration decreased below 20 µg/l as a sign of iron depletion. In these patients oral iron supplementation was doubled (Fe^{2+}-glycine sulfate, 80 mg elemental iron).

Serum transferrin did not change significantly during the trial (initial: 332 ± 139 µg/l; month 12: 327 ± 135 µg/l). HbE and MCV also remained unchanged.

Arterial blood pressure increased in 4 formerly hypertensive CAPD patients on rHuEPO therapy. Statistical analysis of mean arterial blood

Table 1. Hematological data before and on rHuEPO treatment in 14 CAPD patients

	Run-in period −0.5 months	rHuEPO treatment				
		1 month	3 months	6 months	9 months	12 months
Hemoglobin, g/dl	7.7 ± 0.3	8.5 ± 0.2	10.8 ± 0.5**	10.8 ± 0.4**	11.1 ± 0.7**	10.5 ± 0.6**
Erythrocytes, 10^{12}/l	2.58 ± 0.10	2.89 ± 0.08	3.69 ± 0.14**	3.74 ± 0.14**	3.74 ± 0.22**	3.55 ± 0.19**
Platelets, 10^9/l	298 ± 27	305 ± 23	258 ± 20	274 ± 24	296 ± 44	267 ± 36
Leukocytes, 10^9/l	6.04 ± 0.48	5.12 ± 0.63	5.31 ± 0.21	6.12 ± 0.38	5.62 ± 0.58	6.26 ± 0.54
Ferritin, ng/ml	332 ± 139	193 ± 80	123 ± 45*	214 ± 74*	179 ± 64*	327 ± 178

*$p < 0.05$; **$p < 0.03$.

Table 2. Mean arterial blood pressure (MAP), heart rate (HR), and cardiothoracic index in 14 CAPD patients

	Run-in period −0.5 months	rHuEPO treatment				
		1 month	3 months	6 months	9 months	12 months
MAP, mm Hg	102 ± 6	104 ± 7	103 ± 6	103 ± 8	106 ± 7	104 ± 9
HR, beats/min	80 ± 2	80 ± 2	80 ± 2	79 ± 3	79 ± 3	75 ± 3
Cardiothoracic index[1]	0.44 ± 0.06	–	–	0.45 ± 0.05	–	–

[1] Cardiac transversal diameter/thoracic transversal diameter, n = 6.

pressure, heart rate, cardiothoracic index, and body weight in all 14 CAPD patients did not reveal any significant change during 12 months of rHuEPO treatment (table 2).

The serum levels of potassium (initial: 4.84 ± 0.16 mmol/1) and phosphate (initial: 1.49 ± 0.10 mmol/1) increased throughout the first months of the trial (month 6: 5.38 ± 0.27 and 1.84 ± 0.14 mmol/1, respectively; $p < 0.05$) and tended to decrease during the following study time (month 12:

Table 3. Peritoneal ultrafiltration (UF) and solute clearances (Cl) on rHuEPO treatment in 14 CAPD patients

	Run-in period −0.5 months	rHuEPO treatment				
		1 month	3 months	6 months	9 months	12 months
UF, ml/h	41.8 ± 6.2	49.5 ± 9.4*	57.3 ± 9.6**	54.0 ± 5.8*	46.8 ± 7.8*	55.8 ± 11.0*
Cl creatinine, ml/min/1.73 m²	4.11 ± 0.23	4.41 ± 0.28	5.14 ± 0.38*	4.35 ± 0.27	4.39 ± 0.24	4.49 ± 0.35
Cl urea, ml/min/1.73 m²	5.81 ± 0.31	5.80 ± 0.26	6.64 ± 0.45*	5.83 ± 0.26	5.74 ± 0.27	6.00 ± 0.38
Cl phosphate, ml/min/1.73 m²	3.44 ± 0.17	3.99 ± 0.29	4.56 ± 0.30*	4.18 ± 0.38*	3.96 ± 0.34	4.38 ± 0.52*
Cl potassium, ml/min/1.73 m²	5.36 ± 0.37	4.99 ± 0.31	6.11 ± 0.46*	5.43 ± 0.27	5.19 ± 0.20	5.43 ± 0.31

* $p < 0.05$; ** $p < 0.03$.

potassium 5.03 ± 0.30 mmol/l, phosphate 1.52 ± 0.16 mmol/l; n.s. in comparison with initial values). The serum concentrations of sodium, calcium, creatinine, and urea were not affected by rHuEPO.

Peritoneal ultrafiltration (1.5 liters dialysate, 1.5% glucose monohydrate, 4 h dwell time) improved from initially 41.8 ± 6.2 to 57.3 ± 9.6 ml/h after 3 months of rHuEPO. This rise in ultrafiltration continued during the whole following study time (table 3). The augmented peritoneal ultrafiltration also resulted in increased clearance rates of creatinine, urea, potassium (month 3 on rHuEPO treatment), and phosphate (months 3, 6 and 12 on rHuEPO treatment; table 3).

The rise in peritoneal ultrafiltration on rHuEPO treatment was positively correlated with the rHuEPO-induced increase of hematocrit (fig. 2).

The peritoneal release of the eicosanoids PGE_2, 6-keto-$PGF_{1\alpha}$, and TXB_2 into the dialysate was not affected by rHuEPO treatment (table 4).

Discussion

In a recent preliminary study we reported the partial correction of renal anemia and an improved peritoneal ultrafiltration after 12 weeks of subcutaneous rHuEPO treatment [12]. The present results in 14 CAPD patients on rHuEPO for 1 year confirm our former findings.

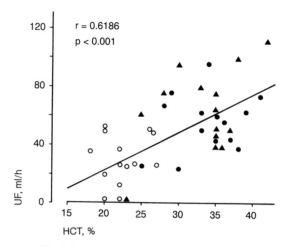

Fig. 2. Relationship between peritoneal ultrafiltration (UF) and hematocrit (HCT) in 14 CAPD patients on rHuEPO treatment. 0 = Run-in period before the onset of rHuEPO; ● = 6 months on rHuEPO; ▲ = 12 months on rHuEPO.

Table 4. Peritoneal release of prostanoids on rHuEPO treatment in 14 CAPD patients

	Before rHuEPO 0.5 months	On rHuEPO treatment			
		1 month	3 months	6 months	12 months
PGE_2, ng/4 h	108 ± 26	105 ± 19	119 ± 24	127 ± 35	118 ± 16
6-Keto-$PGF_{1\alpha}$, µg/4 h	0.44 ± 0.09	0.51 ± 0.17	0.48 ± 0.14	0.41 ± 0.22	0.47 ± 0.13
TXB_2, ng/4 h	42 ± 10	45 ± 8	47 ± 15	39 ± 11	42 ± 12

Subcutaneous rHuEPO 50–100 U/kg twice weekly resulted in a continuous rise in hematocrit from 23 to 35% within 4 months. During the following study period hematocrit remained stable at a mean rHuEPO dose of 48 U/kg BW two times week. In contrast to the observation of several groups on intravenous rHuEPO in hemodialysis patients [18, 19], platelet count was not affected by rHuEPO. The total and differential leukocyte count did not change significantly either.

The rHuEPO-induced rise in hematocrit was positively correlated with an increase in peritoneal ultrafiltration. This finding gains importance since long-term treatment of chronic renal failure by CAPD can be complicated by decreased ultrafiltration and solute clearances [13, 14]. Several groups have noted a rise in peripheral vascular resistance by correction of anemia on rHuEPO therapy [20–22]. This has been attributed to the reversal of compensatory hypoxic vasodilation due to the improvement in tissue oxygenation. No data are available on the effect of anemia on peritoneal vascular resistance. However, if hypoxic vasodilation occurs mainly in the peripheral vascular regions, the rHuEPO-induced rise in vascular resistance may lead to a redistribution of blood flow, resulting in an augmented mesenteric perfusion. Since increased mesenteric blood flow leads to enhanced peritoneal transport [23], it is reasonable to assume that the rHuEPO-induced rise in ultrafiltration and solute clearances is mediated by an improved perfusion of peritoneal capillaries.

Furthermore, rHuEPO treatment was followed by the suppression of baseline plasma renin activity (PRA) and plasma aldosterone [24] and an increase of atrial natriuretic peptide (ANP) [24, 25]. These hormonal changes can be explained by an rHuEPO-induced hypervolemia associated to increased erythropoiesis [24, 25]. This rise in extracellular fluid volume may contribute to enhanced vascular perfusion. Concerning mesenteric blood flow, this may result in an improved peritoneal transport [23].

Since increased local synthesis of prostanoids during CAPD-associated peritonitis results in augmented peritoneal permeability [17, 26] with the result of decreased ultrafiltration, we looked into the effect of rHuEPO treatment on prostanoid generation. During 12 months of rHuEPO the release of the vasoactive prostanoids PGE_2, TXA_2 (determined as its metabolite TXB_2), and prostacyclin (determined as its metabolite 6-keto-$PGF_{1\alpha}$) into the dialysate remained unchanged. From these data, it is unlikely that the rHuEPO-induced rise in ultrafiltration is mediated by a decreased local generation of prostanoids.

In accordance with recent studies on rHuEPO [27, 28] all CAPD patients reported improved physical condition and well-being after correction of anemia. A rise in serum retention products noted in hemodialysis patients on rHuEPO [29–31] could not be observed in our patients on CAPD but serum potassium and phosphate increased within the first months on rHuEPO treatment. This may be attributed to dietary changes since 12 of 14 patients reported improved appetite. After 12 months on rHuEPO, serum electrolytes as well as body weight did not differ significantly from the initial values before the onset of rHuEPO treatment.

During the trial, arterial blood pressure increased in 4 formerly hypertensive patients. The rise in blood pressure could easily be managed by intensified antihypertensive therapy. After 12 months on rHuEPO, the mean arterial blood pressure did not differ from the initial value. No rise in blood pressure was observed in CAPD patients who were normotensive before the onset of rHuEPO treatment. Adequate iron stores are essential for the optimal response to rHuEPO since stimulated erythropoiesis results in an augmented demand on iron [32]. The response to rHuEPO was excellent in iron-overloaded patients. In 3 CAPD patients with initial ferritin concentrations below 50 µg/l, intercurrent evidence of iron depletion developed (ferritin below 20 µg/l) and forced us to increase iron supplementation. In contrast to recent studies on rHuEPO treatment in patients on maintenance hemodialysis [18, 30, 31, 33], intravenous administration of iron was not necessary in our patients. After 12 months of rHuEPO and oral iron supplementation serum ferritin was in the upper normal range.

In summary, subcutaneous rHuEPO treatment in anemic CAPD patients is effective and safe. After 12 months of therapy, the maintenance dose of rHuEPO was 48 ± 2 U/kg BW twice weekly to keep the hematocrit within the target range of 32–35%. No severe adverse effects were observed. The lasting rise in ultrafiltration after rHuEPO-induced partial correction of anemia might improve fluid balance and dialysis efficiency in patients undergoing CAPD. Further studies are required to clarify the mechanism of an rHuEPO-associated rise in peritoneal transport.

References

1 Gurney CW, Jacobson LO, Goldwasser E: The physiological and clinical significance of erythropoietin. Ann Intern Med 1958;49:363–370.
2 McGonigle RJS, Wallin JD, Shadduck RK, Fisher JW: Erythropoietin deficiency and inhibition of erythropoiesis in renal insufficiency. Kidney Int 1984;25:437–444.
3 Caro J, Brown S, Miller O, Murray T, Erslev AJ: Erythropoietin levels in uremic nephric and anephric patients. J Lab Clin Med 1979;93:449–458.
4 Radtke HW, Claussner A, Erbes PM, Scheuermann EH, Schoeppe W, Koch KM: Serum erythropoietin concentration in chronic renal failure: Relationship to degree of anemia and excretory renal function. Blood 1979;54:877–884.
5 Lindsay RM, Burton JA, King P, Davidson JF, Boddy K, Kennedy AC: The measurement of dialyzer blood loss. Clin Nephrol 1973;1:24–28.
6 Meytes D, Bogin E, Ma A, Dukes PP, Massry SG: Effect of parathyroid hormone on erythropoiesis. J Clin Invest 1981;67:1263–1269.
7 Potasman I, Better OS: The role of secondary hyperparathyroidism in the anemia of chronic renal failure. Nephron 1983;33:229–231.
8 Kaiser L, Schwartz KA: Aluminum-induced anemia. Am J Kidney Dis 1985;6:348–352.
9 Shaw AB: Haemolysis in chronic renal failure. Brit Med J 1967;ii:213–216.

10 Blumberg A: Pathogenese der renalen Anämie. Nephron 1989;51:S15–S19.

11 Moncrief JW, Popovich RP: Continuous ambulatory peritoneal dialysis (CAPD) – worldwide experience; in Nolph KD (ed): Peritoneal Dialysis. The Hague, Martinus Nijhoff, 1981, pp 178–212.

12 Steinhauer HB, Lubrich-Birkner I, Dreyling KW, Hörl WH, Schollmeyer P: Increased ultrafiltration after erythropoietin-induced correction of renal anemia in patients on continuous ambulatory peritoneal dialysis. Nephron 1989;53:91–92.

13 Slingeneyer A, Canaud B, Mion C: Permanent loss of ultrafiltration capacity of the peritoneum in long-term peritoneal dialysis: An epidemiological study. Nephron 1983;33:133–138.

14 Wideröe T-E, Smeby LC, Mjaland S, Dahl K, Berg KJ, Aas TW: Long-term changes in transperitoneal water transport during continuous ambulatory peritoneal dialysis. Nephron 1984;38:238–247.

15 Luderer JR, Riley DL, Demers LM: Rapid extraction of arachidonic acid metabolites utilizing octdecyl reverse-phase columns. J Chromat 1987;273:402–409.

16 Steinhauer HB, Lubrich-Birkner I, Bünter B, Schollmeyer P: Response of human platelets to inhibition of thromboxane synthesis. Clin Hemorrheol 1983;3:1–12.

17 Steinhauer HB, Günter B, Schollmeyer P: Stimulation of peritoneal synthesis of vasoactive prostaglandins during peritonitis in patients on continuous ambulatory peritoneal dialysis. Eur J Clin Invest 1985;15:1–5.

18 Bommer J, Alexiou C, Müller-Bühl U, Eifert J, Ritz E: Recombinant human erythropoietin therapy in hemodialysis patients – dose determination and clinical experience. Nephrol Dial Transplant 1987;2:238–242.

19 Grützmacher P, Bergmann M, Weinreich T, Nattermann U, Reimers E, Pollok M: Benefical and adverse effects of correction of anemia by recombinant human erythropoietin in patients on maintenance hemodialysis: in Koch KM, Kühn K, Nonnast-Daniel B, Scigalla P (eds): Treatment of Renal Anemia with Recombinant Human Erythropoietin. Contr Nephrol. Basel, Karger, 1988, vol 66, pp 104–113.

20 Nonnast-Daniel B, Creutzig A, Kühn K, et al: Effect of treatment with recombinant human erythropoietin on peripheral hemodynamics and oxygenation; in Koch KM, Kühn K, Nonnast-Daniel B, Scigalla P (eds): Treatment of Renal Anemia with Recombinant Human Erythropoietin. Contr Nephrol. Basel, Karger, 1988, vol 66, pp 185–194.

21 Steffen HM, Brunner R, Müller R, Degenhardt S, Pollok M, Lang R, Baldamus CA: Peripheral hemodynamics, blood viscosity, and the renin-angiotensin system in hemodialysis patients under therapy with recombinant human erythropoietin; in Baldamus CA, Koch KM, Scigalla P, Wieczorek L (eds): Erythropoietin: From Molecular Structure to Clinical Application. Contr Nephrol. Basel, Karger, 1989, vol 76, pp 292–298.

22 Buckner FS, Eschbach JW, Haley NR, Davidson RR, Adamson JW: Correction of the anemia in hemodialysis patients with recombinant human erythropoietin (rHuEPO): Hemodynamic changes and risks for hypertension (abstract). Kidney Int 1989;35:190.

23 Maher JF: Pharmacologic manipulation of peritoneal transport; in Nolph KD (ed): Peritoneal Dialysis, The Hague, Martinus Nijhoff, 1981, pp 213–239.

24 Kokot F, Wiecek A, Grzeszczak W, Klepacka J, Klin M, Lao M: Endocrine abnormalities in patients with endstage renal failure; in Hörl WH, Schollmeyer P (eds): New Perspectives in Hemodialysis, Peritoneal Dialysis, Arteriovenous Hemo-

filtration, and Plasmapheresis. Advances in Experimental Medicine and Biology. New York, Plenum Press, 1989, vol 260, pp 61–68.

25 Kühn K, Talartschik H, Koch KM, Eisenhauer T, Nonnast-Daniel B, Scheler F, Brunkhorst R, Reimers E: Plasma atrial natriuretic peptide after partial correction of renal anemia by recombinant human erythropoietin (abstract). Nephrol Dial Transplant 1988;3:497–498.

26 Steinhauer HB, Schollmeyer P: Prostaglandin-mediated loss of proteins during peritonitis in continuous ambulatory peritoneal dialysis. Kidney Int 1986;29: 584–590.

27 Mayer G, Thum J, Cada EM, Stummvoll HK, Graf H: Working capacity is increased following recombinant human erythropoietin treatment. Kidney Int 1988;34: 525–528.

28 Lundin AP: Quality of life: Subjective and objective improvements with recombinant human erythropoietin therapy. Semin Nephrol 1989;9:S22–S29.

29 Winearls CG, Oliver DO, Pippard MJ, Reid C, Downing MR, Cotes PM: Effect of human erythropoietin derived from recombinant DNA on the anaemia of patients maintained by chronic haemodialysis. Lancet 1986;ii:1175–1178.

30 Eschbach JW, Ergie JC, Downing MR, Browne JE, Adamson JW: Correction of the anemia of end-stage renal disease with recombinant human erythropoietin. N Engl J Med 1987;316:73–78.

31 Casati S, Passerini P, Campise MR, Graziani G, Cesana B, Perisic M, Ponticelli C: Benefits and risks of protracted treatment with human recombinant erythropoietin in patients having haemodialysis. Br Med J 1987;295:1017–1020.

32 Van Wyck DB, Stivelman JC, Ruiz J, Kirlin LF, Katz MA, Ogden DA: Iron status in patients receiving erythropoietin for dialysis-associated anemia. Kidney Int 1989;35:712–716.

33 Eschbach JW, Downing MR, Egrie JC, Browne JK, Adamson JW: USA multicenter clinical trial with recombinant human erythropoietin (Amgen). Results in hemodialysis patients; in Baldamus CA, Koch KM, Scigalla P, Wieczorek L (eds): Erythropoietin: From Molecular Structure to Clinical Application. Contr Nephrol. Basel, Karger, 1989, vol 76, pp 160–165.

Hjalmar B. Steinhauer, MD, Medizinische Universitäts-Klinik, Abteilung IV, Nephrologie, Hugstetterstrasse 55, D–W–7800 Freiburg i. Br. (FRG)

Differential Indications for Peritoneal Dialysis

La Greca G, Olivares J, Feriani M, Passlick-Deetjen J (eds): CAPD – A Decade
of Experience. Contrib Nephrol. Basel, Karger, 1991, vol 89, pp 224–230

Patient Selection and Dialysis Prescription in Peritoneal Dialysis

Jose A. Diaz-Buxo

Home Dialysis, Metrolina Kidney Center, Charlotte, N.C., USA

The success of dialytic therapy depends on the proper selection of
patients and the formulation of appropriate prescriptions. A multidisciplin-
ary approach is recommended to effectively match these two entities. Our
therapeutic goal in the treatment of uremic patients should be to provide the
most adequate dialytic therapy with minimal infliction of psychological or
physical pain in a convenient and cost-effective manner. This approach
demands knowledge of the patient's psychosocial and medical condition as
well as the capabilities and limitations of therapy.

The experience gathered during the past decade with continuous ambulatory (CAPD) peritoneal dialysis or continuous cyclic peritoneal dialysis
(CCPD) has shown good acceptance of this therapy, effective solute and fluid
removal on a chronic basis, comparable patient survival to hemodialysis and
competitive cost [1–4]. Nonetheless, the rate of transfer to hemodialysis and the
high incidence of certain complications remain a concern and deserve further
analysis. The cumulative probability of transfer to hemodialysis or abandonment of therapy for CAPD patients in the USA is 34% at 2 years and 52% at 4
years [1]. The main reasons for transfer are peritonitis and exit site infections
(36%), individual choice (17%) and inadequate dialysis (8%). The incidence of
all three complications can be reduced by identifying patients at high risk and by
offering them alternative therapy, whether hemodialysis or another modality of
peritoneal dialysis, by providing special assistance (partners, disconnecting
devices, manual aids) or by altering their dialysis prescription.

Table 1. Considerations in selecting patients for dialysis

Psychosocial considerations	*Physical/medical considerations*
Independence/self-care	Peripheral vascular tree
Self-image	Cardiovascular status
Family/social support	Pulmonary function
Phobias	Diabetes mellitus
Activity/work schedule	Visual/neuromuscular disabilities
Compliance	Bleeding diathesis
Hygiene	Hernias
	Gastrointestinal abnormalities
	Back pain
	Body mass
	Residual renal function

Patient Selection

The psychosocial and medical characteristics of the patient materially affect the success of continuous peritoneal dialysis (CPD). Table 1 lists some of the important considerations in the selection of therapy. Among the psychosocial aspects, desire to undergo self-dialysis, acceptance of a rigid schedule for dialysis and the presence of a peritoneal catheter are of prime importance. Phobia of blood and needles turn many patients towards CPD while abdominal catheters have a negative impact on other patients' sexual performance and self-image. Personal and environmental hygiene should also be considered due to the risk of infectious complications.

The physical and medical considerations are, to a great extent, easier to evaluate. The lack of adequate peripheral blood vessels for the creation of an arteriovenous shunt, unstable cardiovascular status and bleeding diathesis favor the selection of peritoneal dialysis. Patients with severe visual and neuromuscular disabilities, commonly present among diabetics, favor the selection of CCPD or CAPD with special disconnecting assist devices. Individuals at high risk of developing hernias, gastrointestinal reflux, back pain and other complications associated with increased intra-abdominal pressure benefit from CCPD with low diurnal dialysate volumes. Small individuals with significant residual renal function may enjoy the convenience of intermittent peritoneal dialysis (IPD) while those with ultrafiltration failure due to increased solute transport rates may require nocturnal peritoneal dialysis (NPD).

Peritoneal Dialysis Prescription

The first step in determining the peritoneal dialysis prescription is to define the required solute and fluid removal necessary for the patient in question. These dialytic needs will be affected by: (1) peritoneal solute transport rate; (2) dietary protein intake (DPI); (3) fluid intake; (4) body mass, and (5) residual renal function. The next step is to adapt a prescription to the available modalities of peritoneal therapy (CAPD, CCPD, NPD, TPD (tidal PD), IPD) and the selection of dialysis solutions, dialysate volume, dwell time and number of exchanges. The specific dialytic needs of the patient will limit the choice of modality and patient predilection will further narrow the choice.

Peritoneal solute transport rates can be adequately characterized with serial timed measurements of peritoneal equilibration using a standard peritoneal equilibration test (PET) [5, 6]. The study can be simplified to include a 4-hour dialysate plasma ratio (D/P) determination for urea and creatinine, D_4/D_0 (dialysate dextrose concentration at 4 h/dialysate dextrose concentration immediately postinfusion) and net ultrafiltration. The experience gathered during the past 3 years with more than 100 patients studied at the start of peritoneal dialysis and periodically thereafter suggests that the PET is a valuable diagnostic and prognostic tool [7].

Based on the results of our PET determinations and their clinical correlation, we have empirically categorized peritoneal permeability as: (1) normal, for D/P and D/D_0 (dialysate dextrose concentration at various times/dialysate dextrose concentration immediately postinfusion) values within the range of the mean ± 1 SD; (2) high, for D/P values $>$ mean ± 1 SD and the $D/D_0 <$ mean -1 SD; and (3) low, for D/P values $<$ mean -1 SD and $D/D_0 >$ mean $+1$ SD [6]. Our experience parallels the results published by Twardowski et al. [5] using the standard PET.

Table 2 summarizes the numerical ranges for D/P_{4h} creatinine, D_4/D_0, drain volume for different peritoneal permeability states, their clinical correlation and therapeutic recommendations. Most patients with PET values within 1 SD of the mean can maintain adequate biochemical control and ultrafiltration with CAPD/CCPD. Patients with mild to moderately increased permeability maintain good solute clearances, but may require transfer to NPD in order to reduce glucose absorption and achieve adequate ultrafiltration. When solute transport is severely impaired (D/P $>$ mean $+2$ SD or $D/D_0 <$ mean -2 SD), ultrafiltration is rarely achieved and transfer to hemodialysis is often needed.

Table 2. Peritoneal equilibration test-differential diagnosis and therapeutic recommendations

	Peritoneal permeability		
	high	normal	low
$D/P_{creatinine\ (4\ h)}$	$> \bar{x} + 1\ SD\ (>0.85)$	$\bar{x} \pm 1\ SD\ (0.72 \pm 0.13)$	$< \bar{x} - 1\ SD\ (<0.59)$
D_4/D_0	$< \bar{x} - 1\ SD\ (<0.26)$	$\bar{x} \pm 1\ SD\ (0.38 \pm 0.12)$	$> \bar{x} + 1\ SD\ (>0.50)$
Drain volume, ml	$< \bar{x} - 1\ SD\ (<2,113)$	$\bar{x} \pm 1\ SD\ (2,385 \pm 272)$	$> \bar{x} + 1\ SD\ (>2,657)$
Clinical findings	low UF	adequate dialysis and UF	progressive azotemia, high UF early and low UF late
Therapeutic recommendations	NPD (short, frequent cycles)	CAPD/CCPD	increase exchange volume, transfer to HD

Conversely, patients with mild to moderately reduced permeability suffer from low solute clearances and develop progressive azotemia. Increments in the dialysate exchange volume help compensate for the reduced rate of solute transport. High ultrafiltration results from decreased glucose absorption and maintenance of a high osmotic gradient in the early stages. However, as the process becomes more severe (peritoneal sclerosis) water transport across the peritoneum ceases. Transfer to hemodialysis is recommended if azotemia cannot be adequately controlled.

Serial application of the PET has identified several patterns of peritoneal transport [8]. The majority of patients exhibit normal permeability at the inception of therapy and remain stable during the course of treatment (>80%). A small proportion of patients begin peritoneal dialysis with normal peritoneal permeability, but subsequently develop high permeability (5–10%). Multiple etiologic factors have been proposed for this development (peritonitis, plasticizers, drugs, acetate), but none has been consistently identified. Among these patients, some have reverted to normal permeability upon temporary discontinuation of peritoneal dialysis while a few have progressed to low permeability states and peritoneal sclerosis [8, 9]. Finally, a small number of patients (5–7%) exhibit high peritoneal permeability on initial evaluation and remain stable after several years on continuous peritoneal dialysis.

The PET has proven valuable as a diagnostic tool in orienting the clinician in the selection of dialytic modality and is a sensitive instrument for monitoring peritoneal transport. However, in the final assessment of adequacy of dialysis we need a quantitative method that allows comparison of patients on various dialysis schedules and that can correlate dietary protein intake (DPI), body mass, solute clearance and nitrogenous waste product concentrations in the blood. Such an approach has been tested in the hemodialysis population using urea kinetic modeling by the National Cooperative Dialysis Study (NCDS) [10]. The NCDS revealed that urea kinetic guided hemodialysis can reduce dialysis-related morbidity. Highly significant differences in morbidity were noted between patients with high time average urea concentrations (TAC_{urea} 100 mg/dl) and those with lower levels (TAC_{urea} 50 mg/dl). It also correlated the impact of the dialytic process (clearance) and diet. The goal of applying this concept is to provide uniform and adequate therapy while maintaining neutral nitrogen balance at a level of urea nitrogen concentration which is not associated with uremic toxicity.

Teehan et al. [11] have recognized the importance of this well-tested model and applied it to CAPD. Among the potential limitations of this method figure the relatively low clearance of urea in CAPD and our inability to compare TAC_{urea} between CAPD and hemodialysis patients. Given the high permeability of the peritoneal membrane, as compared to hemodialysis, one could conceivably expect comparable clinical results with higher TAC_{urea} values.

The basis of urea kinetic modeling in CAPD is that BUN (TAC_{urea} in the stable CAPD patient) is directly proportional to protein intake and inversely proportional to nitrogen removal. Thus, when intake and removal are equal, BUN remains constant and neutral nitrogen balance is maintained.

The urea kinetic model defines dialysis prescription as:

$$KT/V = 1, \text{ or } KT = V, \tag{1}$$

where KT is the total urea nitrogen clearance, or

$$KT = KD + KR, \tag{2}$$

where KD is the urea nitrogen clearance provided by dialysis and KR is the renal urea nitrogen clearance. V is the urea volume of distribution (equivalent to total body water), or

$$V = (0.5 \, ♀, 0.6 \, ♂) \times IBW, \tag{3}$$

where IBW represents ideal body weight in kilograms multiplied by a factor of 0.5 for females and 0.6 for males.

Since in CAPD urea in the drained dialysate is in equilibrium with plasma, drainage volume (DV) is equivalent to dialysis clearance (KD):

$$DV = KD. \tag{4}$$

In order to relate drainage volume to target BUN (T_{BUN}), protein intake (DPI) and residual renal function (KR), we can use the following formula:

$$DV = (N\ intake) - (nonurea\ N\ losses + KR \times T_{BUN})/T_{BUN}. \qquad (5)$$

The necessary DPI to maintain nitrogen balance in CAPD patients should be ≥ 1.2 g/kg/day [12]. This level of protein intake is higher than that necessary for hemodialysis, probably due to the constant peritoneal protein and amino acid losses. These losses are relatively stable and account for 1,290 mg of nitrogen/day from protein and 520 mg/day for amino acids. In addition, 31–32 mg/kg IBW/day of nitrogen are lost from other sources (uric acid, creatinine, etc.). Residual renal function (KR) can be measured as urea nitrogen clearance (ml/min). Thus, equation 5 becomes:

$$DV = (DPI \times 160 \times IBW) - (1,810 + 31\ IBW + KR \times 1,440 \times T_{BUN})/T_{BUN}, \qquad (6)$$

where DPI is expressed in kg, T_{BUN} in mg/ml, 160 is the conversion factor for g protein to mg nitrogen, and 1,440 are the min/day. Assuming a DPI of 1.2 g/kg/day and a target BUN of 70 mg/dl equation 6 can be simplified to:

$$DV = 0.23 \times IBW - (2.6 + 1.44 \times KR). \qquad (7)$$

Indeed, this formula for urea kinetic modeling for CAPD can also be applied to a partial equilibrium system if a 24-hour collection of the drainage volume is obtained and the D/P ratio is calculated. In such case the drainage volume required to achieve the target BUN of 70 mg/dl would be:

$$DV = 0.23 \times IBW - (2.6 + 1.44 \times KR)/D/P. \qquad (8)$$

Conclusions

The last decade of investigation has produced new and improved peritoneal dialysis techniques, simple and reproducible tools to evaluate peritoneal transport and quantitative methods for evaluation of dialysis capable of correlating dialysis efficiency with nutritional parameters. Thus, we have most of the ingredients for a dialysis prescription.

A most important term, however, remains undefined – the adequacy of dialysis. For lack of a better definition we should strive for that amount of dialysis which frees the patient of all possible uremic manifestations and restores the state of normal health. Prescription dialysis promises to both help in quantitating therapy and making possible the comparison of individuals dialyzed by different modalities and in different places, and correlating dialysis with morbidity and mortality. The systematic and scientific application of these concepts may very well reduce the rate of complications and improve the survival time and quality of life of the patient.

References

1 Lindblad A, Novak JW, Nolph KD (eds): Continuous Ambulatory Peritoneal Dialysis in the USA – Final Report of the National CAPD Registry 1981–1988. Dordrecht, Kluwer, 1989.
2 Posen GA, Arbus GS, Hutchinson T, et al: Dialysis in Canada; in LaGreca G, Chiaramonte S, Fabris A, Feriani M, Ronco C (eds): Peritoneal Dialysis. Milano, Wichtig Editore, 1988, pp 207–212.
3 Maiorca R, Cancarini G, Manili L, Brunori G, Camerini C, Strada A, Feller P: CAPD is a first class treatment. Results of an eight-year experience with a comparison of patient and method survival in CAPD and hemodialysis. Clin Nephrol 1988;30:S3–S7.
4 Diaz-Buxo JA: Current status of CCPD. Periton Dial Int 1989;9:9–14.
5 Twardowski ZJ, Nolph KD, Khanna R, et al: Peritoneal equilibration test. Periton Dial Bull 1987;7:138.
6 Diaz-Buxo JA: Peritoneal permeability and the selection of peritoneal dialysis modalities. Perspect Periton Dial 1988;5:6–10.
7 Diaz-Buxo JA: Inadequacy of dialysis – a preventable cause of drop out; in La Greca G, Chiaramonte S, Fabris A, Feriani M, Ronco C (eds): Peritoneal Dialysis. Milano, Wichtig Editore, 1988, pp 177–180.
8 Diaz-Buxo JA: Natural history of abnormal peritoneal permeability states; in La Greca G, Chiaramonte S, Fabris A, Feriani M, Ronco C (eds): Peritoneal Dialysis. Milano, Wichtig Editore, 1988, pp 181–185.
9 Verger C, Larpent L, Dumontet M: Prognostic value of peritoneal equilibration curves in CAPD patients; in Maher JF, Winchester JF (eds): Frontiers in Peritoneal Dialysis. New York, Field Rich, 1986, pp 88–93.
10 Lowrie EG: Cooperative dialysis study. Kidney Int 1983;23:S1–S122.
11 Teehan BP, Schleifer CR, Sigler MH, Gilgore GS: A quantitative approach to the CAPD prescription. Periton Dial Bull 1985;5:152–156.
12 Blumenkrantz MJ, Kopple JD, Moran JK, et al: Metabolic balance studies and dietary protein requirements in patients undergoing continuous ambulatory peritoneal dialysis. Kidney Int 1982;21:849–896.

Jose A. Diaz-Buxo, MD, FACP, Director, Home Dialysis, Metrolina Kidney Center, 928 Baxter Street, Charlotte, NC 28204 (USA)

La Greca G, Olivares J, Feriani M, Passlick-Deetjen J (eds): CAPD – A Decade of Experience. Contrib Nephrol. Basel, Karger, 1991, vol 89, pp 231–236

Choice of Treatment Modality for the Infant, Child and Adolescent with End-Stage Renal Disease

Richard N. Fine[1]

UCLA Center for the Health Sciences, Los Angeles, Calif., USA

Within the past quarter of a century attitudes have changed dramatically regarding the acceptability of pediatric patients with end-stage renal disease (ESRD) for embarking upon the new treatment modalities of dialysis and renal transplantation. In the past the psychosocial and physical trauma of ESRD care was considered so great and the potential benefits so minimal that in many areas of the world, pediatric patients were not considered acceptable candidates for ESRD care. However, there has been sufficient progress in the past two decades in adapting these treatment modalities to the pediatric population and the outcome of utilizing these modalities in children has been sufficiently rewarding that few physicians caring for children in the 'developed' countries would currently deny pediatric patients access to treatment.

Nevertheless, when contemplating initiating a treatment program for the infant, child or adolescent with ESRD there are a number of factors that require consideration. The primary factors are as follows: patient age, mental status, psychosocial status, and primary renal disease. In this presentation I will consider the factors surrounding the patient's age which impact upon the selection of treatment modality.

[1] This manuscript was completed during the time Dr. Fine was recipient of the United States Senior Research Scientist Award of The Alexander von Humboldt Foundation.

Infants (Birth to 2 Years)

The indications for initiating dialysis in the infant differ significantly from those used in the older pediatric patient. These include the following: failure to achieve normal developmental milestones, failure to attain normal statural length and normal weight, and development of progressive bone disease.

Infants who manifest renal failure during the first year of life frequently have concomitant neurologic abnormalities. This was emphasized initially in the report of Rotundo et al. [1]. These authors described profound neurologic abnormalities consisting of developmental delay, microcephaly, hypotonia and seizures in 20 of 23 infants with the onset of renal failure during the first year of life. The precise etiology of these neurologic abnormalities was not apparent; but aluminum (AL) toxicity was somewhat discounted because 4 of the infants had never received AL-containing phosphate binders. However, Freundlich et al. [2] subsequently demonstrated elevated brain AL levels in 2 infants with chronic renal failure (CRF) who died in the first year of life without receiving any AL-containing phosphate binders. The authors implicated the AL content of the infant's formula as the source of the high brain AL levels. Although the incidence of severe neurologic abnormalities in infants with the onset of renal failure during the first year of life has diminished somewhat with the substitution of calcium carbonate as the phosphate binder of choice in infants and children with CRF, it appears that developmental delay remains a significant problem. Uremia in all probability has an adverse impact on the developing brain, although the exact mechanism has not been definitively elucidated.

The major unanswered question is if the earlier initiation of dialysis in the infant with CRF would minimize the adverse impact of uremia on the developing brain. Before such a question can be answered it will be necessary to devise more precise measures of subtle developmental deviation. The tests currently used depend upon the infant's motor skills to indicate developmental progress. Since infants with CRF have delayed motor development, it may not be possible to utilize these tests to accurately assess attainment of development milestones in the uremic infant. Therefore, pre-emptive dialysis to prevent the adverse neurologic consequences of uremia on the infant is not recommended at the present time. However, if the infant demonstrates significant deviation of the attainment of developmental milestones or significant progressive neurologic abnormalities, it may be prudent to consider initiation of dialysis.

Growth retardation is a common occurrence in pediatric patients with CRF. Multiple factors have been implicated, although a precise etiology is unknown [3]. In normal infants there is a rapid period of growth during the first 2 years of life. Therefore, any factors which impact negatively on growth during this period will have profound consequences on the ultimate statural height of the infant. Indeed, Betts and McGrath [4] demonstrated that the growth impairment of infants with CRF during the first 2 years of life adversely impacted on ultimate adult height. Growth velocity lost during this period was rarely regained despite subsequent therapeutic interventions.

The relationship between insufficient caloric intake and growth retardation in infants with CRF remains to be validated; however, it is important to assure that the infant consumes at least the recommended daily allowance (RDA) for age. If this is not possible it has been recommended that a nasogastric (NG) tube be inserted and supplemental nightime NG feedings be prescribed to assure adequate caloric intake.

Recently, recombinant human growth hormone (rhGH) has been shown to be effective in stimulating an acceleration in growth velocity in growth-retarded children with CRF [5]. It is possible that the prophylactic use of rhGH in the future will thwart the development of growth retardation and eliminate this clinical manifestation as an indication to initiate dialysis in the infant with CRF. However, at the present time, it would be judicious to carefully monitor the growth velocity of the infant with CRF, and if significant deceleration occurs, it would be prudent to consider initiation of dialysis. As indicated previously, growth loss during the first 2 years of life is rarely regained subsequently. Therefore, vigorous attempts should be made to minimize the magnitude of the loss.

The last unique indication to initiate dialysis in the infant with CRF is the avoidance of bone disease. Renal osteodystrophy (ROD) in infants can result in severe osseous deformities. Once these develop complicated orthopedic surgical procedures are often required that do not always lead to optimal cosmetic correction. Therefore, prevention is advisable. The judicious use of vitamin D analogues and phosphate binders is usually sufficient to prevent severe ROD; however, if progressive ROD ensues despite these preventative measures it is, at times, advantageous to initiate dialysis in an attempt to curtail progression of ROD and to affect a resolution.

During the past decade the preferred mode of dialysis has changed markedly for the infant with ESRD. Prior to the availability of continuous ambulatory peritoneal dialysis (CAPD) and continuous cycling peritoneal dialysis (CCPD), hemodialysis (HD) was the only modality available. Prolonged HD is rather difficult in infants because of the dietary restrictions required and the limited number of vascular access sites. In contrast, both CAPD and CCPD are feasible long-term dialytic modalities for infants.

Psychosocial factors dictate that CCPD is the optimal dialytic modality for the infant. The requirement for only one connection/disconnection daily with CCPD in contrast to at least 5 or 6 with CAPD is much easier for the working parent(s) or the parent with other young children at home. It is unusual for 4 CAPD exchanges to adequately control the fluid and biochemical abnormalities in the uremic infant; therefore, additional exchanges are required which are cumbersome for the caretaker. The cycler also facilitates delivery of more precise dialysate volumes than that obtainable with the commercially available CAPD dialysate volumes. An additional advantage of CCPD is that it facilitates an empty peritoneum during the day, which may have a salutary effect on the infant's food consumption.

The timing of renal transplantation in infants is dictated by the potential short- and long-term results, and the availability of a donor organ. Cadaver donor transplantation in the first year of life has been universally dismal [6]; whereas, recent data indicated the potential for a good short-term outcome with cadaver donor transplantation during the second year of life [7]. Short-term results of live-related donor transplantation in infancy are acceptable [7, 8]; however, only limited data are available.

Currently, it is generally recommended that transplantation in infants be delayed until approximately 2 years of age when the infant attains a weight of approximately 10 kg. This policy has two advantages. First, it limits the catabolic consequences of transplantation during the period of rapid growth and, second, it minimizes the pressure on parents to make an immediate decision regarding live-related organ donation.

Pre-School-Age Children (2–5 Years)

The unique indications for initiating dialysis in the pre-school-aged child are to maximize growth, improve nutritional status and avoid significant ROD. These are in addition to alleviation of the symptoms of uremia.

Repetitive HD is certainly possible in the pre-school-aged child; however, the necessity for repetitive fistula puncture and severe dietary restrictions in the oliguric child make this dialytic modality less desirable. Both CAPD and CCPD are better tolerated by the pre-school-aged child. Reduction in the parental tasks required with CCPD make that the modality of choice.

The timing of transplantation in the pre-school-aged child is determined by two opposing factors: the potential increased immunologic responsiveness of the young child reducing graft survival rates [8], and the potential for accelerated growth following successful transplantation in children <7 years of age [9]. Currently, the availability of a donor kidney is the primary factor determining the timing of transplantation.

School-Aged Children (6–11 Years)

The indications to initiate dialysis in the school-aged child are similar to those for the adolescent and adult patient with ESRD: clinical manifestations of uremia; glomerular filtration rate <5 ml/min/1.73 m²; progressive ROD despite optimal medical management, and the inability to undertake the usual daily functions. The latter should be observed rather carefully because the school-aged child will deny symptoms in order to avoid initiating dialysis.

The choice of dialytic modality is dependent upon patient and parent preference. With increasing frequency either home dialysis modality of CAPD/CCPD is being chosen. CCPD is usually preferred, if available, because it avoids the requirement for an exchange at school, which limits the exposure of the child to peer scrutiny.

The timing of transplantation is solely dependent upon the availability of a donor kidney. As indicated previously, posttransplant growth appears to be superior in younger children; therefore, there is no justification to delay transplantation in the school-aged child.

Adolescents

The indications for initiating dialysis in the adolescent patient are similar to those used in the adult patient with ESRD. Adolescents tend to deny symptoms and, therefore, it is important to monitor the biochemical parameters of uremia rather closely in order to avoid clinical catastrophes.

In the adolescent patient the choice of dialytic modality is primarily the patient's. With increasing frequency the adolescent patient is choosing a home dialysis modality. This is being motivated by the desire to 'be in control of their own destiny'. CAPD/CCPD offer this possibility. In our experience CCPD is the modality of choice because it eliminates the need for daytime exchanges at school.

The major liability with either CAPD or CCPD in the adolescent is the potential for noncompliance with the therapeutic regimen. Such noncompliance can have catastrophic consequences; therefore, constant surveillance is mandatory when caring for the adolescent undergoing home peritoneal dialysis.

Transplantation can proceed in the adolescent when a donor kidney becomes available. As during the period of dialysis, it is imperative to constantly monitor the adolescent patient following transplantation in order to detect noncompliance at the earliest moment.

References

1   Rotundo, A.; Nevins, T.E.; Lipton, M.; et al.: Progressive encephalopathy in children with chronic renal insufficiency in infancy. Kidney int. *21:* 486 (1982).

2   Freundlich, M.; Zilleruelo, G.; Abitol, C.; et al.: Infant formula as a cause of aluminium toxicity in neonatal uremia. Lancet *ii:* 527–529 (1985).

3   Fine, R.N.: Growth in children with renal insufficiency; in Nissenson, Fine, Gentile, Clinical dialysis, p. 661 (Appelton-Century-Crofts, Norwalk 1984).

4   Betts, P.R.; McGrath, G.: Growth pattern and dietary intake of children with chronic renal insufficiency. Br. med. J. *ii:* 189–193 (1974).

5   Koch, V.H.; Lippe, B.M.; Nelson, P.A.; et al.: Accelerated growth following recombinant human growth hormone treatment of children with chronic renal failure. J. Pediat. *115:* 365–371 (1989).

6   Fine, R.N.: Renal transplantation in children; in Morris, Kidney transplantation: principles and practice; 2nd ed., p. 509 (Grune & Stratton, New York 1984).

7   Kohaut, E.C.; Whelchel, J.; Waldo, F.B.; et al.: Aggressive therapy of infants with renal failure. Pediat. Nephrol. *1:* 150–153 (1987).

8   So, S.K.S.; Nevins, T.E.; Change, P.N.; et al.: Preliminary results of renal transplantation in children under 1 year of age. Transplant. Proc. *17:* 182–183 (1985).

9   Ingelfinger, G.R.; Grupe, W.E.; Harmon, W.E.; Fernbach, S.K.; Levey, R.H.: Growth acceleration following renal transplantation in children less than 7 years of age. Pediatrics *68:* 255–259 (1981).

Richard N. Fine, MD, Department of Pediatrics, State University of New York (Suny) at Stony Brook, Stony Brook, NY 11794–8111 (USA)

La Greca G, Olivares J, Feriani M, Passlick-Deetjen J (eds): CAPD – A Decade of Experience. Contrib Nephrol. Basel, Karger, 1991, vol 89, pp 237–242

CAPD and Systemic Diseases

C. Michel, P. Bindi, P. Dosquet, F. Mignon

Service de Néphrologie, Hôpital Tenon, Paris, France

Systemic diseases with severe renal involvement leading to end-stage renal failure (ESRD) and dialysis set up an uncommon but difficult problem in terms of management [1, 2]. Extrarenal manifestations of the underlying disease may enhance specific complications related to the dialysis method, such as vascular access problems and cardiovascular intolerance on hemodialysis or peritoneal dialysis (PD). On the other hand, the dialysis method may interfere with the progression of the systemic disease. A decade after the introduction of CAPD, controversy still exists about the advantages and drawbacks of CAPD versus hemodialysis in this group of patients.

Mutual impacts of the dialysis method and the systemic disease as well as specific complications are reviewed for systemic lupus erythematosus (SLE), myeloma, systemic amyloidosis and human immunodeficiency virus (HIV) infection, based on our own experiences and the literature.

Systemic Lupus Erythematosus

Since serologic and clinical extrarenal lupus activity has been generally reported to be minimal during hemodialysis in ESRD caused by lupus nephritis, usually no steroid or immunosuppressive therapy is necessary [3–7]. Coplon et al. [8] found only 3 of 28 patients with any evidence of clinical activity after starting hemodialysis, only 2 required prednisone. In the early 1980s, Correia et al. [9] reported a similar outcome in 5 patients on CAPD. More recently, a less favorable outcome was described by Wu et al. [10] in 3 patients who experienced a clinical and serologic reactivation of the SLE while being treated with PD. Rodby et al. [11] confirmed these findings in 8 patients. Less immunodepression by PD has been assumed as the cause of the less favorable outcome [12].

Table 1. Characteristics of SLE patients in a French multicenter study

	Hemodialysis group 1	CAPD group 2
Number of patients	32	13
Age at onset of SLE, years	23.2 ± 7.8	28 ± 13
SLE duration before dialysis, years	5.9 ± 4.4	8.7 ± 9
Active SLE at the onset of dialysis	7	7
Duration of dialysis, years	4.1 ± 2.5	2.4 ± 2

Table 2. Outcome of dialysis of SLE patients in a French multicenter study

	Hemodialysis group 1	CAPD group 2
Number of patients	32	13
Patients without SLE flares and corticoid requirements	22	5
Patients with SLE flares during dialysis	10	8
Duration of dialysis before the first flare, months	1–48	1–36
Mild flares	8	10
Severe flares	4	3
Deaths	0	2

We performed a multicenter retrospective study in 45 patients with ESRD caused by SLE who had been treated with dialysis for at least 6 months between 1980 and 1988. The diagnosis of SLE was according to the definition of the American Rheumatism Association. At the onset of dialysis lupus was classified as 'active' under the following conditions: recent clinical, renal and/or extrarenal, even minor, manifestations (such as skin or joint involvement), immunological and/or histological evidence of activity. The characteristics of the patients are summarized in table 1.

Table 2 shows the outcome of these patients on dialysis. While 22 patients on hemodialysis experienced no flares during the follow-up, 10 experienced 13 flares, which were easily cured with steroid therapy alone. No death related to lupus occurred. Five patients on PD were successfully treated by PD without flares and corticoid requirement during a mean dialysis duration of 4 years. The other 8 experienced 13 flares, 2 of them with active lupus at the initiation of the dialysis died in the first year of lupus cardiovascular flares (1 cardiomyopathy, 1 upperlimb phlebothrombosis with pulmonary embolism). Lupus flares were observed more frequently in each group, when SLE was still active at the onset of dialysis.

Our results are consistent with others [8, 13] who recently reported prolonged predialytic inactivity of clinical SLE being the best criterion for a good prognosis in hemodialysis patients.

Since HD and CAPD patients were significantly different regarding the SLE activity at the initiation of dialysis, no definitive conclusion could be drawn on the role of the dialysis modality. Clinicians, however, should be aware of a less favorable outcome, especially if lupus is active at the initiation of dialysis. Therefore, clinical and immunological data should be sequentially monitored.

Myeloma and Systemic Amyloidosis

Since PD may significantly increase light chain removal, CAPD may enhance reversal of renal failure in patients with nephrotoxic light chain disease. Yet, a superiority of PD over hemodialysis concerning the frequency of renal function recovery, ranging from 0 to 60%, could not be proved [14–17]. Only Cosio et al. [18] reported a more favorable outcome in terms of renal function recovery in patients on PD. However, PD cannot be recommended unless prospective studies have shown its benefits.

Myeloma patients on CAPD appear to have no increased incidence of peritonitis, unless an intensive induction chemotherapy is used. From 1983 to 1989, 5 patients with light chain myeloma were treated with CAPD at the Hôpital Tenon. Three patients suffered from low cell mass myeloma. Duration of treatment was 9.5, 12 and 16 months, respectively. Only 1 patient had a peritonitis episode. One patient recovered from renal failure, the other 2 died. Two patients with high cell mass myeloma undergoing intensive chemotherapy experienced peritonitis episodes very early (gram-negative and fungal). Duration of CAPD was 15 and 65 days, respectively. They had to be switched to hemodialysis.

Hence, the choice of dialysis modality in patients with myeloma-related renal failure should be based on the stage of the disease, the type of chemotherapy and the response to treatment.

In systemic amyloidosis CAPD has several advantages over hemodialysis especially regarding the high incidence of cardiac amyloid involvement and vascular access problems arising from amyloid deposits in large vessels. Nevertheless, malnutrition due to nephrotic syndrome and enteral amyloidosis may be increased by peritoneal protein losses being particularly high in this disease [20].

Human Immunodeficiency Virus (HIV) Infection

ESRD in HIV-infected patients is steadily increasing but there is no general agreement on the best dialysis modality for these patients [21–25]. As during PD treatment the risk of exposure of hospital staff to blood is lower, it has been advocated to be a safer method than hemodialysis. Nevertheless, the risk of HIV infection after documented exposure to the blood of a HIV-positive patient is relatively low. Recently, it was reported to be 0.42% in a cohort of about 1,000 health care workers [26]. The adherence to the guidelines for the care of hepatitis B virus-infected patients appears to be sufficient to prevent transmission of HIV in dialysis units [27]. There is no evidence hitherto that a patient has been infected with HIV during dialysis treatment [28].

On the other hand, several studies have demonstrated HIV antibodies and HIV antigen in PD effluent: Dratwa's group [29] in 1, ourselves in another, and Correa-Roter et al. [30] in 2 patients. Therefore, PD effluent is potentially infective and alertness is advisable for the related persons.

Another problem is the complication rate in these patients. The incidence of peritonitis was described as being extremely high by Kaul et al. [31] (1 episode per 2.7 patient-months) and by Dressler et al. [32] who observed a high incidence of pseudomonal and candidal peritonitis episodes. In accordance, we found in 3 patients a slightly better, but still high, peritonitis incidence of 1 episode per 12.5 patient-months, which occurred in 2 of these 3 patients. Germs isolated were *Pseudomonas aeruginosa* (2 episodes) and *Staphylococcus epidermidis* (1 episode).

On the other hand, according to our experience in 10 HIV patients on hemodialysis, fistula infection was rare, no staphylococcal septicemia occurred and only 2 patients experienced vascular access problems.

No justification remains for a preferred use of PD in HIV infection. Only the nutritional status, the stage of the infection and the personal abilities should be considered in the choice of dialysis treatment.

In conclusion, CAPD may provide a suitable treatment modality for selected patients in the management of systemic diseases with severe renal involvement. However, extrarenal complication of the underlying disease, combined treatment and the patient's choice should also be taken into account.

References

1 Cantaluppi A: CAPD and systemic diseases. Clin Nephrol 1988;30:S8–S12.
2 Michel C, Dosquet P, Viron B, et al: La dialyse péritonéale, méthode de traitement de l'insuffisance rénale terminale: évolution des indications au cours des dix dernières années en fonction de la maladie rénale initiale et des pathologies extrarénales. Néphrologie 1989;10(suppl):15–17.
3 Brown C, Rao T, Maxey R, et al: Regression of clinical and immunological expression of systemic lupus erythematosus consequent to development of uraemia. Kidney Int 1979;16:884.
4 Kimberly RP, Locksin MD, Sherman RL, et al: End-stage lupus nephritis: Clinical course to and outcome on dialysis – experience with 39 patients. Medicine 1981;60: 277–287.
5 Jarret MP, Santhernam S, Del Greco F: The clinical course of end-stage renal disease in systemic lupus erythematosus. Arch Intern Med 1983;143:1353–1356.
6 Ziff M, Helderman JH: Dialysis and transplantation in end-stage lupus nephritis. N Engl J Med 1983;308:218–219.
7 Cheigh J, Stenzel K, Rubin A, et al: Systemic lupus erythematosus in patients with chronic renal failure. Am J Med 1983;75:602–606.
8 Coplon NS, Diskin CJ, Petersen J, et al: The long term clinical course of systemic lupus erythematosus in end-stage renal disease. N Engl J Med 1983;308:186–190.
9 Correia P, Cameron JS, Ogg CS, et al: End-stage renal failure in systemic lupus erythematosus with nephritis. Clin Nephrol 1984;22:293–302.
10 Wu GG, Gelbart DR, Hasbargen JA, et al: Reactivation of systemic lupus in three patients undergoing CAPD. Periton Dial Bull 1986;6:6–9.
11 Rodby RA, Korbet SM, Lewis EJ: Persistence of clinical and serologic activity in patients with systemic lupus erythematosis undergoing peritoneal dialysis. Am J Med 1987;83:613–618.
12 Giacchino F, Pozatto M, Formica M, et al: Improved cell-mediated immunity in CAPD patients as compared to those on hemodialysis. Periton Dial Bull 1984;4: 209–212.
13 Sires RL, Adler SG, Louie JS, et al: Poor prognosis in end-stage lupus nephritis due to nonautologous vascular access site associated septicemia and lupus flares. Am J Nephrol 1989;9:279–284.
14 Johnson WJ, Kyle RA, Dahlberg PJ: Dialysis in the treatment of multiple myeloma. Mayo Clin Proc 1980;55:65–72.
15 Dahlberg PJ, Newcomer KL, Yutuc WR, et al: Myeloma kidney: Improved renal function following long-term chemotherapy and hemodialysis. Am J Nephrol 1983; 3:242–243.
16 Mallick NP: Uraemia in myeloma: Management and prognosis; in Minetti (ed): The Kidney in Plasma Cell Dyscrasies. Dordrecht, Kluwer Academic Publishers, 1988, pp 265–270.

17 Rota S, Mougenot B, Baudouin B, et al: Multiple myeloma and severe renal failure: A clinicopathologic study of outcome and prognosis in 34 patients. Medicine 1987; 66:126–137.

18 Cosio FG, Pence TV, Shapirio FL, et al: Severe renal failure in multiple myeloma. Clin Nephrol 1981;15:206–210.

19 Agostini L, Leon IK, Rojas M: Treatment with CAPD for 54 months of a patient with end stage renal disease due to multiple myeloma. Periton Dial Bull 1986;6:46.

20 Krediet RT, Boeschoten EW, Zuyderhoudt FMJ, Arisz L: Permeability of the peritoneum to proteins in continuous ambulatory peritoneal dialysis patients with systemic disease. Proc Eur Dialy Transplant Assoc 1985;22:405–409.

21 Humphreys MH, Schoenfeld P: Renal complications in patients with the acquired immune deficiency syndrome (AIDS). Am J Nephrol 1987;7:1–7.

22 Ortiz C, Meneses R, Jaffe D, et al: Outcome of patients with human immunodeficiency virus on maintenance hemodialysis. Kidney Int 1988;34:248–253.

23 Berlyne GM, Rubin J, Adler AJ: Dialysis in AIDS patients. Nephron 1986;44: 265–266.

24 Robles R, Lopez-Gomez JM, Muino A, et al: Dialysis in AIDS patients: A new problem. Nephron 1986;44:375–376.

25 Heering PJ, Bach D, Heinzler P, Grabensee B: Dialysis and HIV infection. Nephron 1987;47:158–159.

26 Marcus R, and CDC Cooperative Needlestick Surveillance Group: Surveillance of health care workers exposed to blood from patients infected with the human immunodeficiency virus. N Engl J Med 1988;319:1118–1123.

27 Recommendations for providing dialysis treatment to patients infected with human T-lymphotropic virus type III/lymphadenopathy-associated virus. Ann Intern Med 1986;105:558–559.

28 Perez GO, Ortiz C, De Medina M, et al: Lack of transmission of human immunodeficiency virus in chronic hemodialysis patients. Am J Nephrol 1988;8:123–126.

29 van Beers D, Dratwa M, Sprecher S, Smet L, et al: Peritoneal dialysis (PD) in AIDS – another risky situation? Periton Dial Int 1988;8:S56.

30 Correa-Roter R, Saldivar S, Soto LE, et al: HIV-AG in dialysis fluid of CAPD patients. Kidney Int 1989;35:268.

31 Kaul R, Faber M, Markowitz N, et al: Dialysis options for HIV infected patients. Periton Dial Int 1989;9:S89.

32 Dressler R, Peters AT, Lynn RI: Pseudomonal and candidal peritonitis as a complication of continuous ambulatory peritoneal dialysis in human immunodeficiency virus-infected patients. Am J Med 1989;86:787–790.

C. Michel, MD, Hôpital Tenon, Service de Néphrologie A,
4, rue de la Chine, F–75020 Paris (France)

La Greca G, Olivares J, Feriani M, Passlick-Deetjen J (eds): CAPD – A Decade of Experience. Contrib Nephrol. Basel, Karger, 1991, vol 89, pp 243–247

CAPD in Children with Special Aspects of Renal Transplantation

G. Offner, K. Latta, P.F. Hoyer

Medizinische Hochschule Hannover, Kinderklinik, Hannover, BRD

After the first reports of CAPD in children [1, 2], this method increasingly became the preferred dialysis modality for children [3, 4]. In the children's hospital of the Medical School of Hannover, CAPD and continuous cycling peritoneal dialysis (CCPD) were started in September 1984. Until 1988, a total number of 66 children were treated by this method, 29 with acute renal failure (ARF) and 37 with end-stage renal failure (ESRD). Thirty-one renal transplantations (RTx) were performed in 27 patients. In the following report the results are concentrated on the course and outcome of ARF, the problem of peritonitis in patients with ESRD and the benefit of CAPD/CCPD for RTx (table 1).

Continuous Peritoneal Dialysis for Acute Renal Failure

In case of ARF a removable curled Tenckhoff catheter without cuffs was implanted under general anesthesia. Twenty-nine children (17 male, 12 female) aged 1 day to 17.1 years (median 1.35 years) had to be dialysed for 1–86 days (median 9.0 days). Seventeen children regained renal function, 12 children died, which means a survival rate of 59% (table 1). The most common cause of ARF was the hemolytic uremic syndrome in 10 children who all recovered. Further causes with different outcomes were cardiac surgery, septicemia, dehydration, polytrauma, liver transplantation, rhabdomyolysis, vasculitis and decompensation of nephrotic syndrome. Death in all patients was due to the primary disease and not related to dialysis. Two patients developed peritonitis. No peritoneal leakage occurred, though cuffless catheters, which could easily be removed after recovery of renal function, were used.

Table 1. CAPD/CCPD in children with ARF, ESRD, and RTx (Hannover 1984–1988)

	ARF	ESRD	RTx
Patients, n	29	37	27[1]
Median age, years	1.35	11.6	9.6
Range	0.003–17.1	0.72–22.1	1.7–21.1
Median time on CAPD	9 days	6.6 months	4.0 months
Range	1–86 days	0.3–36 months	0.3–31 months
Patients survived	17 (59%)	34 (92%)	26 (96%)
Functioning grafts	–	–	24 (76%)
Peritonitis	2 patients	1/16.1 months	2 patients
Blood transfusion	–	1/4.7 months	23 patients

[1] 31 graftings (1st = 20, 2nd = 9, 3rd = 2).

Table 2. Blood chemistry of 18 patients with CAPD/CCPD after 6 months (mean ± 1 SD)

Calcium, mmol/l	2.50 ± 0.13
Phosphate, mmol/l	1.44 ± 0.23
Alkaline phosphatase, U/l	402 ± 370
Urea, mmol/l	21.8 ± 3.0

CAPD/CCPD for ESRD

During the same period 37 patients (13 male/24 female) with ESRD were on CAPD (24 patients) and CCPD (13 patients). Median age was 11.6 years and median dialysis time was 6.6 months (table 1). Three patients died, 1 of Wilm's tumor, 1 of septicemia after graft failure, and 1 of cardiac decompensation. Consequently, 34 (92%) patients survived. Blood transfusions were necessary every 4.7 months before we started erythropoietin therapy in June 1988.

The major problem was peritonitis. In 18 patients 28 episodes of peritonitis were observed with 57% culture-positive episodes. The organism mainly isolated was *Staphylococcus epidermidis*. The rate of peritonitis was 1 episode per 16.1 months.

In table 2 the blood chemistry of 18 patients who were on CAPD/CCPD for at least 6 months demonstrate a good control of the calcium-phosphate

Table 3. Growth rates of 13 children with CAPD/CCPD for 1 year

Pubertal stage	n	Age years	Mean growth rate cm/year
Prepubertal	1	0.7	9
Pubertal	8	8.5–12.5	2.5
Postpubertal	4	14.9–19.6	1.6

metabolism and urea. The growth rates of 13 children (1 infant, 8 prepubertal and 4 pubertal children) were reduced (table 3).

Renal Transplantation of Children with CAPD/CCPD

Twenty-seven patients (9 male/18 female), aged from 1.7 to 21.1 years, underwent 31 kidney transplantations (3 living related, 28 cadaveric) after a median time of 4 months. The ratio of 1st, 2nd, and 3rd grafting was 20 to 9 to 2 (table 1). The Tenckhoff catheter was removed after a mean time of 39 days after the beginning of graft function. In June 1989, 26 (96%) patients were alive and 24 (76%) grafts still functioned (table 1). Eleven patients were highly sensitized prior to transplantation due to previous graft loss or frequent blood transfusions. Their mean level of cytotoxic antibodies in the lymphocyte panel set decreased from 93.5 to 19.5% after a period of 8 to 28 months on CAPD/CCPD. Six of these patients have already been successfully transplanted (fig. 1). Two patients without decrease of cytotoxic antibodies had lost ultrafiltration capacity after peritonitis, and one was switched to hemodialysis.

Conclusion

Four years' experience with CAPD/CCPD in children demonstrated good results in ARF and ESRD as well as in RTx. In ARF, peritoneal dialysis enabled treatment of newborns and overcoming of the catabolic state with improved survival rates [5, 6]. In ESRD the problem of peritonitis was evident but the frequency of 1 episode per 16.1 months was tolerable compared to other pediatric CAPD experiences [7]. The blood transfusion

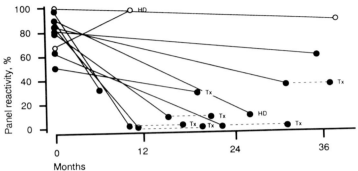

Fig. 1. Decrease of cytotoxic antibodies (panel reactivity) of 9 patients (filled circles) is depicted against the time on CAPD. Tx = Successful kidney transplantation of 6 patients. ○ = 2 patients without decrease of cytotoxic antibodies and with loss of ultrafiltration capacity. HD = 2 patients had to be switched to hemodialysis.

rate was 1 per 4.7 months before erythropoietin was available, which was clearly less than on hemodialysis while results of blood chemistry were comparable [8]. Growth rates were slightly improved compared to children on hemodialysis but still reduced. Therefore, kidney transplantation was the only replacement therapy which provided a satisfying rehabilitation of the children. The observed reduction of cytotoxic antibodies by CAPD/CCPD proved this method to be preferred for transplant recipients [9]. Patient survival of 96% with functioning grafts (76% after 3 years) are encouraging compared to the reported results of pediatric kidney transplantation [10].

References

1 Oreopulos DG, Robson M, Izatt S, Clyton S, DeVeber GA: A simple and safe technique for continuous ambulatory peritoneal dialysis (CAPD). Trans Am Soc Artif Intern Organs 1978;24:484–489.
2 Salusky IB, Kopple JD, Fine RN: Continuous ambulatory peritoneal dialysis in pediatric patients: A 20-month experience. Kidney Int 1983;24(suppl 15):101–105.
3 Bonzel KE, Mehls O, Mueller-Wiefel DE, Diekmann L, Wartha R, Ruder H, Rascher W, Schaerer K: Kontinuierliche ambulante Peritonealdialyse (CAPD) bei Kindern und Jugendlichen. Monatschr Kinderheilkd 1986;134:197–204.
4 Ehrich JHH, Rizzoni G, Broyer FP, Brynger H, Dykes SR, Geerlings W, Fassbinder W, Tufveson G, Selwood NH, Wing AJ: Combined report on regular dialysis and tranplantation of children in Europe, 1987. Nephrol Dial Transplant 1989; 4(suppl 2):33–41.

5 Abbad FCB, Ploos van Amstel SLB: CAPD in acute renal failure: Clinical experience in children; in Fine RN, Schaerer K, Mehls O (eds): CAPD in Children. Berlin, Springer 1985, pp 52–57.

6 Offner G, Brodehl J, Galaske R, Rutt T: Acute renal failure in children: Prognostic features after treatment with acute dialysis. Eur J Pediatr 1986;144:482–486.

7 Novello AC, Lindblad A, Novak JW, Nolph KD: Demographic data on the use of CAPD/CCPD as a primary dialytic therapy in children in the United States; in Fine RN (ed): Chronic Ambulatory Peritoneal Dialysis (CAPD) and Chronic Cycling Peritoneal Dialysis (CCPD) in Children. Dordrecht, Martinus Nijhoff, 1987, pp 13–20.

8 Offner G, Aschendorff C, Hoyer PF, Krohn HP, Ehrich JHH, Pichlmayr R, Brodehl J: Endstage renal failure: 14 years experience of dialysis and renal transplantation. Arch Dis Child 1988;63:120–126.

9 Latta K, Offner G, Hoyer PF, Brodehl J: Reduction of cytotoxic antibodies after continuous ambulatory peritoneal dialysis in highly sensitized patients. Lancet 1988;ii:847–848.

10 Offner G, Hoyer PF, Kron HP, Brodehl J: Cyclosporin A in paediatric kidney transplantation. Pediatr Nephrol 1987;1:125–133.

Dr. Gisela Offner, Medizinische Hochschule Hannover, Kinderklinik,
Konstanty Gutschowstrasse 8, D–W–3000 Hannover 61 (FRG)

La Greca G, Olivares J, Feriani M, Passlick-Deetjen J (eds): CAPD – A Decade of Experience. Contrib Nephrol. Basel, Karger, 1991, vol 89, pp 248–253

Hemodialysis and CAPD in Diabetic Patients

T. Tsobanelis[a], *P. Kurz*[a], *D. Hoppe*[a], *W. Schoeppe*[b], *J. Vlachojannis*[a]

[a]Medical Clinic II, St. Markus Hospital, and [b]Department of Nephrology, University Hospital, Frankfurt/M., FRG

According to 1986 EDTA annual report, the number of patients suffering from diabetic nephropathy has been steadily increasing over the past 10 years. At present, in Europe, 10% of new patients starting dialysis treatment are diabetics. The majority of diabetic patients belongs to the age group of 55–65 years [1]. Unfortunately, vascular alterations in long-term diabetes negatively affect the establishment and long-term duration of an adequate vascular access in treatment [2, 3]. The development of CAPD as an adequate dialysis modality comparable to hemodialysis, gave hope for a better and less complicated treatment of end-stage renal disease in elderly diabetic patients [4]. Specific laboratory data and clinical parameters of 51 selected elderly diabetic patients with end-stage renal disease, treated either with hemodialysis or with CAPD over a period of 8 years will be compared.

Patients and Methods

Twenty-five hemodialysis and 26 CAPD patients, similar in age (60 ± 12 and 62 ± 4, respectively), sex distribution (14 males, 11 females and 15 females, 11 females, respectively), and duration of treatment (25.6 ± 14.7 and 22.8 ± 17.4, respectively) were investigated. Four exchanges of 2 liters of dialysate with glucose concentrations of 1.36 and 3.86% were performed daily by CAPD patients. Hemodialysis patients were dialyzed 3 times a week for a total of 15 h by means of a hollow fiber dialyzer. The glucose concentration in the dialysate was 1.0 or 2.0 g/l. The effect on diabetic metabolism of the two treatment modalities were investigated by comparing biochemical data, arterial blood pressure, patient survival rate and causes of death.

Student's t-test was utilized to analyze the differences between the two groups.

Table 1. Effect of dialysis on biochemical parameters after 6 months of therapy

	Hemodialysis	CAPD	p
Potassium, mmol/l	5.3 ± 0.7	4.6 ± 0.5	<0.001
Sodium, mmol/l	136 ± 2.5	138 ± 2.0	<0.05
Creatinine, mg/dl	9.8 ± 2.0	7.7 ± 1.2	<0.001
Urea, mg/dl	134 ± 34	78 ± 10	<0.001
Calcium, mmol/l	2.3 ± 0.25	2.3 ± 0.2	n.s.
Inorganic phosphate, mg/dl	5.2 ± 1.2	5.1 ± 1.5	n.s.
Alkaline phosphatase, U/l	162 ± 70	146 ± 87	n.s.

Results and Discussion

Table 1 depicts some biochemical data of the two populations after 6 months of therapy

As expected, significantly lower serum levels of creatinine and urea were detected in CAPD patients in comparison with hemodialysis patients. On the contrary, no significant differences between the two groups were found regarding calcium, inorganic phosphate and alkaline phosphatase.

The course of renal anemia did not differ statistically in CAPD and hemodialysis patients (table 2). Hyperlipidemia, a common complication of diabetic patients, was not improved by the treatments. On the other hand, glucose absorption from the dialysate and protein losses across the peritoneal membrane could account for the higher but not significant rise in serum lipids of the CAPD group (table 2).

Mean fasting blood glucose levels ranged between 160 and 180 mg/dl and no significant differences between the two groups were observed (table 2).

In hemodialysis patients major therapeutic changes were not needed in order to control blood glucose levels: only 2 patients were switched to insulin therapy as a consequence of dialysis treatment. On the contrary, the majority of patients treated by diet restrictions or oral antidiabetic medication before the beginning of CAPD treatment, required insulin administration when dialysis was started (table 3).

The influence of the two different dialysis modalities on blood pressure control is depicted in figure 1. The mean values of systolic, diastolic and mean arterial pressure are shown in the upper part of the figure, while the

Table 2. Effect of dialysis on biochemical parameters

	Hb g/dl	Hct %	Triglycerides mg/dl	Cholesterol mg/dl	Fasting glucose mg/dl
Start					
HD	8.7 ± 0.5	25.6 ± 1.0	338 ± 49	202 ± 13	162 ± 9.2
CAPD	8.8 ± 0.4	26.5 ± 1.1	339 ± 61	236 ± 18	146 ± 8.8
6 months					
HD	9.0 ± 1.8	27 ± 1.0	408 ± 92	223 ± 20	159 ± 7.4
CAPD	9.3 ± 1.7	27 ± 1.1	529 ± 72	238 ± 12	199 ± 17.0
12 months					
HD	8.7 ± 0.4	27 ± 1.1	416 ± 64	217 ± 17	148 ± 9.7
CAPD	9.4 ± 0.4	28 ± 1.2	505 ± 102	253 ± 25	174 ± 19.0
24 months					
HD	8.9 ± 0.6	27 ± 1.8	321 ± 61	213 ± 18	149 ± 11.5
CAPD	9.3 ± 0.7	28 ± 1.6	421 ± 110	247 ± 20	160 ± 16.4

$\bar{x}$ ± SE, p = n.s.

Table 3. Blood glucose control before and during dialysis

	CAPD (n = 26)		Hemodialysis (n = 25)	
	before	during	before	during
Dietary treatment	8	1	5	1
Antidiabetic medication	4	3	8	10
Insulin dependent	14	22	12	14

lower part illustrates the number of patients needing antihypertensive medication for satisfactory control of blood pressure.

CAPD treatment led to a better control of hypertension and consequently antihypertensive medication could be reduced. After 6 months of treatment, blood pressure was nearly within the normal range. The percentage of patients with antihypertensive medication dropped from 85 to 28%. In hemodialysis, despite the adjustment of therapy, blood pressure was

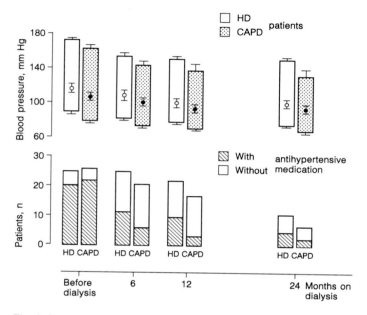

Fig. 1. Control of blood pressure in diabetic patients on regular dialysis treatment.

slightly higher and 44% of the patients still required antihypertensive medication.

The survival rate of both groups of patients is shown in figure 2; 96% of the hemodialysis patients survived the first year of treatment, compared to 82% of the CAPD patients. After 2 years the percentages fell to 70 and 65%, respectively, and reached 64 and 58%, respectively, after 3 years. However, no statistically significant difference between the two groups were found.

The various causes of death in diabetic hemodialysis and CAPD patients are given in table 4. Cardiovascular complications accounted for the majority of deaths in both groups. Peritonitis is a common complication in CAPD treatment, while fistula occlusion frequently occurs in hemodialysis patients. Comparing both types of events, the rate of peritonitis was 1/12 months and the rate of fistula revisions was 1/13 months. While in our population the drop out rate was 42% after 3 years, other authors report a higher drop out rate [4–6].

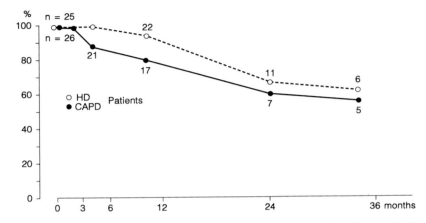

Fig. 2. Patient survival rate of diabetic patients on hemodialysis and CAPD treatment.

Table 4. Causes of death in diabetic patients on hemodialysis and CAPD treatment

	Hemodialysis	CAPD
Myocardial infarction	4	3
Peripherovascular diseases	2	4
Cerebrovascular complications	1	1
Gastrointestinal complications	1	2
Marasmus	1	1
Total	9	11

Conclusion

The number of patients in this study is too small to allow statistically acceptable conclusions. However, it can be stated that, when the two dialysis methods are compared in elderly diabetic patients, neither seems to be superior in survival rate [7–9]. Despite differing influences on the studied parameters by the applied dialysis method, clinical and biochemical data are similar in both groups. Neither hemodialysis nor CAPD can be considered to be a totally satisfactory modality of treatment for diabetics. The availability of different types of renal replacement therapy in diabetics provides a larger range of alternatives. The patients' individual needs could be the best guidelines for the choice of treatment.

References

1   Combined Report on Regular Dialysis and Transplantation in Europe, vol XVII EDTA. Hospal Ltd., Basel, 1986.
2   Vlachojannis J, Kurz P, Hoppe D: CAPD in elderly patients with cardiovascular risk factors. Clin Nephrol 1988;30(Suppl 1):13–17.
3   Vlachojannis J, Pyriki P, Hoppe D, et al: Kontinuierliche ambulante Peritonealdialyse (CAPD) als Alternative zur Hämodialyse (HD) bei der Behandlung der chronischen Niereninsuffizienz insulinpflichtiger Diabetiker. Verh Dt Ges Inn Med 1982;88:883–886.
4   Khanna R, Oreopoulos D: Continuous ambulatory peritoneal dialysis in end-stage diabetic nephropathy; in Diabetic Nephropathy – Strategy for Therapy. Boston, Martinus Nijhoff, 1986, pp 105–138.
5   Wu C, Oreopoulos D: Prolonged survival of type I diabetics on CAPD with end-stage renal disease. Diabet Nephropathy 1985;4:190.
6   Nolph K, Steinberg S, Cutler S, et al: Diabetic nephropathy and the CAPD registry. Diabetic Nephropathy 1985;4:161–162.
7   Nolph K: Comparison of continuous ambulatory peritoneal dialysis and hemodialysis. Kidney Int 1988;33(suppl 24):123–131.
8   Mejia G, Zimmermann S: Comparison of continuous ambulatory peritoneal dialysis and hemodialysis for diabetics. Periton Dial Bull 1985;5:7–11.
9   Charytan C, Spinowitz B, Galler M: A comparative study of continuous ambulatory peritoneal dialysis and center hemodialysis: Efficacy, complications and outcome in the treatment of end-stage renal disease. Arch Intern Med 1986;146:1138–1143.

Dr. T. Tsobanelis, II. Medizinische Klinik, St. Markus Krankenhaus,
Wilhelm Epstein Strasse 2, D–W–6000 Frankfurt/Main 50 (FRG)

La Greca G, Olivares J, Feriani M, Passlick-Deetjen J (eds): CAPD – A Decade
of Experience. Contrib Nephrol. Basel, Karger, 1991, vol 89, pp 254–259

Cardiac Status and Differential Indication for Renal Replacement Methods

V. Wizemann[a], *W. Kramer*[b]

[a]Georg Haas Dialysezentrum, Giessen, und [b]Zentrum für Innere Medizin der
Justus-Liebig-Universität Giessen, BRD

One often neglected aspect of dialysis therapy is the fact that dialysis per
se influences the cardiovascular system comparable to cardiovascular drugs.
These effects occur in a subset of patients who – in addition to chronic renal
failure – often suffer from cardiovascular diseases. Thus, the selection of a
primary renal replacement method should be based on detoxification properties, social effects and, additionally, on the individual cardiovascular status
considering the expected cardiovascular responses of an individual renal
replacement method. This review will describe the acute and chronic effects
of dialysis methods on the heart and will describe cardiac diseases commonly
identified in patients with chronic renal failure.

Acute Effects of Hemodialysis

Hemofiltration, hemodialysis, and hemodiafiltration are characterized
by their intermittent application. One consequence of this mode of therapy is
the constant absence of equilibrium. Varying body fluid states influence
cardiac loading conditions, varying ionized calcium concentrations in the
plasma can interfere with cardiac contractility as does varying degree of
metabolic acidosis. Shifts in plasma potassium may influence inotropism as
well as the electric stability of the heart. In addition, patients on maintenance
hemodialysis are often under antihypertensive medication or digitalis therapy [1, 2], which might be influenced in its effects during dialysis.

Three main effects of dialysis on the heart can be identified. The first is
due to ultrafiltration rate and the projected dry weight of a patient. Ultrafiltration leads to an unpredictable reduction of plasma volume [3] by the range

of 0–25%. Although plasma volume decrease is inversely related to the degree of interstitial fluid volume, clinical estimation of appropriate dry weight is a crude parameter which allows a span of several kilograms between hypovolemic shock and congestive symptoms. A consequence of unpredictable reduction of plasma volume by ultrafiltration is a disproportionated reduction in cardiac preload. It has been shown that ultrafiltration reduces central venous and thereby left ventricular (LV) end-diastolic pressure [4]. The subsequent effect on LV stroke volume reduction is more pronounced in patients with normo- or hypohydration than in patients with hyperhydration [5].

The second cardiac effect of dialysis is dependent on whether acetate is used as a dialysis buffer. In dialysis patients with invasive assessment of cardiovascular function, infusion of acetate in a concentration comparable to those measured during hemodialysis, predominantly results in a reduction of end-diastolic LV pressure [6]. In the face of many discrepant published observations on the cardiac actions of acetate, the cardiac preload lowering effect was solely due to acetate, since influences of dialysis on cardiac parameters were excluded. Thus, the influence on acetate plasma concentrations of 3–5 mmol/l may be compared to the response of an infusion of nitroglycerin. Consequently, influx of acetate during hemodialysis amplifies the action of ultrafiltration on cardiac preload.

The third cardiac effect of hemodialysis, hemofiltration as well as hemodiafiltration results from the necessary electrolyte corrections. It was shown by several dialysis maneuvers that the increase of ionized calcium in the plasma has a positive inotropic effect, which is enhanced by a simultaneous decrease in plasma potassium concentration [7]. Since systolic function in dialysis patients without coronary heart disease is usually normal, the benefits of increasing myocardial contractility by luxury inotropism are rather doubtful. It has been shown that stimulation of LV systolic function by catecholamines like dobutamine in dialysis patients interferes with diastolic function. Thus, several dialysis-imminent stimuli influence the filling properties of the left ventricle by a high incidence of pre-existing diastolic dysfunction [8].

Long-Term Effects of Dialysis on the Heart

Replacement of renal function by dialysis varies largely throughout the world with respect to technology and methods applied, duration, clinical assessment of dry weight, and in the extent of drug therapy. Arterial hypertension, e.g. the most powerful risk factor for developing coronary artery disease in patients with renal failure, was reported to be absent in centers using long-duration dialysis (24 h or more/week) and, consequently, atherosclerotic disease seems to be only the minor problem [9]. In contrast, in centers with a different dialysis strategy, arterial hypertension affects the majority of dialysis patients [1, 2] and death from cardiovascular diseases is the major cause of mortality in the dialysis population. Arterial hypertension might be influenced by the choice of renal replacement method. The concept that CAPD often leads to a better control of hypertension and allows a reduction or a discontinuation of antihypertensive drug therapy [10], however, has been challenged by French observations demonstrating a high prevalence of arterial hypertension in a CAPD population of 139 patients (C. Jacobs, Hôpital de la Pitié-Salpétrière, Paris, personal communication). As reported in patients on peritoneal dialysis, who were pretreated by IPD and transferred to CAPD, amelioration of hypertension is related to the absence of volume overload [11].

Cardiac Status of Chronic Dialysis Patients

Independent of the dialysis methods used, LV hypertrophy is one of the most frequent echocardiographic findings in chronic dialysis patients. Functionally, the left ventricles are primarily hyperdynamic due to arteriovenous shunts, renal anemia, intermittent hyperhydration and a dialysis-induced increase in LV contractility. In about 40% of dialysis patients, secondary hypertrophic cardiomyopathy is present as shown by invasive LV characterization [8]. While systolic function is usually normal or even enhanced, the main adverse effect concerns diastolic function.

Ventricular arrhythmias may be a symptom of LV hypertrophy but more frequently of ischemic heart disease in dialysis patients [12]. Significant ischemic heart disease proven by coronary angiography, has a varying prevalence of 30–50% in the dialysis population. Low sensitivity and specificity of symptoms such as angina pectoris and noninvasive tests like ECG exercise tests or thallium perfusion imaging represent considerable diagnostic difficulties and may over- or underestimate the true prevalence. Impaired LV systolic function and a high incidence of complex ventricular ectopies are often associated with significant ischemic heart disease. Although a variety of further morphological abnormalities can be demonstrated in dialysis patients, this review is restricted to cardiomyopathy and ischemic heart disease since they imply general therapeutic consequences for a nephrologist.

Differential Indications Dependent on Cardiac Status

The first and most important therapeutic consequence is the notion that technology cannot replace medical intelligence. The patient has to be diagnosed first and in a second step an adequate therapy has to be applied. Taking into account unexplainable discrepancies between different centers in prescription of dialysis therapy and in definition of the goals of that therapy, standardization according to technical, economical and habitual criteria appears to guideline dialysis therapy rather than rational individualization. Secondly, pre-existent cardiovascular disease in the majority of patients and cardiac effects of hemodialysis characterize dialysis as an aggressive mode of treatment. In patients with established diastolic dysfunction of the left ventricle and/or ischemic heart disease the potentially adverse cardiac effects of dialysis can be easily attenuated by applying low ultrafiltration rates (slow reduction of cardiac preload) as well as small dialyzers and blood flows. Thus, dialysis becomes less aggressive and the individual safety margin in preventing hypotension and probably sudden death (in hypertrophic cardiomyopathy) might be enlarged. The same strategy can be applied to ischemic heart disease, although cardiac preload reduction by ultrafiltration is a desirable effect of dialysis in this subset of patients. Low ultrafiltration rates will allow lower dry weights and thereby a reduced cardiac preload. Furthermore, prevention of arrhythmias by potassium and calcium shifts, prevention of critical blood pressure decrease and tachycardia – a further determinant of myocardial perfusion – might be more effective. Thirdly, technical and method-related considerations can be helpful. Control of ultrafiltration resulting in a predictable reduction of circulating blood volume and thereby decrease in cardiac preload is nonexistent, since individual factors determining blood volume and compliance are unknown. However, technical control of ultrafiltration can at least prevent sudden changes in ultrafiltration rate. Hyperacetatemia reduces cardiac preload as does ultrafiltration. As long as arterial hypotension is excluded, acetate dialysis might be indicated in ischemic heart disease. In contrast, in secondary hypertrophic cardiomyopathy, enhanced reduction of cardiac loading conditions might be hazardous and bicarbonate dialysis should be preferred. CAPD does not necessitate an arteriovenous fistula, which, besides anemia, is one of the main causes of hypercirculation in dialysis patients. Since cardiac output can be lower without an arteriovenous shunt, CAPD might be indicated in patients suffering from ischemic heart disease. The same holds for patients with hypertrophic cardiomyopathy and diastolic dysfunction, where constant reduction of cardiac preload without dramatic shifts in end-diastolic pressure are preferable. Furthermore, drug therapy in ischemic heart disease or hypertrophic cardiomyopathy might be more predictable during constant hyperhydration conditions and slow dialysis.

The many subjunctives in the therapeutical recommendations might have been noticed. The reasons why one technique is preferable over another is by far more dependent on the human user than on the technique actually used. The example of CAPD might elucidate the problem: If CAPD ensures a continuously low hydration state, hypertrophy will regress as does arterial hypertension and ischemic heart disease patients will profit from improved myocardial perfusion. If CAPD – on the other hand – is associated with a continuously high hydration state, nearly all cardiovascular effects of the methods result into the opposite.

References

1   Anderson RJ: Polypharmacy in the dialysis center. Int J Art Organs 1982;5:289.
2   Schaefer K, Jahnke J, von Herrath D: Medikamentöse Therapie bei Dialysepatienten. Nieren- Hochdruckkrankh 1986;15:509–513.
3   Koomans HA, Geers AB, Dorhout Mees J: Plasma volume recovery after ultrafiltration in patients with chronic renal failure. Kidney Int 1984;26:848.
4   Kinet JP, Soyeur D, Balland N, et al: Hemodynamic study of hypotension during hemodialysis. Kidney Int 1982;21:868.
5   Leunissen KML: Dry weight in dialysis patients. Dialysejournal 1989;27:24–37.
6   Wizemann V, Kramer W, Soetanto RW, Thorman J, Schütterle, G: Action of acetate infusion on myocardial function in dialysis patients. XXIVth Congr EDTA-ERA, Berlin, 1987.
7   Kramer W, Wizemann V, Thormann J, Bechthold A, Schütterle G, Lasch H-G: Mechanisms of altered myocardial contractility during hemodialysis: importance of changes in the ionized calcium to potassium ratio. Klin Wochenschr 1985;63:272.
8   Kramer W, Wizemann V, Laemmlein G, Thormann J, Kindler M, Schlepper M: Cardiac dysfunction in patients on maintenance hemodialysis. II. Systolic and diastolic properties on the left ventricle assessed by invasive methods. Contr Nephrol 1986;52:110.
9   Charra B, Calemard E, Cuche M, et al: Control of hypertension and prolonged survival on maintenance hemodialysis. Nephron 1983;33:96.
10 Khanna R, Oreopoulos DG, Dombros N et al: CAPD after three years: Still a promising treatment. Periton Dial Bull 1981;1:24.

11 Leenen FH, Smith DL, Khanna R, Oreopoulos DG: Changes in left ventricular
    hypertrophy and function in hypertensive patients started on continuous ambula-
    tory dialysis. Am Heart J 1985;110:102.
12 Wizemann V, Kramer W, Thormann J, Kindler M, Schütterle G: Cardiac arrythmias
    in patients on maintenance hemodialysis: causes and management. Contr Nephrol.
    Basel, Karger, 1986, vol 52, p 42.

Prof. Dr. V. Wizemann, Georg Haas Dialysis Center,
Johann Sebastian Bach Strasse 40, D–W–6300 Giessen (FRG)

Psychological, Social and Economic Aspects of Peritoneal Dialysis

La Greca G, Olivares J, Feriani M, Passlick-Deetjen J (eds): CAPD – A Decade of Experience. Contrib Nephrol. Basel, Karger, 1991, vol 89, pp 260–264

CAPD with Three Bag Exchanges and One Day Rest

Results of a New Protocol

J.P. Contreras, J.M. Gas, M.C. Prados, A. Franco, L. Jiménez,
F. Picazo, C. de Santiago, J. Olivares

Sección de Nefrologia, Hospital del SVS, Alicante, Spain

The patient's acceptance of CAPD is, in our opinion, one of the major causes that has limited the growth and expansion of this technique as a treatment for end-stage renal failure.

Successful experiences with the reduction of the number of exchanges from 28 to 21 per week without reducing the total weekly amount of administered dialysate have previously been reported [1–3].

Encouraged by these results and in order to obtain some improvement in the patient's quality of life and a better acceptance of CAPD as an alternative to hemodialysis, a new protocol with 3 two-liter exchanges per day and a complete day off treatment each week has been established in our unit [4].

Patients and Method

In November 1986, 11 CAPD patients (3 male, 8 female; mean age 55.3 years, range 30–71) were enrolled in the new protocol as described in table 1.

A significant urine volume, a well-controlled blood pressure, an adequate biochemistry on dialysis and the support of relatives were the essential criteria for the inclusion in the trial.

Two 1.5% glucose and one 4.25% glucose two-liter exchanges with a dwell time of 8 h were performed 6 days a week. The day without exchanges was fixed on Sundays, the last 1.5% glucose exchange was performed on Saturday at midnight to avoid a long period of abdominal distension. No further exchanges took place until Monday morning. Once patients had been selected they and their relatives were interviewed. Patients gave verbal consent to participate in the trial.

Weekly clinical (weight, diuresis, blood pressure, edemas, peritonitis) and biochemical (hemoglobin, hematocrit, glucose, urea, creatinine, residual creatinine clearance,

Table 1. Rest protocol

Three two-liter exchanges per day
Last exchange: Saturday midnight (two-liter, 1.5% glucose bag)
No further exchange until Monday morning, 8 a.m. (two-liter, 4.25% glucose bag)
Four weekly and then monthly clinical and biochemical controls

Table 2. Description of the 5 patients on the rest program after 30 months

Sex	4 female, 1 male
Age, years	51.6 ± 15.1
Time on CAPD, months	5.6 ± 4.6
Primary renal disease	2 unknown cause
	1 pyelonephritis
	1 diabetic nephropathy
	1 polycystic disease
CAPD schedule	3 two-liter exchanges
	(one 4.25% glucose bag)

dialysate/plasma creatinine ratio, sodium, potassium, bicarbonate, uric acid, calcium, phosphorus, total proteins, albumin, cholesterol and triglycerides) parameters were recorded on Monday for the first 4 weeks and then monthly. After a few weeks patients were allowed to choose the day without exchanges.

In the first week 2 patients abandoned the trial, one because of anxiety and the other because of congestive cardiac failure after 42 h without exchanges (a longer interval than recommended). Several months later 3 patients were transplanted and one was switched to hemodialysis due to recurrent peritonitis.

In April 1989, 30 months after the beginning of this protocol, 5 patients were still carrying on the trial.

Table 2 gives details of these patients. For statistical analysis the Wilcoxon test was used. Only values of $p < 0.05$ or less were considered significant.

Results

Table 3 depicts the clinical results of these 5 patients. After 30 months, no changes in the clinical condition except for a not significant decrease in diuresis due to a decline in residual renal function were observed. In

Table 3. Clinical results

	Initial (mean ± SD)	Final (mean ± SD)	Wilcoxon test p
Systolic blood pressure, mm Hg	130 ± 18.7	132 ± 13	NS
Diastolic blood pressure, mm Hg	74 ± 10.8	70 ± 7.1	NS
Weight, kg	58.8 ± 6.2	58.8 ± 6.1	NS
Diuresis, ml	770 ± 740.4	400 ± 454.1	NS
Edema	no	no	–
Peritonitis (n/patient-month)	1/28	1/30	NS

Table 4. Analytical results of the 5 patients on the rest program after 30 months

	Initial (mean ± SD)	Final (mean ± SD)	Wilcoxon test p
Hemoglobin g/dl	11.3 ± 3.5	9.5 ± 2.6	NS
Hematocrit, %	34.4 ± 10.6	28 ± 8	0.04
Glucose, mg/dl	109.8 ± 35.3	98 ± 13.6	NS
Urea, mg/dl	101.2 ± 23.3	123.6 ± 6.3	0.04
Creatinine, mg/dl	7.3 ± 1.6	10.7 ± 1.9	0.04
Residual creatinine clearance, ml/min	4.2 ± 3.4	0.7 ± 0.7	0.04
Dialysate/plasma creatinine ratio	0.8 ± 0.1	0.9 ± 0.1	NS
Sodium, mEq/l	143 ± 1.4	143 ± 6	NS
Potassium, mEq/l	4.5 ± 0.6	5.5 ± 0.8	0.04
Bicarbonate, mEq/l	22.8 ± 1.3	20.1 ± 1.9	NS
Uric acid, mg/dl	6.4 ± 1.1	6.8 ± 0.8	NS
Calcium, mg/dl	9.3 ± 0.6	9.1 ± 0.3	NS
Phosphorus, mg/dl	4.4 ± 0.4	5.9 ± 1.2	0.04
Total proteins, g/dl	6.2 ± 0.5	6.7 ± 0.4	NS
Albumin, g/dl	3.1 ± 0.3	3.5 ± 0.4	NS
Cholesterol, mg/dl	249.8 ± 36.9	217.2 ± 26.6	0.04
Triglycerides, mg/dl	231.2 ± 143.4	193 ± 124.9	NS

particular, well-controlled blood pressure, unchanged weight and no edema were recorded.

The incidence of peritonitis varied from 1 episode/28 patient-months for the patients without a day's rest to 1 episode/30 patient-months for the patients included in the trial; the difference was not statistically significant.

Table 4 depicts the biochemical data of the patients. Serum urea, creatinine, potassium and phosphorus rose significantly during the study, while hematocrit, total cholesterol and residual creatinine clearance showed a significant decrease. There were no significant differences in the other biochemical parameters including the dialysate/plasma creatinine ratio.

Discussion

Although 11 patients entered the study, only 5 of them are still on this program for the above-mentioned reasons. It is important to note that only 1 patient experienced clinical side effects with this new regimen, due to a longer rest period than the one originally recommended. Though the low number of patients does not allow definite conclusions, some general impressions can be given.

The deterioration of several biochemical parameters is probably due to both the decline in residual renal function and the reduction of the administered dialysate. Although the exact share of each variable cannot be determined, a biochemical deterioration due to a decrease in residual renal function has been observed in several patients without a day's rest after few years of treatment, in accordance with other authors [5, 6]. The residual creatinine clearance of our patients changed from 4.2 ± 3.4 ml/min to 0.7 ± 0.7 ml/min during the study. These findings suggest that the observed biochemical deterioration was mainly due to the decline in residual renal function.

Although a decrease in peritonitis rate as a consequence of a reduced number of CAPD exchanges has been reported [3] and was expected by us, no significant reduction of peritonitis episodes occurred in our study in which only 18 exchanges per week were performed.

In addition, with our protocol a lower incidence of peritoneal ultrafiltration loss and a decrease in serum triglyceride levels due to a minor glucose load should be expected after a longer period of treatment.

This new protocol reduces the costs of treatment and, what is most important, enables an improvement in the patient's psychosocial condition, allowing not only a better quality of life, but also a better compliance to the CAPD program.

Although further studies (a control group and a study of peritoneal mass transfer) are required to reach definite conclusions, we think that this protocol could provide clinical stability with a mild biochemical deterioration completely overcompensated by a great improvement in the patient's quality of life. We have recently added three new patients to this program believing that this schedule could provide an improvement in the well-being of the CAPD patient.

References

1   Forbes AMW, Reed VL, Goldswith HJ: The adequacy of six-litre continuous ambulatory peritoneal dialysis. Proc Eur Dial Transplant Assoc 1980;17:276–280.
2   Twardowski Z, Janicka J: Three exchanges with a 2.5 liter volume for continuous ambulatory peritoneal dialysis. Kidney Int 1981;20:281–284.
3   Kiw D, Khanna R, Wu G, et al: Continuous ambulatory peritoneal dialysis with three-liter exchanges: A prospective study. Periton Dial Bull 1984;4:82–85.
4   Clemente P, Picó I, Peral F et al: Improvement of psychosocial conditions in patients on continuous ambulatory peritoneal dialysis when introducing a complete day off dialysis treatment every week. Aspects Renal Care 1987;2:112–114.
5   Kurtz SB, Johnson WJ: A four-year comparison of continuous ambulatory peritoneal dialysis and haemodialysis: A preliminary report. Mayo Clin Proc 1984;59:659–662.
6   Maiorca R, Cancarini G, Manili L, et al: CAPD is a first class treatment: Results of an eight-year experience with a comparison of patient and method survival in CAPD and hemodialysis. Clin Nephrol 1988;30:S3–S7.

Dr. J.P. Contreras, Hospital Alicante Insalud,
Nefrologia, C/Maestro Alonso 109, E–03012 Alicante (Spain)

La Greca G, Olivares J, Feriani M, Passlick-Deetjen J (eds): CAPD – A Decade of Experience. Contrib Nephrol. Basel, Karger, 1991, vol 89, pp 265–273

Quality of Life of Patients with End-Stage Renal Failure

A Comparison of Hemodialysis, CAPD, and Transplantation

F. A. Muthny, U. Koch[1]

Department of Rehabilitation Psychology, University of Freiburg i. Br., FRG

Traditionally, rehabilitation after illness was mainly understood to be medical and vocational rehabilitation. Further aspects of psychosocial rehabilitation (e.g. emotional well-being, partnership and family life, treatment satisfaction, and leisure time activities) have only rarely been taken into account.

The recently introduced concept of 'quality of life' places increasing emphasis on a broad spectrum of chronic diseases, mainly cancer [1] but also including different treatments of end-stage renal disease (ESRD).

In most of the studies comparing different treatments of ESRD, renal transplantation (RT) proved to be the superior treatment in terms of medical rehabilitation, but also in terms of quality of life [2]. But Kalman et al. [3] failed to find significant differences between hemodialysis (HD) and RT. Comparisons of hemodialysis and peritoneal dialysis, especially continuous ambulatory peritoneal dialysis (CAPD), have yielded contradicting results [4].

One of the reasons why psychosocial aspects in treatment of ESRD have been discussed for two decades, might be the existence of 3 alternative treatment modes, which are only partially indicated by medical criteria. Furthermore, even experienced clinicians find it difficult to predict which patient will do well with which treatment in terms of psychosocial adaptation and quality of life. The following investigation was conducted to obtain more basic information about psychosocial impacts and indication criteria in order to improve medical treatment and counseling.

[1] The authors wish to express their gratitude to all cooperating institutions and persons for their support of the study.

To allow for some generalizing conclusions, a multicenter study was designed, including 11 HD, CAPD and transplantation centers spread throughout the Federal Republic of Germany.

Patients and Methods

The investigation was conducted anonymously, applying a *clinical questionnaire* covering the following main issues:
- Patient's history of ESRD and treatment.
- Somatic complaints and medical complications.
- Life satisfaction in different areas (present time and changes in comparison to the time before ESRD).
- A broad spectrum of rehabilitation and quality-of-life criteria: emotional well-being, vocational situation, partnership/family life, leisure time activities.
- Sociodemographic data.

More than 1,100 patients with ESRD completed the questionnaire (approximately 50% had replied):
- 761 transplanted patients (4 centers: Berlin, Hannover, Heidelberg, Munich).
- 290 HD patients (7 centers: Berlin, Brühl, Freiburg, Trier, Hannover, Heidelberg, Munich).
- 68 CAPD patients (5 centers: Karlsruhe, Düsseldorf, Munich, Offenburg, Stuttgart).

Table 1 demonstrates that some significant differences between the treatment groups do exist and this should be kept in mind regarding the results. The transplant group has the lowest mean age and a high percentage of male patients; a similar trend is to be seen in the other groups, especially the CAPD patients.

The CAPD group shows the highest percentage of patients living with a partner and the highest educational level. As expected, CAPD patients also have the shortest mean duration of illness in terms of time from first symptoms as well as time from start of dialysis.

Results

Because of the different male/female ratios of the 3 treatment groups (as demonstrated above) gender was included in the two-way analysis of variance. Effects of age, education and duration of illness were taken into account in the statistical analyses by including them as covariates in the 'ANOVA' design and thus partializing out variance due to these variables (program SPSS9).

Comparing the 3 treatment groups (RT, HD, and CAPD) with respect to *life satisfaction*, RT showed the most favorable results with respect to 9 of the 12 areas of life considered. Only 3 areas did not show any treatment-related

Table 1. Description of patients

		RT (n = 761)	HD[1] (n = 290)	CAPD[2] (n = 68)
Age	mean	43.5	50.1	51.8
	(range)	(17–77)	(14–85)	(22–77)
Gender	male	59%	57%	68%
	female	41%	43%	32%
Living situation	with partner	70%	68%	79%
	without partner	30%	32%	21%
Education	primary level	62%	70%	64%
	secondary level	27%	21%	20%
	college	11%	9%	16%
Duration of illness, years	mean	14.7	13.1	9.8
Renal failure since, years	mean	7.5	5.9	2.7

[1] 54% center dialysis, 24% limited care dialysis, 22% home dialysis, about 40% on the transplant list.
[2] Approximately 30% on the transplant list.

differences: financial situation, interpersonal relationship with partner, and role in the family (table 2).

While 30% of the HD patients were not satisfied with their life in general, this percentage is only 17% in the CAPD group and 5% in the transplanted sample. With reference to the whole sample, physical performance, sex life, as well as vocational and financial situation are the life areas with which patients are mainly dissatisfied. Family life and interpersonal relationships are the areas relatively least affected by illness and treatment.

Only one gender-related difference could be found in these two-way analyses of variance: female patients expressed a higher satisfaction with (remaining) sex life.

Somatic and Psychosomatic Complaints

As depicted in table 3, the highest percentage of patients was found to be suffering from blood pressure disorders, fatigue, thirst, arthritic pains and some psychosomatic complaints such as restlessness/nervousness and fears (approximately 20% of each).

For most of the complaints, treatment-related differences still remain, despite the influences of gender, age, education and duration of illness being

Table 2. Present life satisfaction in different areas (comparison of RT, HD, and CAPD)

Areas of life	Percentage with low satisfaction (scale values 1–2)[1]				Results of the two-way analyses of variance[2]	
	total (n = 1,119)	RT (n = 761)	HD (n = 290)	CAPD (n = 68)	gender-related differences	treatment-related differences[3]
Physical performance	28	18	51	47	n.s.	RT > HD, CAPD[3]
Intellectual functioning	19	17	27	12	n.s.	HD < RT, CAPD
Assertiveness	12	10	16	12	n.s.	RT > HD
Working situation	20	17	29	20	n.s.	RT > HD
Financial situation	21	21	23	18	n.s.	n.s.
Interpersonal relationship with partner	9	9	12	6	n.s	n.s.
Sexual performance	29	25	39	32	F > M	RT > HD, CAPD
Family life	6	6	9	14	n.s.	HD < CAPD
Role in the family	6	6	7	9	n.s.	n.s.
Number of friends, acquaintances	10	7	18	5	n.s.	HD < RT, CAPD
Hobbies, free-time	17	11	33	20	n.s.	RT > HD, CAPD
General quality of life	13	5	30	17	n.s.	RT > HD, CAPD

[1] Referring to a 5-point scale; 1 = applies not at all; 5 = applies very strongly.
[2] SPSS program 'ANOVA', factors: gender/treatment; covariates: age, education, duration of illness.
[3] a > b means: a is more favorable than b.

Table 3. Somatic and psychosomatic complaints of HD, CAPD and transplanted patients

		Percentage with marked complaints (scale values 4–5)[1]				Results of the two-way analyses of variance[2]	
		total (n = 1,119)	RT (n = 761)	HD (n = 290)	CAPD (n = 68)	gender-related differences	treatment-related differences
1	Nausea, loss of appetite	9	6	13	21	F > M	RT < HD, CAPD
2	Blood pressure disorders	28	25	36	28	n.s.	RT < HD
3	Drowsiness, fatigue	26	20	43	32	n.s.	RT < HD, CAPD
4	Circulatory and cardiac complaints	14	12	20	13	n.s.	RT < HD
5	Skin disorders and itching	15	8	32	15	n.s.	RT < HD, CAPD
6	Digestive problems	12	9	19	15	F > M	RT < HD
7	Arthritic pains	21	19	29	12	n.s.	HD > RT, CAPD
8	Muscle cramps, restless legs	13	7	24	35	n.s.	RT < HD, CAPD
9	Headaches	10	9	11	9	F > M	HD > CAPD
10	Disturbed sleep	18	12	31	14	F > M	HD > RT, CAPD
11	Strain from required dietary limitations	10	8	17	11	n.s.	HD > RT, CAPD
12	Thirst	23	12	51	20	n.s.	HD > CAPD > RT
13	Irritability	18	16	23	14	n.s.	HD > RT, CAPD
14	Disturbances in memory and concentration	15	15	18	9	n.s.	HD > RT > CAPD
15	Nightmares	7	6	8	11	F > M	n.s.
16	Restlessness, nervousness	23	22	26	26	n.s.	HD > RT, CAPD
17	Discomfort with changes in external appearance	13	15	7	6	F > M	RT < HD, CAPD
18	Fear of medical complications	17	19	13	17	F > M	RT > HD
19	Apprehension towards side effects from medication	20	22	17	15	F > M	RT > HD
20	Fear of the future	20	18	35	23	F > M	n.s.
21	Depressive mood	13	10	13	15	F > M	HD > RT, CAPD
22	Disinterest	8	5	13	15	n.s.	HD > RT

[1] 5-point scale with 1 = applies not at all, 5 = applies very strongly.
[2] SPSS program 'ANOVA', factors: gender/treatment; covariates: age, education, duration of illness.

under control. The transplant group usually shows the most favorable results, the hemodialysis patients the least favorable – with two exceptions: transplant patients score the highest values in 'fear of medical complications' and 'apprehension towards side effects from medication'.

Regarding the extent of complaints within the groups: (1) The transplant group predominantly reports blood pressure problems, restlessness and nervousness as well as fears of medical complications and side effects of medication; (2) The hemodialysis patients mainly complain about thirst, fatigue, blood pressure problems and fear of the future, while (3) CAPD patients suffer mostly from restless legs and muscle cramps, followed by blood pressure problems, restlessness/nervousness and fear of the future.

Thus, a mixture of somatic and psychosomatic/psychological complaints are present in all groups, although the kind and extent of symptoms differ considerably between the groups.

In comparison to males, female patients report not only suffering more from psychological complaints (nightmares, discomfort with changes in external appearance, anxiety and depression), but also from headaches, digestive problems, nausea and sleep disturbances.

Vocational Rehabilitation

As expected, the transplant group has achieved the highest vocational rehabilitation rate, but even 39% 'on job' do not look very impressive (table 4). If those patients certified as ill and those with part-time occupations are eliminated, there are only approximately 30% of patients with full-time jobs remaining in the transplant group, and less than 20% in the dialysis groups. Accordingly, a high percentage of at least 50% has retired prematurely (only patients under 61 considered).

Satisfaction with Partnership, Sex Life, and Family Life

As already demonstrated above, relatively high contentedness was reported with respect to family life, partnership, and role in the family. Less than 10% score marked dissatisfaction with these areas, results being almost independent of treatment mode. In contrast to this picture, almost 30% reported marked dissatisfaction with sex life, the highest rate being almost 40% in the hemodialysis group. 23% of the RT, 43% of the HD and 56% of the CAPD patients reported that they had had no sexual intercourse in the past 4 weeks (only patients under 61 years were included in the analysis). The results are fraught with a high missing-data rate: approximately 30% did not answer the question, although the investigation was conducted anonymously.

Table 4. Vocational status in the 3 treatment groups (only patients not older than 60 years included): percent values

	RT (n = 675)	HD (n = 207)	CAPD (n = 43)	
On job				
Yes	39	27	23	
No	57	70	77	
(No answer)	(4)	(3)	(0)	$\chi^2 = 4$ $p < 0.001$
Present vocational status				
Full-time job	31	16	19	
Part-time job	11	11	5	
Certified as ill	3	4	9	
Application for retirement	2	4	7	
Retired	50	57	51	
(No answer)	(3)	(8)	(9)	$\chi^2 = 25$ $p < 0.001$

Influence of Duration of Illness, Age, Gender, and Education on the Quality of Life Scores

Education yielded the most frequent effects (5 of 6 scores showed significant relationships): Higher education level is related to a higher extent of positive moods and less complaints, depression and anxiety.

Elder patients on average report more marked complaints, less general life satisfaction, but higher satisfaction with partnership and family life.

Women report more marked complaints, anxiety and depression than *men* do, but no gender-related differences are found with respect to positive moods and general life satisfaction.

Duration of illness did not show correlation coefficients higher than $r = 0.10$ with the quality of life scores and will therefore not be interpreted (although some are statistically significant because of the big sample size).

Discussion

The study confirms the favorable outcome of renal transplantation in terms of medical and vocational rehabilitation, but also with respect to emotional well-being, complaints and satisfaction with different life areas (especially satisfaction with physical performance, intellectual functioning, partnership, family life, sex life and leisure time activities). Thus, the results confirm the findings by Evans et al. [2] and are in conflict with those of Kalman et al. [3], who did not find differences between the treatment groups. Even after controlling gender, age, education and duration of illness by partializing out variance due to these influencing factors, the effects still remain and therefore cannot be explained sufficiently by selection effects [4].

Besides this superiority of the renal transplantation in terms of quality of life, the global anxiety score does not discriminate between the three groups, thus pointing to a similar level but different objects of fear in the groups: HD patients are primarily afraid of shunt complications and side effects of dialysis; CAPD patients realize the risk of peritonitis, and transplant patients are afraid of the final rejection of the graft and side effects of the immunosuppressive drugs. CAPD shows a middle position between transplantation and hemodialysis with respect to many quality-of-life criteria.

Referring to the *vocational rehabilitation*, the transplant group has the highest percentage of patients on full-time jobs (31%) in comparison to HD and CAPD, but still a rather poor result in comparison to other western industrial countries [5].

The better results of the RT group with respect to sex life might be due to the better medical rehabilitation [6, 7], but should also be seen in the context of increased emotional well-being and self-confidence after transplantation [8]. *Family life* and *partnership* are not very much affected by illness and treatments as reported by the patients themselves. These findings might reflect a disconnection of sex life from partnership and family life, but might also be interpreted by the great importance of social support in the coping with chronic diseases or in the light of harmonizing tendencies of patients with ESRD [9].

The findings with respect to treatment-related differences in quality of life do look rather impressive, but it must nevertheless be pointed out that they are weakened by certain methodological problems:

(a) The testing could not be done between randomized groups (and the method of analysis of covariance is only good for eliminating linear effects of age, education and duration of illness).

(b) The HD group has a large portion of center-dialysis patients (in a worse medical precondition).

(c) The CAPD group has the shortest duration of illness and (as social psychologists know from minority groups in general) a high motivation to justify and demonstrate the advantages of their method.

Of course we do not know how results would have turned out if we had had 20% (instead of less than 5%) on CAPD or a percentage of 50% treated by RT (instead of less than 20%). But it can be stated that it appears useful to reconsider and discuss indication criteria for the three treatments of ESRD in the FRG. Particularly, the low transplantation rate in the FRG should be regarded in relation to the practice in other western industrial nations and from the background of the outcome in terms of medical and psychosocial rehabilitation.

References

1   Aaronson NK, Beckmann J: Quality of Life of Cancer Patients. New York, Raven Press, 1987.
2   Evans RW, Manninen DL, Garrison LP, Hart L, Blagg CR, Gutman RA, Lowrie EG: The quality of life of patients with end-stage renal disease. N Engl J Med 1985;312:553–559.
3   Kalman TP, Wilson PG, Kalman CM: Psychiatric morbidity in long-term renal transplant recipients and patients undergoing hemodialysis. JAMA 1983;250:55–58.
4   Soskolne V, Kaplan De-Nour A: Psychosocial adjustment of home hemodialysis, continuous ambulatory peritoneal dialysis and hospital dialysis patients and their spouses. Nephron 1987;47:266–273.
5   European Dialysis and Transplant Association (EDTA): Combined Report on Regular Dialysis and Transplantation in Europe, 1984. Basel, Hospal Ltd, 1985.
6   Levy NB: Sexual dysfunction of hemodialysis patients. Clin Exp Dial Apheresis 1983;7:275–288.
7   Procci WR, Goldstein DA, Kletzky OA, Campese VM, Massry SG: Impotence in uremia; in Levy NB (ed): Psychonephrology 2. New York, Plenum Press, 1983, pp 235–256.
8   Muthny FA, Koch U: Psychosocial rehabilitation after renal transplantation. 17th Eur Conf Psychosomatic Res., Marburg, 1988.
9   Speidel H, Koch U, Balck F, Kniess J: Empirical questionnaire survey of the education of hemodialysis patients and their partners in various dialysis settings; in Levy NB (ed): Psychonephrology, vol I. New York, Plenum Press, 1981, pp 147–167.

F.A. Muthny, MD, Department of Rehabilitation Psychology,
University of Freiburg, D–W–7800 Freiburg i. Br. (FRG)

La Greca G, Olivares J, Feriani M, Passlick-Deetjen J (eds): CAPD – A Decade of Experience. Contrib Nephrol. Basel, Karger, 1991, vol 89, pp 274–281

Analysis and Comparison of Treatment Costs in Peritoneal Dialysis and Hemodialysis

Michael Nebel, Klaus Finke, Eckehard Renner

Department of Medicine, Städtisches Krankenhaus Köln-Merheim, FRG

The problem of rising costs in the health services along with a simultaneous reduction of financial resources is well known to the public in the Federal Republic of Germany and is also being controversially discussed in the journalistic media. For this reason, and as long-term cost analyses of CAPD treatment are not available in the Federal Republic of Germany, it was considered to be necessary to analyse and compare the costs of the various methods of dialysis treatment.

On the one hand, CAPD is regarded as being the least expensive dialysis method; on the other hand, increased costs due to complications have often been neglected. Cost calculations arising from dialysis treatment have already been published [1–5]; however, expenses were only based on cost of materials and physician fees without taking into account hospital treatment and technical complications [1, 3, 5].

In this analysis, costs for dialysis treatment, hospital care due to dialysis complications or other diseases of home hemodialysis patients (HHD), center hemodialysis patients (CHD), or CAPD patients were determined retrospectively. Costs for ambulatory treatment of peritonitis in CAPD patients were also included.

Patients and Methods

Thirty-four HHD patients, 22 CHD, and 32 CAPD patients were included in the study. Each patient was observed from the start of treatment with observation periods up to 194 months.

HHD patients were studied as of August 31, 1984 until December 31, 1987, CHD patients as of August 1, 1984 being on dialysis at the same center for at least 3 years or having been treated with dialysis for a period of 3 years until December 31, 1987, CAPD patients having been dialyzed for more than 2 years after August 1, 1984 or before December 31, 1987.

The following data were studied and calculated for each individual patient group:

Net Dialysis Costs

Cost calculation was based on the fees being reimbursed by the health insurance to the dialysis center in Cologne-Merheim. Costs were split up for material, physician fees and laboratory testing.

Technical Complications during Dialysis

(1) Number of days of hospital treatment due to dialysis access complications. Dialysis access was denoted as A-V fistula for hemodialysis patients and as peritoneal catheter for CAPD patients. The following complications occurred: HD: A-V fistula thrombosis or infection; CAPD: peritonitis episodes, exit site or tunnel infections and different catheter-related problems.

(2) Costs based on the fees for hospital care valid at the time of hospitalization. At the beginning of the analysis in 1974, the daily charges amounted to DM 131 while they increased to DM 330 in 1987. Treatment costs were calculated for each patient according to the number of treatment days. The entire costs for all patients in each group were added and divided by the months of treatment.

Diseases Not Associated with Dialysis Treatment

(1) Number of days of hospital treatment due to diseases not related to dialysis treatment.

(2) Individual costs for hospital care calculated as above.

Out-Patient Care of CAPD Patients (Peritonitis Episodes, Exit Site and Tunnel Infections)

Calculations for the CAPD patients were based on a peritonitis rate of 1 episode per 19 patient months (during 1,486 treatment months 78 peritonitis episodes occurred). Calculated costs included antibiotics, bacteriological tests and transportation to the dialysis center. The costs for antibiotics were assessed according to the official pharmacy selling price. Therapy costs for the necessary antibiotics (cephalotin, cefotiam, cefuroxim, cefotaxim, amikacin, gentamycin, dicloxacillin, mezlocillin, azlocillin, clindamycin, vancomycin) varied between DM 11.50 (gentamycin) and DM 61.90 (vancomycin) per day. Bacteriological tests for 2 culture flasks (anaerobe and aerobe with resistance determination) amounted to DM 96.60 for each out-patient peritonitis diagnosis.

Transportation Costs

Expenditures for the transportation of patients to the dialysis center were based on the actual expenses. CAPD and HHD patients in general needed only 1 transportation every 6 weeks for an out-patient control check-up. The average transportation costs for 12 representative HD patients were determined, and the costs for transportation to and from the dialysis center were fixed at DM 76.70. For driving to the dialysis center by private car, a rate of DM 10 was fixed. Calculated transportation costs for CAPD patients were DM 360 per annum but, since the necessary transportation to out-patient peritonitis therapy has to be included, costs were fixed at DM 480.

Table 1. Demographic data and number of patients: HHD, CHD and CAPD patients

	HHD	CHD	CAPD
Number of patients	34	22	32
Average age, years (range)	41.9 (20–63)	48.2 (22–72)	47.1 (24–63)
Total treatment months	3,542	1,904	1,486
Average treatment months (range)	104.5 (51–194)	86.5 (36–168)	46.3 (24–97)

Excluded Costs

Costs for hospital care at the beginning of dialysis treatment were not taken into consideration as diagnostic measures in certain patients exceeded those of most of the other patients. Likewise, costs of training for home dialysis (CAPD or HHD) were excluded, since they were only a small part of the expenditure. The average length of out-patient training for HHD patients amounted to 3 months; the hospital training for CAPD patients took 2 weeks. Apart from antibiotics, pharmaceutical therapeutics, e.g. antihypertensive, cardiovascular agents, etc., were not included in the cost analysis.

New CAPD Systems

New systems now available for CAPD treatment (i.e. disconnect system) have the advantage of decreasing the peritonitis rate and relieving patients from carrying the empty dialysate bag. The disadvantages of these systems are the considerably higher costs. In our calculations additional costs of DM 15 per day for these systems were fixed.

Results

Demographic data and number of patients included are shown in table 1. As demonstrated in figure 1, primarily younger patients are treated with home hemodialysis in contrast to CHD and CAPD patients.

The total costs for hospital treatment for dialysis-associated complications and for other diseases not associated with dialysis, as well as out-patient care of CAPD patients are given in table 2.

A total of 805 out-patient and 762 in-hospital days were necessary for peritonitis therapy and for peritoneal catheter-related problems. During the 805 days of CAPD out-patient care total costs of DM 16,236 arose from antibiotics and DM 6,568 from bacteriological examinations. The total sum of DM 22,804 equals costs of DM 15.34 per patient-month. Altogether the costs in CAPD treatment arising from out-patient and hospital peritonitis therapy, exit site or tunnel infections or catheter problems amounted to DM 281.7 per patient and month.

Table 2. Days in hospital and treatment costs due to dialysis access complications, to other diseases and to out-patient therapy of CAPD patients

	HHD	CHD	CAPD
Total patient months	3,542	1,904	1,486
Days in hospital a.c. (total number)	100	248	762
Days in hospital a.c./patient-month	0.03	0.13	0.51
Costs (DM) a.c./patient-month	7.11	30.99	154.90
Days in hospital o.d. (total number)	1,085	940	420
Days in hospital o.d./patient-month	0.31	0.49	0.28
Costs (DM) o.d./patient-month	85.25	149.73	111.48
Outpatient treatment days (total) a.c.			805
Costs/patient-month			15.34
Total costs/patient-month (DM)	92.36	180.72	281.7

a.c. = For treatment of access complications; o.d. = for treatment of other diseases.

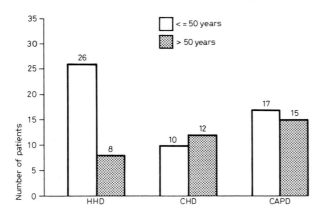

Fig. 1. Age distribution of HHD, CHD and CAPD patients.

Table 3 depicts net dialysis costs, including all dialysis access complications, e.g. peritonitis treatment, physician fees and transportation costs. Thirty of 34 HHD patients came to the out-patient control examinations by private car, 4 patients came by taxi, while only 5 of 22 CHD patients used their own cars and 17 came by taxi; 15 CAPD patients drove to the clinic by themselves and 17 came by taxi.

Table 3. Net dialysis costs per patient including all dialysis access complications and transportation costs (in DM)

	HHD	CHD	CAPD
Material/month	3,175	4,199	2,863
Physician/month	460	499	393
Dialysis treatment/month	3,635	4,698	3,256
Dialysis access/month	7	31	170
Other diseases/month	85	150	111
Total treatment/month	3,727	4,879	3,537
Total transportation/month	8	750	40
Treatment and transportation/year	44,820	67,548	42,924

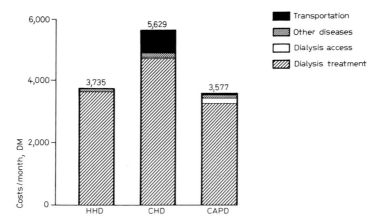

Fig. 2. Treatment and transportation costs. Costs for dialysis treatment, dialysis access complications, treatment of other diseases and transportation of HHD, CHD and CAPD patients in DM per month.

The total treatment costs were calculated from the expenditure for (1) pure dialysis treatment; (2) clinical care due to problems on dialysis access; (3) clinical care due to diseases not associated with dialysis; (4) outpatient care for CAPD patients; (5) transportation to dialysis center (table 3). For a better comparison, monthly costs are shown in figure 2.

Table 4. Dialysis treatment costs per patient in different reviews for 1 year of treatment (in thousand DM)

Author	Year	HHD	CHD	CAPD
Mahoney and Kachel Australia [2]	1982	12.4	n.d.	11.0
Nolph USA [3]	1983	26.7	50.4	32.9*
Renner and Renner FRG [6]	1983	49.6	63.1	n.d.
Gokal UK [1]	1984	31.1	49.0	35.2*
Prowant et al. USA [4]	1986	n.d.	82.0	47.6
Prichard CDN [5]	1988	n.d.	43.8	32.5*
Nebel et al. FRG [this work]	1989	42.9	67.5	44.8

*Complications not analysed. n.d. = Not determined.

If the material costs for CAPD increase due to new transfer sets, we would estimate that costs of DM 4,033 per month or DM 48,396 per year will arise.

Discussion

Many discussions on the costs of different dialysis modalities have arisen in the past few years. In several countries CAPD is used preferably because of the presumed or real financial advantage, while in the Federal Republic of Germany only approximately 5% of all dialysis patients are treated with CAPD. The – to some extent – controversial opinions about the financial situation of CAPD in Germany and the missing cost analysis led to the submitted study. In several studies in the USA, Canada, Great Britain and Australia [1–5], analyses and comparisons of the treatment costs of CAPD and HD were carried out (table 4).

These cost analyses are comparable with our results only to a certain extent, due to the different structures of the health services. In addition, the costs of hospital treatment for complications related to dialysis or to other diseases were only partly taken into account [1, 3 , 5]. All in all, cost levels for CAPD are low compared to center hemodialysis, whereas costs for home hemodialysis and CAPD hardly differ.

At our center the costs for CAPD were nearly as high as those for HHD (DM 42,924 and 44,800), whereas CHD (DM 67,548) was distinctly more expensive. If a more expensive transfer set, which may be used more often in the future, is taken into account, the costs for CAPD are even higher than the costs for HHD (DM 48,396 as against DM 44,820), but the difference to CHD still remains obvious.

In our study published in 1983 [6], the costs for HHD (DM 49,656) are slightly higher than the calculations in the present analysis, possibly as a result of the smaller patient groups in that study. The costs for CHD (DM 63,114) were somewhat lower in the previous calculations.

Surprisingly, the analysis of the individual groups shows that in HHD patients only minor costs are related to dialysis access problems and to other diseases. The reason for this certainly is the selection of patients for home hemodialysis. In our study 76% of the HHD patients were under 50 years of age, while in the CHD and CAPD group the proportion of patients above or below 50 years hardly differed. Therefore, due to the high percentage of younger patients in HHD, a lower percentage for diseases not related to dialysis could have been expected. Moreover, HHD patients seem to take better care of their A-V fistula, as is demonstrated by the low number of shunt problems (100 days of hospital treatment in 3,542 treatment months).

In contrast, CAPD patients needed 762 days of hospital treatment for peritonitis and catheter-associated problems at costs of DM 230,175. The number of days in hospital per patient month (0.51 and 0.03, respectively) also stresses the high rate of technical complications in comparison to HHD. In addition, the costs for out-patient peritonitis therapy with 805 days of treatment have to be taken into account, but they are relatively low (DM 22,804) and amounted to only 1/10 of the hospital therapy costs. This demonstrates the necessity for out-patient care as frequently as possible. However, the possibility of out-patient care depends on the selection of patients on the one hand, and on the availability of staff and medical facilities at a CAPD unit on the other.

Our study shows that despite the considerable number of additional costs of treatment, CAPD together with HHD belongs to the less expensive dialysis methods. However, CAPD is – in contrast to many suppositions – not considerably cheaper than HHD.

Unfortunately, the frequency of HHD in the Federal Republic of Germany has been decreasing in the past few years. Yet, a wider use of CAPD as an alternative method of home dialysis for patients who cannot be treated with HHD for medical or psychosocial reasons, could save costs considerably. For example, an increase in the frequency of the home dialysis methods, CAPD and HHD, of only 10% in a group of 20,000 dialysis patients would amount to savings of DM 40 millions per year in the Federal Republic of Germany.

In future, a reduction of complications in peritoneal dialysis will be necessary to obtain a better prognosis and to reduce treatment costs. This could be achieved by better training of the patients, further education of nursing staff and of physicians, as well as by better CAPD transfer sets and catheters. In addition, selection of CAPD patients is still a problem. If, particularly, patients suffering from diabetes mellitus, cardiovascular or cerebrovascular problems are put on this dialysis method, higher complication rates could be expected.

References

1   Gokal R: World-wide experience, cost effectiveness and future of CAPD; in Gokal R (ed): Continuous Ambulatory Peritoneal Dialysis. London, Churchill-Livingstone, 1986, pp 349–369.
2   Mahoney JF, Kachel G: Comparative costs of dialysis; in Atkins RC, Thomson NM, Farrell PC (eds): Peritoneal Dialysis. London, Churchill-Livingstone, 1982, pp 418–423.
3   Nolph KD: Dialysis and transplantation in the USA and impact of CAPD; in Parson F, Ogg C (eds): Renal Failure – Who Cares? Lancaster, MTP Press, 1983, pp 75–87.
4   Prowant BF, Kappel DF, Campbell A: A comparison of inpatient and outpatient medicare allowable charges for continuous ambulatory peritoneal and center hemodialysis: A single center study. Am J Kidney Dis 1986;8:248–252.
5   Prichard SS: The cost of dialysis; in Khanna R, Nolph KD, Prowant BF, et al (eds): Advances in continuous ambulatory peritoneal dialysis 1988. Toronto, Peritoneal Dialysis Bulletin Inc, 1988, pp 66–72.
6   Renner E, Renner H: Ökonomische und gesundheitspolitische Aspekte in der Versorgung terminal niereninsuffizienter Patienten. Internist 1983;24:517–524.
7   Wing AJ, Broyer F, Brunner FP, et al: Demography of dialysis and transplantation in Europe in 1985 and 1986: Trends over the previous decade. Nephrol Dial Transplant 1988;3:714–727.

Dr. Michael Nebel, Medizinische Klinik I, Städtisches Krankenhaus, Ostmerheimer Strasse 200, D–W–5000 Köln 91 (FRG)

Subject Index